SOUND ADVICE—AND SURPRISING FACTS—
FROM THE EXPERTS

CELLULITE: What you can—and cannot—do to get rid of those troubling dimpled thighs, including the latest medical procedures. Page 86.

EATING DISORDERS: These common but often overlooked warning signs can tell you when food has become a dangerous obsession. Page 195.

MENOPAUSE: The best-kept secret that can actually have you looking forward to this turning point in your life as a woman. Page 329.

YEAST INFECTIONS: How to assess and reduce your personal risk factors and what you can do to remedy the situation if all else fails. Page 591.

STEPFAMILIES: This simple, seven-stage plan can ease conflicts, open communication, and help you come together as a family. Page 508.

MISCARRIAGE: These medical and emotional tips can help you make it past the pain and regain your hope for the future. Page 345.

WOMEN'S ENCYCLOPEDIA OF HEALTH &
EMOTIONAL HEALING

WOMEN'S

ENCYCLOPEDIA
OF HEALTH
& EMOTIONAL
HEALING

Top Women Doctors Share Their Unique Self-Help Advice on Your Body, Your Feelings and Your Life

BY DENISE FOLEY, EILEEN NECHAS
and the Editors of *PREVENTION* Magazine

MEDICAL ADVISER LILA A. WALLIS, M.D.
Founder of National Council on Women in Medicine

BANTAM BOOKS
New York   Toronto   London   Sydney   Auckland

This edition contains the complete text
of the original hardcover edition.
NOT ONE WORD HAS BEEN OMITTED.

WOMEN'S ENCYCLOPEDIA OF HEALTH & EMOTIONAL HEALING
A Bantam Book / published by arrangement
with Rodale Press, Inc.

PUBLISHING HISTORY
Rodale Press edition published 1993
Bantam edition / April 1995

The questions in "Could You Become an Addict?" on page 166 are reprinted
with permission from *Holistic Medicine*, September/October 1989, The American Holistic Medicine Association.

The questions in "Advice for Consent" on page 412 are reprinted with permission from *The Sexes at Work*, © 1983 by Lois B. Hart and J. David Duke,
Leadership Dynamics, 875 Poplar Avenue, Boulder, CO 80304.

ISBN 0-553-56987-2

Published simultaneously in the United States and Canada

PRINTED IN THE UNITED STATES OF AMERICA
OPM   0   9   8   7   6   5   4   3   2   1

MEDICAL ADVISER: LILA A. WALLIS, M.D.
CONTRIBUTING WRITERS AND EDITORS: ALICE FEINSTEIN, ELLEN MICHAUD
RESEARCH CHIEF: ANN GOSSY
RESEARCH AND FACT-CHECKING: CHRISTINE DREISBACH, MELISSA DUNFORD,
JEWEL FLEGAL, MELISSA GOTTHARDT, ANNE IMHOFF, KAREN LOMBARDI INGLE,
DEBORAH PEDRON, BERNADETTE SUKLEY
ILLUSTRATOR: VIVIENNE FLESHER

CONTRIBUTING PHYSICIANS AND PROFESSIONALS

We thank the following physicians, psychologists, educators and other professionals for sharing their expertise, advice and professional opinions in the making of this book.

Constance Ahrons, Ph.D., is a family and marital therapist in private practice, professor of sociology and associate director of the Marriage and Family Therapy Program at the University of Southern California in Los Angeles and coauthor of *Divorced Families: Meeting the Challenge of Divorce and Remarriage.*

Elizabeth Auchincloss, M.D., is a psychiatrist at Cornell University Medical College in New York City.

Nancy Balaban, Ed.D., is director of the Infant and Parent Development Program at New York City's Bank Street College Graduate School of Education and author of *Learning to Say Goodbye: Starting School and Early Childhood Separations.*

Mary Lou Ballweg is the cofounder and president of the Endometriosis Association in Milwaukee and author of *Overcoming Endometriosis: New Help from the Endometriosis Association.*

Lonnie Barbach, Ph.D., a psychologist and sex therapist, is an assistant clinical professor of medical psychology at the University of California, San Francisco, School of Medicine and author of *For Yourself: the Fulfillment of Female Sexuality* and *For Each Other: Sharing Sexual Intimacy.*

Laura Barbanel, Ed.D., is a professor and head of the graduate program in school psychology at Brooklyn College of the City University of New York.

Dorothy Barbo, M.D., is a professor of obstetrics and gynecology at the University of New Mexico School of Medicine and medical director of the university's Center for Women's Health in Albuquerque.

Rosalind C. Barnett, Ph.D., is director of the Adult Lives Project and a clinical and research psychologist at the Center for Research on Women at Wellesley College in Massachusetts.

Linda J. Beckman, Ph.D., is director of research at the California School of Professional Psychology in Alhambra and an adjunct professor in the Department of Psychology at the University of California, Los Angeles.

Victoria Hilkevitch Bedford, Ph.D., is a psychologist at the University of Indianapolis.

Stephanie DeGraff Bender is clinical psychology director of The PMS Clinic in Boulder and author of *PMS: Questions & Answers*.

JoAnne Bitner, Ph.D., is a psychotherapist and a member of the San Diego Family Institute in California.

Gisela Booth, Ph.D., is a clinical psychologist and assistant clinical professor of psychology at Northwestern University in Chicago.

Linda Brubaker, M.D., is director of the Section of Urogynecology, Rush Presbyterian–St. Luke's Medical Center in Chicago.

Dedra Buchwald, M.D., is an assistant professor of medicine at the University of Washington and director of the Chronic Fatigue Syndrome Clinic at Harborview Medical Center in Seattle.

Penny Wise Budoff, M.D., is director of the Women's Pavillion of Northshore University Hospital in Bethpage, New York, and author of *No More Menstrual Cramps and Other Good News*.

Kathryn L. Burgio, Ph.D., is a behavioral psychologist, a research assistant professor of medicine at the University of Pittsburgh School of Medicine and coauthor of *Staying Dry: A Practical Guide to Bladder Control*.

Angela Burke, Ph.D., is a clinical psychologist and director of the Psychology Clinic at North Texas State University in Denton.

Carol Ann Burton, M.D., is a clinical instructor of obstetrics and gynecology at the University of Southern California School of Medicine in Los Angeles.

Trudy L. Bush, Ph.D., is an associate professor of epidemiology at the Johns Hopkins University School of Hygiene and Public Health in Baltimore.

Jean Carter, M.D., is an obstetrician at Wilkerson Obstetrics and Gynecology, Professional Associates, in Raleigh, North Carolina, and coauthor of *Sweet Grapes*.

Barrie Cassileth, Ph.D., former director of psychological programs at the University of Pennsylvania Cancer Center, is a professor of medicine at Duke University in Durham and the University of North Carolina.

Joanne Cipollini, R.N., is a cancer clinical nurse specialist at Montgomery Cancer Center of the Fox Chase Cancer Center in Norristown, Pennsylvania.

Nora W. Coffey is president of Hysterectomy Educational Resources and Services (HERS) in Bala Cynwyd, Pennsylvania.

Diane Courney, R.N., is a clinical specialist in childbirth education and assessing problem pregnancies at the University of Texas Health Science Center in San Antonio.

Chris Courtois, Ph.D., is a psychologist in private practice in Washington, D.C., and author of *Healing the Incest Wound*.

Rebecca Curtis, Ph.D., is a professor of psychology at Adelphi University in Garden City, New York, and author of *Self-Defeating Behaviors*.

Constance V. Dancu, Ph.D., is an anxiety disorder specialist, a professor in the Department of Psychiatry and the director of the Crime Victims Program at the Medical College of Pennsylvania in Philadelphia.

Barbara De Angelis, Ph.D., is a therapist in Los Angeles.

Sally Faith Dorfman, M.D., an obstetrician and gynecologist, is Commissioner of Health for Orange County, New York.

Linda Dunlap, Ph.D., is an assistant professor of psychology at Marist College in Poughkeepsie, New York.

Adele Faber of Roslyn Heights, New York, is coauthor of *Siblings without Rivalry* and *Between Brothers and Sisters*.

April Fallon, Ph.D., is an assistant professor in the Department of Psychiatry at the Medical College of Pennsylvania in Philadelphia.

Jacqueline Fawcett, R.N., Ph.D., is a researcher in maternity nursing and a professor at the University of Pennsylvania School of Nursing in Philadelphia.

Helen Fisher, Ph.D., is an associate in the anthropology department of the American Museum of Natural History in New York City and author of *The Sex Contract: The Evolution of Human Behavior*.

Deborah Foley, M.D., is a staff physician at the Vein Clinics of America in Chicago.

Jacqueline Darroch Forrest, Ph.D., is vice-president of research at the Alan Guttmacher Institute, a nonprofit organization that does research in reproductive studies, in New York City.

Marion Frank, Ph.D., is a psychologist in private practice at Marion Frank and Associates in Philadelphia.

Mary Froning, Psy.D., is a clinical psychologist in private practice in Washington, D.C.

Ellen Galinsky is co-president of the Families and Work Institute in New York City and coauthor of *The Preschool Years*.

Linda Gannon, Ph.D., is a professor of psychology at Southern Illinois University at Carbondale.

Ann Garber, Dr.P.H., is a reproductive geneticist at Cedars-Sinai Medical Center in Los Angeles.

Jane Gaunt is a certified addictions counselor and clinical supervisor of the women's unit at the Betty Ford Center in Rancho Mirage, California.

Diane Gerber, M.D., is a plastic and reconstructive surgeon in private practice in Chicago.

Mary M. Gergen, Ph.D., is an associate professor of psychology at Pennsylvania State University.

Matti Gershenfeld, Ph.D., is a professor at Temple University in Philadelphia and director of the Couples Learning Center in Jenkintown, Pennsylvania.

Lucia A. Gilbert, Ph.D., is a professor in the Department of Educational Psychology at the University of Texas in Austin and author of *Sharing It All: The Rewards and Struggles of Two-Career Families.*

Cynthia Gillespie is a Seattle attorney and author of *Justifiable Homicide: Battered Women, Self-Defense and the Law.*

Leslie Hartley Gise, M.D., is a psychiatrist and director of the Premenstrual Syndromes Program at Mount Sinai Medical Center in New York City.

Shirley Glass, Ph.D., is a clinical psychologist in private practice in Owings Mills, Maryland, and a member of the American Association for Marriage and Family Therapy.

Deborah T. Gold, Ph.D., is a senior fellow and assistant professor of psychiatry and sociology at the Center for the Study of Aging and Human Development at Duke University Medical Center in Durham, North Carolina.

Deborah Gowen is a certified nurse-midwife with the Harvard Community Health Plan in Wellesley, Massachusetts, Brigham and Women's Hospital in Boston and WomenCare at Malden Hospital.

Michelle Harrison, M.D., is assistant professor of psychiatry at the University of Pittsburgh School of Medicine and author of *Self-Help for Premenstrual Syndrome.*

Marion Hart, M.D., is a psychoanalyst in Scarsdale, New York, and a professor of psychiatry at Cornell Medical Center in Westchester, New York.

Renee Hartz, M.D., is a cardiothoracic surgeon and associate professor of surgery at Northwestern University Medical School in Chicago.

Penny Hitchcock is an epidemiologist and acting chief of the Sexually Transmitted Diseases Branch of the National Institute of Allergy and Infectious Diseases in Bethesda, Maryland.

Ellen Hock, Ph.D., is a professor of family relations and human development at Ohio State University.

Jimmie Holland, M.D., is chief of psychiatry services at Memorial Sloan-Kettering Cancer Center in New York City.

Marsha Hudnell is a registered dietitian and nutritional consultant for Green Mountain at Fox Run, a women's weight-management facility in Ludlow, Vermont.

Mardy Ireland, Ph.D., is a clinical psychologist in Oakland, California, and adjunct faculty member at Santa Clara University in Berkeley.

Marla Beth Isaacs, Ph.D., is a psychologist in private practice in Philadelphia and author of *Difficult Divorce: Therapy for Children and Parents*.

Margaret Jensvold, M.D., is the director of the Institute for Research on Women's Health in Washington, D.C.

Karen Johnson, M.D., is in private practice and is an assistant clinical professor of psychiatry at the University of California, San Francisco, and co-sponsor of a movement to include a women's health specialty in medical education.

Rosemary Johnson, Ph.D., is an assistant professor at the University of Southern Maine School of Nursing in Portland.

Florence Kaslow, Ph.D., is director of the Florida Couples and Family Institute in West Palm Beach and past president of the International Family Therapy Association.

Susan Kayman, Dr.P.H., is a registered dietitian in Oakland, California, and nutritionist and weight-maintenance specialist for the Kaiser Permanente Medical Group.

Bonnie Kin, Ph.D., is a psychologist at California State University.

Abby King, Ph.D., is a senior research scientist at the Stanford University School of Medicine's Center for Research in Disease Prevention.

Diana Kirschner, Ph.D., is a clinical psychologist in private practice in Gwynedd Valley, Pennsylvania.

Ronette Kolotkin, Ph.D., is a clinical psychologist at the Duke University Diet and Fitness Center in Durham, North Carolina.

Mary Koss, Ph.D., is a professor of psychiatry at the University of Arizona.

Terry Kriedman, M.D., is director of the Obstetrics and Gynecology Department at Chestnut Hill Hospital in Philadelphia.

Judith Lasker, Ph.D., is a sociology professor at Lehigh University in Bethlehem, Pennsylvania, and coauthor of *When Pregnancy Fails*.

Maureen Lassen, Ph.D., is a clinical psychologist in Phoenix.

Jeannette Lauer, Ph.D., is dean of the College of Liberal Studies at the United States International University in San Diego and coauthor of *Til Death Do Us Part*.

Caryn Lerman, Ph.D., is director of behavorial oncology at Fox Chase Cancer Center in Cheltenham, Pennsylvania.

Paula Levine, Ph.D., is a psychologist and director of the Agoraphobia Resource Center in Coral Gables, Florida.

Linnea Lindholm, Ph.D., is a research manager in the Department of Medicine, Division of Cardiology of the University of Florida.

Dorothy Litwin, Ph.D., is a psychologist in private practice in New York City and suburban Larchmont.

Sharon A. Lobel, Ph.D., is an assistant professor of management in the Albers School of Business and Economics at Seattle University.

Wende Logan-Young, M.D., is director of the Breast Clinic in Rochester, New York, and a consultant to the Roswell Park Cancer Institute in Buffalo.

Susan Love, M.D., is director of the Faulkner Breast Center in Boston, clinical assistant professor of surgery at Harvard Medical School and author of *Dr. Susan Love's Breast Book*.

Suzanne McClure, M.D., Ph.D., is an assistant professor of medicine in the Division of Hematology-Oncology at the University of Texas Medical Branch in Galveston.

Kay McFarland, M.D., is an endocrinologist and professor of medicine at the University of South Carolina School of Medicine in Columbia.

Kerry McGinn, R.N., of San Francisco is author of *Keeping Abreast: Breast Changes That Are Not Cancer*.

Ellen McGrath, Ph.D., is executive director of the Psychology Center in Laguna Beach, California, chairperson of the American Psychological Association National Task Force on Women and Depression and author of *Women and Depression: Risk Factors and Treatment Issues*.

Kathleen MacPherson, R.N., Ph.D., is a professor of nursing at the University of Southern Maine School of Nursing in Portland.

Maria Mancusi, Ph.D., is a psychologist and unit director of the Mount Vernon Center for Community Mental Health in Springfield, Virginia.

Linda Mangels, Ph.D., is a behavioral psychologist and president of the American Academy of Risk Management in Longwood, Florida.

Judith Martindale is a financial planner and host of a radio talk show and TV segment on money issues in San Luis Obispo, California, and author of *Creating Your Own Future: A Women's Guide to Retirement Planning*.

Diane Martinez, M.D., is a psychiatrist at the University of Texas Health Science Center in San Antonio.

Midge Marvel is senior program specialist for the Widowed Persons Service of the American Association of Retired Persons in Washington, D.C.

Mary Jane Massie, M.D., is an associate attending psychiatrist at Memorial Sloan-Kettering Cancer Center in New York City.

Jane Mattes is a psychotherapist in private practice in New York City and founder of Single Mothers by Choice.

Diane Medved, Ph.D., is a psychologist in private practice in Santa Monica, California, and author of *The Case against Divorce*.

Diane Meier, M.D., is co-director of the Osteoporosis and Metabolic Bone Disease Program at Mount Sinai Medical Center in New York City and associate professor of geriatrics and medicine at Mount Sinai School of Medicine of the City University of New York.

Susan Mikesell, Ph.D., is a psychologist in private practice in Washington, D.C.

Pamela Murray, M.D., is director of adolescent medicine at the Children's Hospital of Pittsburgh.

Joyce Nash, Ph.D., is a psychologist in private practice in Woodside, California, and author of *Maximize Your Body Potential*.

Annette Natow, Ph.D., is a registered dietitian and nutrition consultant at Nutrition Consultants, Inc., in Valley Stream, New York, and a professor emerita of nutrition at Adelphi University in Garden City.

Elizabeth Harper Neeld, Ph.D., of Houston is a grief researcher and author of *Seven Choices: Taking the Steps to a New Life after Losing Someone You Love.*

Christiane Northrup, M.D., is an assistant clinical professor of obstetrics and gynecology at the University of Vermont College of Medicine, a gynecologist at Woman to Woman in Yarmouth, Maine, and co-president of the American Holistic Medical Association.

Renae Norton, Ph.D., is a clinical psychologist at the Montgomery Center in Cincinnati.

Nancy Norvell, Ph.D., is a clinical psychologist who specializes in behavioral medicine at the University of South Florida.

Michele Paludi, Ph.D., is coordinator for the Women's Studies Program at Hunter College in New York City.

Jeanne A. Petrek, M.D., is a breast cancer surgeon at Memorial Sloan-Kettering Cancer Center in New York City and author of *A Woman's Guide to the Prevention, Detection, and Treatment of Cancer.*

Kathleen Pike, Ph.D., is a psychologist at the New York State Psychiatric Institute at Columbia Presbyterian Medical Center in New York City.

Suzanne Pope, Ph.D., is director of the Colorado Institute for Marriage and the Family in Boulder.

Robin Post, Ph.D., is a clinical psychologist in private practice in Denver.

Jill Maura Rabin, M.D., is an assistant professor of obstetrics and gynecology in the Division of Urogynecology at Long Island Jewish Medical Center in New Hyde Park, New York.

Janice Rench is a national consultant on physical abuse and rape and former director of the Cleveland Rape Crisis Center in Ohio.

Virginia Revere, Ph.D., is a psychologist in private practice in Alexandria, Virginia.

Joyce Roberts, Ph.D., is a certified nurse-midwife, professor and head of the Department of Maternal-Child Nursing at the University of Illinois College of Nursing in Chicago.

Beatrice Robinson, Ph.D., is a psychologist in private practice and an assistant professor of psychology at the University of Minnesota Medical School in Minneapolis.

Lillian B. Rubin, Ph.D., is a psychologist, alumni professor of interpretive sociology at Queens College of the City University of New York, senior research associate at the Institute for the Study of Social Change at the University of California in Berkeley and author of *Erotic Wars: What Happened to the Sexual Revolution?*

Reva Rubin is a Pennsylvania pregnancy researcher and the author of *Maternal Identity and the Maternal Experience.*

Linda Tschirhart Sanford is a social worker and psychotherapist in Quincy, Massachusetts, coauthor of *Women and Self-Esteem* and author of *Strong at the Broken Places: Overcoming the Trauma of Childhood Abuse.*

Iris Sanguiliano, Ph.D., is a psychologist in private practice in New York City.

Rosemarie Schultz, Ph.D., is a clinical psychologist in private practice in Chicago, specializing in issues of women and money.

Ruth Schwartz, M.D., is a clinical professor of obstetrics and gynecology at the University of Rochester School of Medicine and Dentistry in New York and serves on the American College of Obstetricians and Gynecologists' task force on hysterectomy.

Judith H. Seifer, R.N., Ph.D., is an associate clinical professor of psychiatry and obstetrics and gynecology at Wright State University School of Medicine in Dayton, Ohio.

Marjorie Hansen Shaevitz is a family and marriage counselor at the Institute of Family and Work Relationships in La Jolla, California, and author of *The Superwoman Syndrome.*

Barbara B. Sherwin, Ph.D., is an associate professor of psychology and obstetrics and gynecology at McGill University in Montreal.

Donna Shoupe, M.D., is an associate professor of obstetrics and gynecology at the University of Southern California in Los Angeles.

Judith Siegel, Ph.D., is an associate professor in the School of Social Work at New York University in New York City and a marital therapist in private practice in Westchester County.

Lisa Silberstein, Ph.D., former clinical director of Yale University Eating Disorder Clinic, is in private practice in New Haven, Connecticut.

Judith Sills, Ph.D., is a clinical psychologist in private practice in Philadelphia.

Judith Slater, Ph.D., is a clinical psychologist in private practice in Buffalo.

Felicia Stewart, M.D., is a gynecologist at the Valley Center for Women's Health in Sacramento, California, and coauthor of *Understanding Your Body: Every Woman's Guide to Gynecology and Health*.

Nia Terezakis, M.D., is a clinical professor of dermatology at Tulane University School of Medicine and a practicing dermatologist in New Orleans.

Sandra Thomas, R.N., Ph.D., is director of the Center for Nursing Research at the University of Tennessee College of Nursing at Knoxville.

Yvonne S. Thornton, M.D., is an associate professor of obstetrics and gynecology at Cornell University Medical College in New York City.

Sarah Ullman, Ph.D., is a psychologist at the University of California, Los Angeles.

Emily Visher, Ph.D., a Lafayette, California, clinical psychologist and family therapist, is cofounder of Stepfamily Associates of America in Lincoln, Nebraska.

Victoria Vitale-Lewis, M.D., is a plastic surgeon with Plastic and Reconstructive Surgery Associates in Melbourne, Florida.

Lenore E. Walker, Ed.D., is a clinical and forensic psychologist with Walker and Associates in Denver and author of *The Battered Woman Syndrome*.

Marsha Walker, R.N., is president of Lactation Associates in Weston, Massachusetts, and an international lactation consultant.

Lila A. Wallis, M.D., is clinical professor of medicine at Cornell University Medical College in New York City, past president of the American Medical Women's Association and founder and first president of the National Council on Women in Medicine.

Michele Weiner-Davis is a therapist in private practice in Woodstock, Illinois, and author of *Divorce Busting: A Revolutionary and Rapid Program for Staying Together*.

Carol Weiss, M.D., is a clinical assistant professor of psychiatry and public health at Cornell University Medical College in New York City and a psychiatrist in private practice.

Nanette K. Wenger, M.D., is a professor at Emory University School of Medicine and director of the cardiac clinics at Grady Memorial Hospital in Atlanta.

Deborah White is spokesperson for and co-director of the National Coalition against Domestic Violence in Washington, D.C.

Kristene E. Whitmore, M.D., is a clinical associate professor of urology at the University of Pennsylvania, director of the Incontinence Center and chief of the Department of Urology at Graduate Hospital in Philadelphia and coauthor of *Overcoming Bladder Disorders* and *Staying Dry: A Practical Guide to Bladder Control.*

Midge Wilson, Ph.D., is an associate professor of psychology and women's studies at De Paul University in Chicago.

Bonnie Worthington-Roberts, Ph.D., is a professor and director of the Nutritional Sciences Program at the University of Washington.

Camille Wortman, Ph.D., is a researcher at the University of Michigan.

Judith Wurtman, Ph.D., is a nutrition researcher at the Massachusetts Institute of Technology.

Ellen L. Yankauskas, M.D., is director of the Women's Center for Family Health in Atascadero, California.

Shirley Zussman, Ed.D., is a marital and sex therapist in New York City.

CONTENTS

PREFACE

The last half-century has seen fundamental changes in the demographic structure of American society. The explosion in medical knowledge and technology, and its impact on the health habits of Americans, have contributed to longer life expectancy. We live longer and enjoy better health than at any time in history. Women now spend a third of their lives in the post-menopausal state, and that has created new health problems and calls for new approaches.

Changes in the family structure also have generated new challenges and health issues for women. First there was the "extended family," which was superseded in midcentury by the "nuclear family." Since then it has undergone a further and even more consequential transformation into the two-wage-earner family.

A powerful instrument of change has been the expansion of the role women play in our society and the massive entrance of women into the workforce. Women now assert themselves in many spheres, and the societal attitudes, values and structure are now in a fluid state of creative readjustment to this change.

The consumer movement, along with women's awareness about themselves, gave rise to a new doctor/patient relationship, a partnership based on the patient's education, knowledge, sophistication and demand "to know." Women want to have their health demystified. No longer do we see a docile submission to the recommendation of experts—doctors included. Women want to "take back their bodies" and be the ultimate decision-makers in their individual health matters. Doctors are seen as concerned advisers, educators and teachers, as skillful detectives and contributors of expert opinions. But it is the woman who decides.

Women's relationship to health and medicine has also been affected by the breakthroughs in medical research and high technology. The availability of many new medications for old and new ills, the development of the mammogram, application of ultrasonography to studies of fertility and pregnancy, prenatal genetic testing—including amniocentesis and chorionic villus sampling—have transformed everybody's care, but especially that of women.

The *Women's Encyclopedia of Health & Emotional Healing* is a compendium of health problems women *today* encounter throughout their lives. While accurate scientifically, it is not a cut-and-dried exposition of facts. It is a lively account of problems and solutions, a broad panorama of contemporary women's health. Its pages are peopled by scores of women with health problems who for the most part found ways to solve their problems, with or without the help of experts. In addition, this book presents opinions of M.D.'s, Ph.D.'s and Ed.D.'s—all women, all credible and all outstanding authorities.

Entertaining and optimistic, the *Women's Encyclopedia of Health & Emotional Healing* stresses common sense but clearly refers individuals to contact their physicians for perplexing problems. Its anecdotes and vignettes are witty, picturesque and practical.

The consumer's point of view of health care is clear but not abrasive. This is *the* women's health book for the 1990s.

LILA A. WALLIS, M.D.
*Clinical Professor of Medicine, Cornell
University Medical College; Past President,
American Medical Women's Association; Founder
and First President, National Council on
Women in Medicine
New York, December 1992*

INTRODUCTION

THE *WOMEN'S* BOOK OF WOMEN'S HEALTH

A few years ago I asked a psychiatrist friend of mine for some advice on how to get out of a particularly unpleasant situation I found myself in. Her response made a major impression on me. Not because she had a quick solution to my problem (she didn't), but because of an offhand remark she made about the way professional counselors counsel female patients.

"Men doctors and women doctors counsel women patients differently," she commented. "They may end up getting the same results, but they approach the problem in totally different ways."

I get to meet and talk to a lot of doctors in my job as a health editor, and I found myself relating this story time and again to other doctors I'd meet—both male and female. Yes, they told me, men doctors and women doctors *are* a lot different in the way they relate to women patients. Not that one is right and the other wrong. Their approach is just . . . different.

It got me thinking. Since statistics say that 84 percent of all women are treated and counseled by men physicians, then interviewing *women* doctors about the issues that are closest to a woman's medical and emotional well-being might give us a brand-new look at ourselves.

And that's exactly what the *Women's Encyclopedia of Health & Emotional Healing* offers: a unique, refreshing, positive point of view. The authors of this book spent more than a year interviewing hundreds of *women* professionals—physicians, psychiatrists, psychologists, nurses, midwives, counselors and others—for their personal perspective and advice on a whole range of women's concerns: from aging, birth control and cancer to thyroid problems, virginity and widowhood. After all, who better understands the fright of discovering a breast lump, the despair of infertility, the misery of PMS, the happiness of motherhood—who better than other women? Especially other women who've been there.

And that brings me to another benefit that makes this book a standout in the burgeoning field of women's self-help advice. Authors Denise Foley and Eileen Nechas spent countless hours talking with women who have actually experienced the problems and concerns this book addresses. Many of their stories are retold here. They are all real stories—of rape, stillbirth, adultery, sibling rivalry, low self-esteem, fears and sickness. Because their stories are so revealing, we agreed to disguise their identities behind masked names. And we thank them for their candidness and honesty.

"Some of the stories were so difficult for some of these women to discuss that I often had to get up and walk away from my writing when I was trying to put their stories on paper," Eileen told me. "That's how hard it hit *my* emotions."

But what makes many of their stories so poignant is why they decided to share their lives with our readers. "Many women told me that if their stories would make it easier for others to get through what they went through, it would be worth it," says Eileen.

And that's why you won't find any pessimism or unresolved hopelessness in this book. The *Women's Encyclopedia of Health & Emotional Healing* shows you how to take charge of your health and control your emotions. It tells you what to expect—both physically and mentally—from an illness, personal problem or just the vagaries of getting older. And there is plenty of woman-to-woman advice that will help you make the right decisions for yourself. This is *the* book about women, from women and by women. And one no woman should be without.

DEBORA TKAC
Executive Editor
Prevention Magazine Health Books

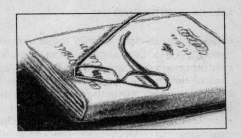

AGING

IT'S ONLY A STATE OF MIND

*T*he transition between young and old can begin in the blink of an eye.

It can begin the moment you come in from the beach, shower off a sprinkling of sand, glance in the mirror and discover a whole sketchbook of vertical lines.

It can begin the moment you bury your last parent, glance down at the age spots on your hands and realize that you're the head of the family. How did *this* happen?

Or it can begin the moment you glance in a shop window and notice—with a double take that drops your jaw—that the woman looking back is *not* your mother.

A MOMENT OF DISCERNMENT

The realization that finishes your youth, marks the midpoint of life and launches you firmly toward becoming what the French call a woman of "a certain age" is frequently triggered by a moment of startled discernment. It's a moment that can propel you into months or even years of self-examination and evaluation: "What have I done with my life so far?" "Where am I going?" "What do I want to do with the rest of my life?" But it's also a moment that can—and *should*—launch you into an energizing time of self-discovery and personal growth.

When does it start? Some women develop a sense of their own aging and begin the transition from youth into middle age in their thirties. Some begin in their forties, some even as late as their fifties, says Mary M. Gergen, Ph.D., an associate professor of psychology at Pennsylvania State University. And although we generally refer to the transition from young to old as midlife, the timing is different for everyone.

"My daughter is 29 and already checking the mirror for wrinkles," says Dr. Gergen. She's looking for the physical signs of aging that will tell her whether she still looks youthful or is getting old. Because, generally speaking, that's how most women judge themselves. Most mark the end of youth and the beginning of old age by physical changes.

The mirror, of course, is where most women approaching middle age seem to spend an inordinate amount of time. Like Dr. Gergen's daughter, we're checking for wrinkles, looking for sags, investigating skin tone. None of us wants to enter middle age lined and bagged—not of our own free will.

Lena Borovitz is a case in point. A tall, slender, strawberry blond with soul-searching eyes, Lena is concerned with the fate of the world, the fate of her soul and the trajectory of her career. How she looks—beyond intelligent to her boss and sexy to her husband—has never been a major concern.

Yet even Lena is not happy with the physical changes she sees happening to her 44-year-old body. It's not so much the graying hair, which she describes as looking like it's been frosted, but the crinkles at the corners of her eyes, the bags under her eyes, her tendency to now gain weight— these things bother Lena.

"I try to be philosophical but it doesn't work," she says candidly. "I catch a little glimpse of myself in a shop window as I walk downtown and think, 'My God! When did *that* happen?'"

FEAR OF AGING

Unfortunately, explains Dr. Gergen, the cultural imperative that how we look determines how valuable we are—to

WHO'S AFRAID OF THE BIG 4-0?

You are. At least you are if you haven't reached it.

"Turning 40 is pivotal," says Cornell Medical Center professor Marion Hart, M.D. "Decades mark off a piece of life, and turning 40 is the decade in which you really begin to realize that half your life is over." Fear of 40 is really fear of getting old.

But once they get there, most people actually find out they really *like* being 40.

"I dreaded turning 40 like you wouldn't believe," admits Melanie Anderson, a child-free by choice career woman. "The weekend of my 40th birthday, my husband and I went on a sailing trip because I wanted to be away from it all when 'it' happened. I also knew I wouldn't be around a mirror. I don't know what I expected to happen when I woke up on my birthday, but I can tell you what I felt was great relief. Waiting around for 40 to happen was the worst part. I didn't look any different or feel any different—except maybe a little stupid for making such a big deal out of it."

It's common to approach a 40th birthday with some degree of angst, says Dr. Hart, especially since society tends to make such a to-do of it.

But you should keep it on the same level as the greeting cards: It's just something to smile about.

ourselves, our men, our world—is what makes women so inordinately sensitive to the physical signs of aging.

Still? Yes, still. Despite women in the surgical suite, the cockpit and the boardroom, psychologists have found that most women still think that how they look rather than what they do is what gives them value.

At some primitive level, women equate being beautiful with being sexually appealing, says Laura Barbanel, Ed.D., professor and head of the graduate program in school psychology at Brooklyn College of the City University of New York.

Maybe it's an extension of the old "If . . . then . . ." equation: *If* aging reduces our beauty, *then* it also reduces our sex appeal. *If* we have less sex appeal, *then* we won't attract mates. *If* we don't attract mates, *then* we won't have babies. *If* we have no babies, *then* we have no function. *If* we have no function, *then* we have no value. Is this logic? Is the value of a woman really in her ability to reproduce?

Obviously, no. Yet that's what a fear of aging basically comes down to, says Dr. Barbanel. To a woman, as one of her colleagues puts it, aging is nothing less than "a humiliating process of sexual disqualification."

THE JANE FONDA EFFECT

Complicating the issue is the 1990s awareness that we have the power to postpone at least the obvious signs of aging. Exercise can firm flabby thighs, tummy tucks can tighten sagging bellies, eye-lifts can eliminate bags, moisturizers can fill in the crow's feet. Clearly the way *we* look at 40 is not how our mothers did.

Ironically, says Dr. Gergen, our ability to look young as we approach midlife may actually perpetuate the you're-only-as-good-as-you-look myth. It's what she calls the Jane Fonda effect.

The problem, she explains, is that if Jane can look good at 44 or 54, we feel that we should, too. And pretty soon it becomes another cultural imperative. It's something society expects of us, something we expect of ourselves. We become so obsessed with pinning things up, smoothing things out or erasing them altogether that we continue to believe a woman with lines on her face, spots on her hands or gray in her hair is losing her value, or at least a part of her self. But, in truth, just the opposite is happening. Midlife can actually be a time of tremendous personal growth because it's the time we look in the mirror and ask: "What have I done with my life?" "What am I going to do with the rest of it?"

GIVING BIRTH TO YOURSELF

This is what aging is *really* all about.

Midlife is similar to the time during childhood called

DOUBLE STANDARD: MARRIAGE MAKES A DIFFERENCE

It's a theory as old as time itself and it goes something like this: Men age well—they actually become *more* attractive as they age. Their lines add character, their gray hair wisdom. But women? In them, lines are wrinkles and gray is matronly. Women become less attractive as they age.

What does the 1990s woman think?

To find out, researcher Carol B. Giesen, Ph.D., of the Division of Human Development at St. Mary's College of Maryland in St. Mary's City asked 32 women ranging in age from 28 to 63 to share their definitions of attractiveness, femininity and sexual appeal.

She found that the old double standard still exists—at least in the minds of middle-aged and older married woman. All the women agreed that men are at their most attractive and are most sexually appealing in their early forties to late fifties. The married women, however, said they felt their peak years of attractiveness and sex appeal occurred during their early twenties to early thirties. Single and young married women, however, felt a woman's peak years to be from the early thirties to the early fifties. Single women also tended to downplay the definition of attractiveness and preferred to think of themselves as "growing more attractive and sexually appealing over the years."

Middle-aged and older married women blamed age-related changes such as gray hair, wrinkles and weight gain as the cause of their diminished attractiveness and sexual appeal. Single women—particularly middle-aged ones—said these things added to their attractiveness. Interestingly, she says, both groups attributed their divergent views to the same thing—a greater acceptance of themselves.

What gives here? Perhaps, speculates Dr. Giesen, her findings "reflect qualitatively different life experiences for single and married women."

rapprochement when a child—usually around the age of 18 months—first realizes that she is not omnipotent, explains Elizabeth Auchincloss, M.D., a psychiatrist at Cornell University Medical College in New York City.

That realization makes the child feel vulnerable, says Dr. Auchincloss, and she responds with a burst of rich personal growth so intense that at least one psychologist has labeled it a second, psychological birth. A woman's response to the awareness of her mortality is almost the same. In fact, you might even think of midlife as a time of giving birth yet again—this time to yourself.

So how does a woman giving birth to herself react? Every woman is different, scientists agree. One woman buys herself a Mercedes. Another goes back to school. A third quits her job, sells her house and spends six months in Spain. A fourth goes on a crusade protesting the development of nuclear power. A fifth takes up sailboarding. A sixth takes a six-month leave of absence to play with her son in the Gulf of Mexico, hike with her husband in Vermont and plant a rose garden for her mother-in-law in Philadelphia.

The common thread that seems to pull all of these women together is that each woman is discovering a particular facet of herself. The woman who bought a Mercedes is discovering that she can earn her own luxuries instead of waiting around for Prince Charming to hand her the keys. The woman who gets political is discovering that she has the strength to stand up to the powerful and tell them that she thinks what they're doing is wrong. And the woman who takes up sailboarding is discovering a physical prowess that she never even suspected she possessed.

Each of these women is also doing something that she's wanted to do for a long time but somehow never got around to doing. In effect each woman is saying, "Hey! I'm not going to be here forever. I have to make some choices. I have to set my priorities and concentrate on what's important."

DEVELOP YOUR SKILLS

Midlife choices can sometimes cause a degree of emotional pain because frequently, when you choose to do one thing, you're also relinquishing the ability to do another. The woman who chooses to write a book, for example, may have to give up her dream of getting a Ph.D.—simply because there's only enough time to do one or the other.

Fortunately, the amount of pain you experience as you make midlife choices is—as with any birthing process—directly related to the amount of preparation you've done in advance.

How can you prepare for this particular birth? Well, if you're cruising into middle age solely on a pretty face, you're in trouble, says Dr. Auchincloss bluntly. But if you enter midlife with a lot of skills—skills that give you a sense of competence and independence—midlife can be a period of great creativity and growth.

The woman who knows how to do things—whether she knows how to stretch a dollar, teach children, write a book, organize a barbecue or conduct laboratory tests—is a woman who will think well of herself and use her skills as a basis for further development. Essentially, her skills will provide the raw material from which she will build a new infrastructure of herself.

That's why a lot of women return to school at midlife, adds Dr. Auchincloss. They realize the need for additional skills before they can get on with the building. It's so common that the beauty queen who becomes a homemaker, raises her kids, then goes for her Ph.D. in mathematics is almost a cliché.

DEVELOP A SENSE OF YOURSELF

For the most part, how you experience midlife depends on having a healthy attitude toward life, says Marion Hart, M.D, a psychoanalyst and professor of psychiatry at Cornell Medical Center in Westchester, New York. If you already have one, then dealing with midlife could be easier. If you haven't, you need to retool.

A positive mental attitude depends on having developed a good sense of self, says Dr. Hart. Know who and what you are, who and what you value. Establish full, rich relationships with friends and family—particularly with other women. Aging can be an enriching process with a strong network of support.

Surround yourself with loving, positive, active people, urges Dr. Gergen. Decide who the important people are in your life and make time for them. Pick friends who will enhance your life, friends who want to go and do and be, friends who are as excited about personal growth as you are.

"Let your joy reverberate through your social group," adds Dr. Gergen. It will be reflected back to you 100-fold and enrich your life immeasurably.

BUY A SPORTS CAR

Do things for yourself, says Dr. Barbanel, especially things that are fun.

Sarah Rogers had always wanted a sports car, for example, but she had always bowed to her husband's more practical choices. As a result, every car they ever bought was great on fuel, great on price, great on repairs. But to her, they were also boring, boring, boring!

Eventually, says Sarah, "I realized that there were probably only a few more cars to be bought before I rode in a hearse." So when her old car broke down, she hauled her husband off to the showroom, looked him straight in the eye, pointed to the shiny silver two-seater and said, "That's the car I'm getting."

"Perfect!" chuckled Dr. Barbanel when she heard Sarah's story. Midlife is a time to do this kind of stuff. Experiment. Try new things. Satisfy yourself rather than somebody else.

Just don't do something that involves more work, she cautions. "We women have made a mistake in liberating ourselves to work," she says only half facetiously. "Now we're up to our ears in work, and we're working too hard."

Explore different parts of yourself and try on different aspects of your personality the way you would a new hat, urges Dr. Barbanel.

Remember how you walked through the hat department in a store as a little girl? If your mother stopped to chat with one of her friends, you'd drift away to the mirror and try on one hat after another. The black fedora pulled down over one eye made you look like a spy, didn't it? And the little wisp of black velvet with the short veil that tickled your nose turned you into a *femme fatale*, right? And what about the broad-brimmed straw hat with the velvet ribbons? Didn't you look like a Gibson Girl from the early 1900s? How did you feel when you looked at your Gibson Girl-self in the mirror? Soft? Vulnerable? A little delicate?

All of us have a whole wardrobe of hats inside ourselves just waiting to be worn, says Dr. Barbanel.

The point of midlife is to try them all on.

See also Wrinkles

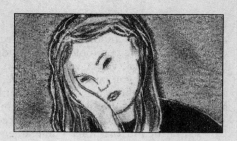

ANEMIA

WHEN YOUR BLOOD RESERVES GO BROKE

*C*heryl Henry always considered herself a low-energy person, but the weakness and fatigue she started to feel after she lost "that last 10 pounds" had her wanting to crawl back into bed by noon.

"It's a good thing I worked at a job where I could sit most of the time," says the 33-year-old secretary and mother of two, "because I wouldn't have made it through the day in a job requiring more physical exertion."

As it was, Cheryl would have to lie down on the sofa as soon as she got home from work. "My husband would fix dinner while I rested," she says, marveling now at his patience, "and then after dinner I'd put on my pajamas and get into bed. No matter how much sleep I got, I would still be wiped out by the end of the day. Forget taking walks together. I couldn't even make it once around the mall without having to sit down. I had no life."

Cheryl says that she was frequently short of breath and felt light-headed, too. "One time I fainted in church—flat out on the pew. When I came to, I heard organ music playing and saw all these people standing over me. I thought I was dead."

It was enough of a scare to send her to the doctor. A simple blood test was all it took to uncover the reason for Cheryl's symptoms: She had iron-deficiency anemia, the "tired blood" disease that's a threat to all women.

IRON DRAIN

"No blood"—that's what anemia literally means. A bit of an exaggeration, but if you asked Cheryl, she probably wouldn't think so. Besides feeling tired and light-headed, she also had the symptoms indicative of a severe case of anemia—her pulse rate went up, her blood pressure went down and she often felt dizzy and weak.

Why? The body's energy levels are taxed when it doesn't get enough iron, the mineral essential to the production of hemoglobin in red blood cells. Hemoglobin carries oxygen through the blood. Without sufficient iron, hemoglobin levels drop and tissues and organs don't get enough oxygen to energize you.

For women, the problem is common. Women's iron reserves can be strained by menstruation, especially for those with a heavy flow. On top of that, a woman's penchant for watching her weight adds to the risk of reduced iron stores. Pregnant women are also at risk. They need more iron because they're sharing their supply with a growing baby. In fact, experts estimate that 5 to 15 percent of menstruating women and 30 percent of pregnant women have iron-deficiency anemia.

Cheryl says that not only were her periods very heavy, but after giving birth to two children, they became even worse. "At first I thought this extreme exhaustion was from caring for two little kids and holding down a part-time job. And I'm sure that contributed to it. But I soon realized that I wasn't just tired, I was dysfunctionally tired, and I had to find out why."

ROBBING THE RESERVES

Iron-deficiency anemia in itself isn't a disease but a symptom that there's something else awry in the body, explains Suzanne McClure, M.D., Ph.D., assistant professor of medicine in the Division of Hematology-Oncology at the University of Texas Medical Branch in Galveston. "It's important to get to the root of the problem. For most women it's a case of too much blood loss from menstruation and not enough iron in the diet to replace what's lost. But if you're past menopause and no longer bleeding every month, then your doctor needs to do a little investigating."

Severe iron loss could be caused by a whole host of ailments, from a bleeding ulcer or hemorrhoids to a more serious condition such as gastrointestinal cancer, although this is rare.

And iron-deficiency anemia doesn't always come on with three-alarm symptoms as Cheryl's did. In fact, you may not even be aware that you have a problem until a routine blood test points it out, says Dr. McClure. In fact, you can be iron deficient without having full-blown anemia.

"Anemia can come on very gradually," says Dr. McClure. "You lose some blood each month, you go through a pregnancy or two over a few years and your iron stores

IRON GOES DOWN IN SMOKE

Getting a blood test on a routine basis is the best way to guard against anemia—unless you're a smoker.

If you smoke you could be anemic even though your levels of hemoglobin, which carries oxygen through the blood, appear to be within the normal range, according to researchers from the Division of Nutrition at the Centers for Disease Control in Atlanta.

Here's why. The carbon monoxide in cigarettes bonds to hemoglobin to form a substance called carboxyhemoglobin. This is an inactive form of hemoglobin that has no oxygen-carrying capacity. "To compensate for the decreased oxygen-delivery capacity, smokers maintain a higher hemoglobin level than nonsmokers," say the researchers. What's more, the more cigarettes you smoke, the higher your hemoglobin reading will be, masking a possible anemia.

The researchers suggest that when screening smokers for anemia, the cutoff level for normal hemoglobin should be adjusted upward depending on the number of cigarettes smoked each day. So if you smoke, make sure you discuss this with your doctor.

slowly diminish," she explains. Or you diet, diet, diet, constantly avoiding the foods—meat, for one—you should be getting.

"If you're not a particularly active person and you have a healthy heart and lungs, you won't feel the effects of iron-poor blood until your iron stores are quite low," notes Dr. McClure. "It's actually amazing how well the body can compensate."

On the other hand, if you're used to being physically active—you run or swim routinely, for example—you may notice a decrease in stamina more quickly, she points out. "Or if the anemia comes on suddenly—a rapid blood loss from a bleeding ulcer, for example, or particularly heavy menstrual periods—your symptoms will be much more pronounced."

THE PROBLEM OF DIET

Because of the nature of their bodies—and, in some cases, the way they treat their bodies—it's almost impossible for most women to get anywhere near the iron they need from their diets, points out Annette Natow, Ph.D., professor emerita of nutrition at Adelphi University in Garden City, New York, and registered dietitian at Nutrition Consultants in Valley Stream. "If a woman is on a 1,000-calorie-a-day diet, for example, she's probably only taking in 6 milligrams of iron—pitifully less than the Recommended Dietary Allowance of 15 milligrams. Even if she eats 2,000 calories a day, which is generally much more than health-conscious women allow themselves, her iron intake will average only about 12 milligrams."

Add to that the fact that if a woman chooses iron-poor foods, such as cottage cheese, yogurt, salad and fruit juice, for a good percentage of her daily intake, iron deficiency becomes even more likely.

Even mild anemia, experts say, is an advanced symptom of iron deficiency, since your body will deplete its store of iron before your blood cells feel the effects. When this happens your doctor most likely will recommend a six-month course of iron supplementation. You should also have your hemoglobin level checked periodically. If increasing your iron does not boost your blood level, your doctor may have to check for other causes of anemia.

"Since you only absorb about a third of the iron in the supplements," says Dr. McClure, "you need to take them for that long, even though you generally notice a difference in how you feel within a month or two. Patients will often comment to me that they didn't realize just how bad they felt until they started to regain their old energy."

IRON QUALITY

Of course, for the average woman, eating a diet rich in iron can help prevent an anemia problem in the first place. But getting enough iron isn't as simple as eating enough iron-rich foods. It's also the quality of the iron you're getting that you need to consider. This is because iron comes in two forms—heme, which is more easily absorbed, and nonheme. Also, certain combinations and components of foods can actually stand in the way of your body's ability to absorb iron.

Here's a dietary checklist to help keep you in iron balance.

Eat lean meats. Meats are your chief source of heme iron. In fact, heme iron is found only in animal products. And you don't have to lean toward fatty cuts to get it. A 6-ounce portion of lean sirloin steak, for example, will give you 5 milligrams of iron.

Eat vegetables and grains along with lean meat. Many grains and vegetables are good sources of nonheme iron. Although the body only absorbs a small percentage of this form of iron, eating these foods along with meat can help boost the iron absorption, says Dr. Natow.

Eat iron-rich legumes. Dried beans and peas are good plant sources of nonheme iron, so get plenty of them in your diet. Eating them along with lean meat will also help iron absorption.

Beware the calcium effect. The high calcium and phosphate content of milk and cheese can slightly inhibit iron absorption. If you're taking iron and calcium supplements, take them at different times of the day.

Combine iron-rich foods with foods high in vitamin C. Vitamin C enhances the absorption of nonheme iron in vegetables, beans grains, fruits and nuts. Drinking a glass of orange juice with your iron-rich meal can more than double the amount of iron your body absorbs.

Avoid drinking tea or coffee with your meals. And don't wash down an iron supplement with a mug of coffee, either. The tannins in these beverages bind with iron, making less of it available for absorption.

Cook foods in a cast-iron pot whenever practical. In one study, spaghetti sauce simmered in a cast-iron pot for about 20 minutes increased its iron content ninefold. Granted, the iron that leaches from the pot is nonheme, but it can make a big difference in your diet.

Eat iron-fortified foods. Iron-fortified or enriched breakfast cereals and other foods can help boost your iron intake. But you shouldn't rely on them exclusively, because the iron in them isn't always very absorbable.

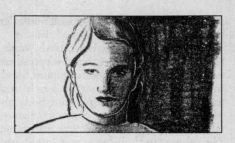

ANGER

ITS EFFECT ON *YOUR* HEALTH

*K*eep it in or spit it out? Suppress it or ventilate it? Slow burn or boil over? Any way you phrase it, anger and its various forms of expression are part of everyone's life.

But not until recently have women—at least "polite" women—had much choice in the matter. Historically, girls have always learned that showing anger is not ladylike, that anger disrupts relationships, that it can ruin your chances of getting a man. But that was yesterday's woman.

How does the woman of today express anger? The same way as a man. Recent research shows that women get angry as often as men, as intensely as men and for much the same reasons as men, says Sandra Thomas, R.N., Ph.D., director at the Center for Nursing Research at the University of Tennessee College of Nursing at Knoxville. Unfair treatment, frustration in their homes and professional lives and unmet expectations in general are just a few of the things that can ignite anger.

And what do they get in return for venting anger like a man? A bad bill of health. Just like a man.

According to research, women's anger has been implicated in a variety of health problems, including depression, high blood pressure, heart disease, arthritis, stress, drug and alcohol abuse and obesity. Women who extremely inhibit or vent their anger have higher rates of breast cancer than women who don't. Women who get angry also have unhappier marriages.

And it seems to be that extreme anger—whether vented or suppressed—is creating the problems for women.

"This goes against one commonly held belief that venting your anger will make you feel better," says Dr. Thomas, one of the researchers. But she found that expressing anger only creates more anger. And suppressing anger isn't necessarily good for you, either. In a study that spanned 18 years, researchers found that women who suppressed their anger over a long period of time were two times more likely to die prematurely than those who directly expressed their anger.

GETTING YOUR COOL

"Given the current state of science," says Dr. Thomas, "the best advice we can offer women is to get rid of their anger. Reflect on the triggers that create anger."

Instead of letting problems fester, she says to address anger-causing problems right away. If it's a person and you can't approach the instigator, then at least discuss it with a trusted friend or relative. Other advice from experts:

Keep an anger diary. In other words, become an expert on your own anger. Write down each episode and note what triggered it, who else was present, what you were thinking, how long it lasted and how you reacted, says Maureen Lassen, Ph.D., a clinical psychologist in Phoenix. You also need to record how you were feeling before the event. After a few weeks, look over your diary and see if any patterns emerge.

Keeping an anger diary also demystifies the emotion, showing you that it isn't an uncontrollable force, adds Carol Tavris, Ph.D., a social psychologist and the author of *Anger: The Misunderstood Emotion.*

Count to 10. Maybe even 20. And then use a technique the experts call reflective coping—trying to solve the underlying problem or source of anger. If the problem can't be solved, then other methods of coping should be used.

Reappraise the situation. When we're provoked by someone, we're likely to inflame the situation even more by saying to ourselves, "What a thoughtless clod!" or "The nerve of that witch!" Instead, try to empathize with the rude person or find justifications for her actions by thinking, "She must have some real problems to behave that way." This is what people who are slow to anger do naturally, says Dr. Tavris.

Sweat it out. Vigorous exercise, says Dr. Thomas, is an excellent outlet for powerful emotions, including anger.

Cut you losses. If there's no possibility of effecting a change, then remove yourself from the anger-provoking situation.

CHAPTER 4

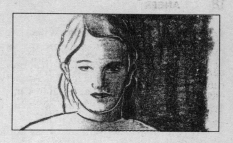

ANXIETY

FROM FEAR TO PHOBIA

*B*eing afraid of the Big Bad Wolf is one thing. But having an anxiety attack—sudden sheer terror for seemingly no reason at all—is something else altogether.

"It was a tidal wave of anxiety and fear that just came out of the blue," is how Philadelphia native Marian Baker recalls her first attack. "I was in college at the time, and a group of friends had gotten together in one of the dorm rooms to have a few beers. Suddenly my heart began racing for no apparent reason, and I was having trouble breathing. I bolted from the room and ran outside to try and get some air.

"I didn't know what was happening to me," adds Marian, "but I was terrified. I felt like I was dying."

Marian's anxiety attack—actually a particular kind of anxiety state called a panic attack—lasted less than an hour. But for the next few days she still felt light-headed and dizzy. "Every day I lived in fear of another attack," she says. "And eventually I had one. I felt like I was going crazy."

Marian is not alone in her experience. Repeated panic attacks—a condition known as panic disorder—are twice as common among women as among men, possibly, researchers suspect, because fluctuations in the female hormone progesterone may help trigger the brain mechanisms involved in the attack.

LIVING ON HOLD

We all feel anxious on occasion, says Paula Levine, Ph.D., a psychologist and director of the Agoraphobia Resource Center in Coral Gables, Florida. Anxiety is a normal part of living. But anxiety that escalates into a panic attack is not normal. In fact, in some women, it can become so severe that it *interferes* with living.

"If you picture a violin or a bass fiddle, we're all strung in the same way," explains Dr. Levine. "We all have the same nervous system, the same adrenaline pump and the same heart that can race too quickly. It's that old fight-or-flight response that kicks in when we perceive ourselves to be in mortal danger.

"Back in caveman times," she adds, "it happened when we were being chased by bears. Today our hearts might race, our palms sweat and our stomachs churn when we're about to give a speech in front of 200 people. Or when we have to take an exam. Or if a police car pulls up behind us and signals us to the side of the road. But that's all part of the normal response to a stressful event, which every human being is capable of feeling."

Those symptoms can occur before, during or after a feared or dreaded event, says Dr. Levine, but as long as you can identify the situation that precipitated the symptoms and they are not incapacitating, they remain normal responses.

"Symptoms of normal anxiety usually subside within a few minutes, too," she says. Fifty seconds into your piano recital, for example, your heart slows down and you're feeling fine. Or three minutes into your exam, you're sailing along with no problem.

ARE YOU A NERVOUS NELLIE?

But some women don't settle down once the cause of a particularly anxious moment is gone. Instead, they seem to stay anxious, experiencing what psychologists call a generalized anxiety disorder.

"It's a constant feeling of excessive fear, worry and apprehension that's unfounded," explains Constance V. Dancu, Ph.D., an anxiety disorder specialist at the Medical College of Pennsylvania in Philadelphia.

It's normal, for example, to be concerned if your teenager is late getting home from a date. Who wouldn't worry at least a little? But a woman who has a generalized anxiety disorder would have images of her daughter being in a car crash every time she went out, when in reality, the probability of that happening is relatively low.

"What's considered normal anxiety becomes an anxiety disorder when even simple, benign events elicit the fight-or-flight response," Dr. Levine explains. "In other words, the response is not appropriate to the situation." There is no bear there—there is no exam two minutes away, no police car signaling you to pull over, no imminent threat to anyone's safety—and yet your body reacts as if there were.

IN A PANIC

A panic attack is an intense type of anxiety disorder in which your body seems to be *trying* to fight a bear.

A full-blown panic attack occurs when—seemingly without cause—your anxiety levels shoot through the roof and trigger at least 4 of the following 12 symptoms: racing or pounding heart, breathing difficulty, dizziness, tingling fingers and feet, chest pain or tightness, a smothering sensation, faintness, sweating, trembling, hot or cold flashes, a sense of unreality and the ultimate whopper, a fear of dying. Symptoms typically last from 5 to 20 minutes, doctors report, during which time many women feel as though they're going crazy.

Although the panic attack is usually short-lived, lasting for only a few minutes, it leaves a nerve-racking residue of anxiety that can last for hours or even days. And even though an attack can actually be an isolated event and never occur again, you can become so frightened of having another attack that the appearance of even one symptom— maybe you feel faint while you're gardening, for example— can trigger a full-blown attack.

Psychologists estimate that 2 percent of American women and 1 percent of men will experience panic disorder during their lifetime. Dr. Levine believes that figure grossly underestimates the prevalence of the problem.

Unfortunately, no one knows for sure what causes panic attacks, says Dr. Levine. But current evidence suggests that it runs in families and that heavy-duty stressors such as major life transitions—job changes, bereavement, surgery, illness, separation from a loved one, difficulty at school—seem to trigger the initial attack.

OF MICE AND WOMEN

Then there is another kind of fear that most women know something about. A fear of creepy, crawly things. If you shiver every time you walk near the snake display at the local zoo—and flatly refuse to get too close—you could very well have a simple phobia about snakes.

Scientists say a simple phobia is a persistent, unrealistic fear that will disrupt normal activity. You may never want to go to a zoo or for a hike. It's not clear how phobias develop. One idea is that this type of fear is a learned response: Something terrible happened in your past—your brother put a snake under your pillow, for example—so now every time you go near a snake, you're afraid.

Another idea is that since many of us have the same phobias—snakes, small skittery animals and insects are the top three for both men and women—a phobia may actually be genetically inherited. It may be that at some time in our past, it was beneficial for us to fear something like a snake so intensely that we avoided it like the plague. We didn't inherit the fear itself, scientists emphasize, but we were somehow prepared on a biological level to learn it very easily.

Wherever it comes from, a phobia can be so mild that it hardly affects your life or so intense that it controls it. "Suppose that you're afraid of heights and bridges," says Dr. Dancu. "If you lived in a place where you never had to cross a bridge, it would never become debilitating. But if you had to cross several high bridges to get to work or go shopping, then your phobia would present a severe problem: It would interfere with your social and occupational functioning."

GETTING PROFESSIONAL HELP

Fortunately, anxiety disorders, including panic attacks and phobias, are very treatable, says Dr. Levine. "Sometimes counseling is all that's needed. Sometimes a combination of counseling and a limited course of medication works best. Whichever, any woman with one of these problems will usually feel much better within three to six months, give or take a little."

With panic disorder, for example, the prescription medication alprazolam (Xanax) has been so successful that your doctor will likely give you a prescription right away. It's probably the reason Xanax is the most popularly prescribed drug on the market today. Another medication used successfully in panic disorder is small dosages of the antidepressant Elavil. Drug treatment has not been successful for most phobias, however.

But for the long term, counseling is your best bet. "We can't promise women that they'll never feel anxious again, because some anxiety is normal," says Dr. Levine, "but a psychologist can teach you how to control it—instead of it controlling you."

Counseling may include learning coping strategies to better understand and manage your anxiety symptoms, says Dr. Dancu. "I ask my patients, 'What is the evidence that you're going to die during a panic attack? You've had 20—or maybe 100—and you haven't died yet.'

"It's a way of examining what's based on fact and is logical," she explains, "and what's based on faulty beliefs or myths and is not logical."

In fact, logic may be a major weapon. "Even if you are never able to identify what triggers a panic attack, you can still change your response to it," says Dr. Levine. "You don't have to think it's going to blind you or make you faint or drive you insane. You can break that catastrophic spiral of thinking and examine the symptoms for what they are—symptoms of an anxiety disorder, not a life-threatening illness.

Treatment also includes reassuring women that they are not going crazy, emphasizes Dr. Dancu. So many patients have been told that their symptoms are all in their minds. But just because there isn't a physical ailment causing their symptoms doesn't make them any less real.

"Panic attacks are a documented physiological phenomenon," stresses Dr. Levine. "Your heart really does race, your vision really can blur, your stomach really churns. This is not psychosomatic. It's not all in your head. Just understanding that something real is indeed happening to

AGORAPHOBIA: HOUSEWIFE'S DISEASE

Panic attacks can be so frightening that any woman who experiences them may begin to avoid situations or places where they've occurred. That's how agoraphobia—literally a "fear of the marketplace"—begins.

It's the number one phobia among women, says Paula Levine, Ph.D., director of Agoraphobia Resource Center in Florida. And, despite its name, it's really a fear of being alone in any public place from which you think escape may be difficult during a panic attack. The National Institute of Mental Health estimates that nearly 8 percent of American women will experience it during their lifetime—more than double the rate at which it affects men.

"At first any woman who's had several random panic attacks over a number of months tries to make sense of what's happening," explains Dr. Levine. "The woman looks around and says to herself, 'I've had attacks in the car. This must happen when I drive' or 'I've had attacks at the supermarket. This must happen when I shop.' So the woman stops driving and shopping. She slowly restricts where she thinks it's safe to go, until eventually she becomes completely housebound. That's why it's known as the housewife's disease."

Fortunately, agoraphobia is highly treatable, doctors agree. Psychotherapy and returning to any place you've experienced a panic attack can eliminate the entire problem.

COOL, CALM AND COLLECTED

If you're experiencing an excessive amount of anxiety, and particularly if you're experiencing panic attacks, here's how the experts say you can lessen anxiety's impact on your life.

Burn up the adrenaline. Excess adrenaline brought on by a fight-or-flight response is what causes some of the most distressing symptoms of panic attacks. To dissipate that adrenaline, try going for a short, brisk walk, running in place or dancing, says Paula Levine, Ph.D., a Florida psychologist.

Slow your breathing. Cool it down to 8 to 12 breaths per minute: Take a deep breath, hold for a count of 4, then exhale slowly.

Distract yourself. Instead of focusing on your physical symptoms, start talking with somebody or start people-watching. Or try splashing cold water on your face or applying a cold washcloth.

Look up. Research indicates that we have more intense feelings, positive or negative, when we are looking down, according to Ruth Dailey Grainger, R.N., Ph.D., clinical director of the Therapy Research Institute in Miami. Looking up can be a powerful interrupter of anxiety.

Lower your shoulders. When you are tense, you almost always raise your shoulders, according to Dr. Grainger, and lowering them can trigger instantaneous relief. If this seems unnatural to you, you might want to practice it.

Slow the pace of your thoughts. Anxious thoughts are usually fast and scattered. By slowing thoughts and making them complete sentences, you may help diminish anxiety in some cases and give yourself a greater feeling of control.

Alter your voice. Making your voice slower, lower in pitch and softer will signal to others and to yourself that you are in control.

Change your facial expression. If you tend to furrow your brow when anxiety strikes, then try smoothing out your forehead and turning the corners of your mouth up instead. Even though you may not be smiling at the moment, says Dr. Grainger, a turned-up mouth sends a physiological message to your mind to lighten up.

your body is a great relief. Sometimes it's all the education people need." For others, muscle relaxation techniques, deep-breathing exercises, imagery or even hypnosis can help reduce anxiety to manageable levels.

FACE-TO-FACE WITH FEAR

Once you can mentally get a handle on your fear, your psychologist will likely want you to put it to a test. "It's the old get-back-up-on-the-horse theory," says Dr. Levine. That is, you must not allow yourself to avoid situations where heightened anxiety or panic attacks occur. On the contrary, you must face them. Doctors enlist a therapy called graduated in vivo exposure; it very slowly reintroduces you to the feared places or situations while you learn to talk yourself through whatever symptoms crop up.

"Suppose, for example, that you haven't been able to go to the grocery store because you're afraid of having a panic attack and embarrassing yourself," says Dr. Dancu. "First, we would have you go to the store with a friend with whom you feel safe. Maybe you'd just walk around the store for 30 minutes or so. After you can accomplish that with little or no anxiety, the next step is to have your friend walk one aisle away from you. After that, perhaps your friend would wait outside for you, and then in the car. With each exercise you build up your courage, and ultimately, your freedom from fear and anxiety.

"The most important thing to remember," adds Dr. Dancu, "is that if you start to get anxiety symptoms, *you must stay in the situation and let that anxiety decrease on its own*. By not running away to a 'safe' place as soon as symptoms appear, you will learn to manage your anxiety and fears."

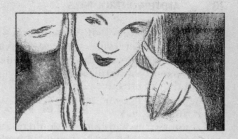

BIRTH CONTROL PILLS

THEY'RE STILL NUMBER ONE

*O*ral contraceptives—synthetic hormones that override the natural hormones that control reproduction—are now so safe that experts say you're ten times more likely to die driving to the drugstore to pick them up than you are from taking them.

That's a pretty good safety score, considering they've become the birth control method of choice among women who intend to have children in the future—but who don't want them now.

First-place status is an achievement that should be expected from the drug that, tablet by tablet, led us into the Sexual Revolution. After all, it was only a little more than a generation ago that most women were so terrified of getting pregnant that they avoided sex until there was a ring on their finger.

Oral contraceptives changed that attitude completely and ripped apart the social structure that supported it. By removing the probability of pregnancy, oral contraceptives also removed the need for a lifetime commitment before women could express their sexuality.

PLUS AND MINUS

How do oral contraceptives work? Essentially, scientists report, they leave no stone—or reproductive function—unturned. They suppress ovulation, change the composition of cervical mucus so that sperm have a difficult time penetrating it, interfere with the transport of an egg though the fallopian tube and change the uterine lining to inhibit implantation of a fertilized egg.

And they're effective. Only 3.8 to 8.7 percent of women taking the Pill become pregnant, most often because they use it incorrectly.

Of course, as with any drug, there are side effects and risks. Spotting and breakthrough bleeding are the most common problems, doctors report, largely because of the low-dose estrogen pills. The less estrogen in a pill, the more likely you are to experience spotting.

Breakthrough bleeding isn't pleasant, of course, but it's a trade-off that allows you to avoid what some women felt were even more unpleasant side effects from the high-dose estrogen pills initially prescribed back in the 1960s: nausea, weight gain, swollen breasts, headaches and changes in skin color. Those side effects are now pretty much a thing of the past, researchers say, as are many of the cardiovascular problems that sometimes accompanied the original pills.

WHEN YOUR PROTECTION GOES UP IN SMOKE

Actually, it's a miracle that the Pill—as it is commonly called—became so overwhelmingly popular considering its debut was marked by reports of such intimidating side effects. In fact, at one point, newspapers carried frequent warnings that oral contraceptives caused strokes and heart attacks.

Originally scientists suspected that the cardiovascular problems reported by oral contraceptive users were simply a side effect of playing around with hormones. Today, however, some feel that many of the problems may have been caused by the interaction among cigarette smoke, the Pill, and age, says Jacqueline Darroch Forrest, Ph.D., vice-president for research of the Alan Guttmacher Institute, a nonprofit organization that does research in reproductive studies, in New York City.

Studies have demonstrated that the combined effect of birth control pills and smoking can increase your risk of a heart attack no matter what your age. And the older you are—possibly because you're more likely to weight the equation with high blood pressure or high cholesterol as well—the more your risk increases.

By age 40, for example, women who take oral contraceptives but do not smoke can expect ten times the heart attack rate per 100,000 women than women who use another method of birth control. But for women who smoke and take the Pill, the risk of heart attack jumps 4,000 percent.

The same kind of relationship seems to exist among smoking, oral contraceptives and stroke, researchers report. By age 40, nonsmokers who take the Pill will experience seven times the stroke rate per 100,000 than those who use other forms of birth control. But by age 30, heavy smokers increase their risk more than 1,000 percent.

Clearly, doctors agree, the added risk of cardiovascular disease for Pill users who are young and do not smoke is very low.

THE PILL AND CANCER

Perhaps the biggest health concern among women is the link between oral contraceptives and breast cancer—a link that seems more confusing with every study that's done. One study seems to indicate that, yes, birth control pills do cause breast cancer. Then another, equally well-conducted study suggests that, no, birth control pills do not cause breast cancer.

What's the bottom line? Well, the Centers for Disease Control in Atlanta conducted a study involving 10,000 women that may explain these seemingly opposite results. The problem, and possibly the source of all the confusion, may be that Pill use seems to *increase* a woman's risk of getting breast cancer under age 35 but *decrease* a woman's risk when she is 45 or older.

One theory that may explain the seemingly odd link between the Pill and breast cancer in younger women is

CONTRACEPTION UNDER YOUR SKIN

The levonorgestrel implant is the first major new contraceptive method introduced in the United States in many years. Best known by its trade name Norplant, the contraceptive consists of six small capsules containing progestin, the same synthetic hormone that is used in oral contraceptives to suppress ovulation. Implanted just under the skin in a woman's arm, these capsules will continually release progestin into the body and prevent pregnancy for up to five years. Fertility is restored once the capsules are removed.

Before it was approved by the Food and Drug Administration in 1990, Norplant was tested on more than 50,000 women worldwide and proved to be highly effective. Statistically, your chance of getting pregnant with the implant is roughly 1 percent, which makes it as effective as oral contraceptives.

The biggest drawback of the implant seems to be menstrual irregularities. Most women using it either stop menstruating altogether, begin to develop heavy periods or experience spotting. Some of these problems resolve themselves after the first year, and acceptance of the method is quite high—in one study 94 percent of women said they would use the implants again even though 95 percent of them had experienced some side effects. Side effects other than menstrual irregularities are headaches, acne, hair loss and weight gain. Another drawback is that the implant may not be as effective in women who weigh more than 154 pounds at the time of insertion or for women who gain weight afterward. Effectiveness goes down as weight goes up. It's also very expensive, costing $500 or more.

Although little is yet known about the major health effects of using only progestin for birth control, experts say you are unlikely to run an increased risk of cardiovascular disease since estrogen is the hormone linked to heart problems. And, as with oral contraceptives, you are likely to be protected from pelvic inflammatory disease, benign breast disease and ovarian cysts. Progestin use has been linked to a rise in blood pressure, however, which is a risk factor for stroke.

that the Pill's hormones don't cause cancer in and of themselves but merely speed up the growth of a cancer that wouldn't be diagnosed until later, says Dr. Forrest. Another theory is that women on the Pill are screened more frequently and therefore a cancer is detected at an earlier stage. Still another theory is that the Pill, by mimicking pregnancy, increases breast cancer risk in the short term, but decreases it over the long term in the same way pregnancy does.

THE PILL PROTECTS

Although the relationship between oral contraceptives and breast cancer is still somewhat up in the air, studies have found that the Pill clearly protects women from other kinds of cancer.

Women who have used oral contraceptives are 40 percent less likely to develop either ovarian or endometrial cancer, scientists report, and, in the case of ovarian cancer at least, the Pill's protective effects can last for 15 years or more after you stop taking it.

Moreover, the longer you take the Pill, the higher the degree of protection it offers. A woman who has taken the Pill for 4 years or less, for example, reduces her risk of ovarian cancer by 30 percent. A woman who has taken the Pill for between 6 and 11 years reduces her risk by 60 percent. And, believe it or not, a woman who has taken the Pill for 12 or more years reduces her risk of ovarian cancer by an astounding 80 percent.

The Pill protects you so effectively that one researcher actually made an educated guess at the number of cancers it prevents: 2,000 cases of endometrial cancer and 1,700 cases of ovarian cancer a year.

But the Pill's protective effects don't stop with cancer. If researchers are correct, each year the Pill may also prevent 51,000 cases of pelvic inflammatory disease, 27,000 cases of iron-deficiency anemia, 20,000 cases of benign breast tumors, 9,900 ectopic pregnancies and 3,000 ovarian cysts.

MAKING A DECISION

Any decision regarding birth control should always be made in consultation with your doctor, says Dr. Forrest. Not just because you need a prescription, but because medical knowledge is evolving so quickly that each of us has a different configuration of possible risk factors at any given moment.

Most doctors agree, for example, that if you're over 35, a heavy smoker, suffering from high blood pressure or other cardiovascular disease or if you have or are suspected to have breast cancer, you should steer clear of oral contraceptives. But what if you have a family history of ovarian cancer? In that case, says Dr. Forrest, some of those negatives might not weigh so heavily.

There are lifestyle considerations as well, adds Linda J. Beckman, Ph.D., director of research at the California School of Professional Psychology in Alhambro who has done several studies on women's contraceptive choices.

If you're not having sex regularly or have multiple partners, birth control pills are probably not the wisest choice, says Dr. Beckman, also an adjunct professor in the Department of Psychology at University of California, Los Angeles. In those cases, you'll need a method that can be used as needed and one that will protect you against sexually transmitted diseases—AIDS, herpes, precancerous genital warts and the like—which can affect your life and future fertility. If you do choose oral contraceptives, you should still use a condom to protect yourself from sexually transmitted disease.

But if you're married and don't want children for a while, says Dr. Beckman, you may find that the Pill is just what the doctor should order.

The choice, she adds, is yours.

See also Contraception, Pregnancy

CHAPTER
6

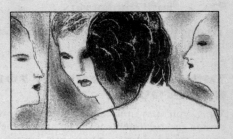

BLEMISHES

FACING UP TO IMPERFECTIONS

*A*cne has never been strictly a teenage scourge. In fact, if you're past 30 and still battling blemishes, you're far from alone. Ask any dermatologist.

"It's no picnic facing the world with a bad complexion," admits Amy Miller, a 31-year-old accountant. "When I was a teenager, I was called pizza face by other kids. I'd wear gobs of makeup and try to ignore the insults, but it was a painful experience nonetheless. Now, even if I get just one pimple on my face, it brings back the old horrors."

An overreaction from an oversensitive woman? Hardly. "We live in an extremely visual society," says Nia Terezakis, M.D., clinical professor of dermatology at Tulane University School of Medicine and a practicing dermatologist in New Orleans. "Skin problems, especially those on the face, make you feel that the world is looking at you as imperfect. Of course, you'd like to think that people will love you for what's on the inside, and the fact is, most do. But there's that insecurity that's built into so many of us."

Dr. Terezakis often sees both the physical and emotional scars that a bad complexion can leave. "I've been treating one woman over a period of years for extreme acne scarring, some of the worst I've ever seen," she says. "She looked like an old woman at 20 because deep scarring winds up resembling wrinkles. If you saw her today, you would see a beautiful young woman with beautiful skin.

Yet, she is so insecure about her appearance that she absolutely will not let me show her off."

THE BREAKTHROUGH FOR BREAKOUTS

What you may not realize is that knowledge about the causes and treatments for acne have come a long way since you were a kid battling your first pimple. Scientific studies over the past 15 years have proven that it's *not* what you eat that causes your face to break out. Heredity is the most important factor determining whether you'll have blemishes.

Stress, on the other hand, is thought to be a perpetrator in a predisposed person, although, as one researcher points out, it would be pretty hard to prove this in controlled studies. After all, who is willing to be placed under extreme stress to find out if their face breaks out? Nevertheless, dermatologists have thousands of patients whose incidence of skin flare-ups can be linked to stressful times in their lives.

Julie Sandburg, a 25-year-old computer programmer, knows what stress can do. "I used to break out before finals when I was in college," she says. "I was so self-conscious that when I'd talk to people, I'd turn my face so the better side was showing. Or I'd keep moving my fingers through my hair to take the focus off my face. My biggest worry was that a date would try to touch my face and he'd feel the pimples." Julie sought help from a dermatologist and also signed up for a stress-management course offered by her college. She says the combination did wonders for her psyche *and* her skin.

THE ANTI-ACNE ARSENAL

Today dermatologists have many weapons in their anti-acne arsenal. Dr. Terezakis often recommends the drug Accutane for the worst cases. "This drug is absolutely sensational for acne. I've had patients so afraid that it will be snatched off the market, they're willing to march to Washington. They tell me they'd like to store a supply in their freezers so their children will never have to go through what they did," she says.

Accutane is controversial, however, because it can cause birth defects. Doctors caution that you should not use it if there is any chance, however remote, that you might be pregnant. Also, you should not start treatment until after the first normal menstrual period following a negative pregnancy test. It also carries side effects, such as decreased night vision and pinkeye.

Once the acne has cleared up, Dr. Terezakis says that Retin-A, the topical form of Accutane, can maintain your new clear complexion. "If deep scarring is left by acne, injections of collagen may help smooth out the skin."

PERFECT PORE PERFORMANCE

Since adult acne is a chronic condition, you'll need to follow a regular program of preventive maintenance to loosen oil plugs and acne-causing bacteria that clog your pores. This means keeping the pores as clean as possible. Doctors recommend using a soft washcloth or your hands and a mild soap such as Dove, Purpose or Neutrogena. Harsh scrubbing to clear out pores can irritate your skin and make the condition worse. Julie's doctor also recommended she use a cleanser that contains salicylic acid, which helps loosen plugs of debris relatively gently.

To discourage new blemishes from forming and limit the severity of pimples if they do form, use an antibacterial lotion containing benzoyl peroxide. And don't forget coverups that hide blemishes while they work to dry them up.

Julie says that after trying just about everything, including Retin-A and antibiotics, she finally found a system that has worked to keep her skin virtually blemish-free. It includes washing her face twice a day with a mild soap and using an over-the-counter cleanser that contains salicylic acid and a cream containing benzoyl peroxide at night.

That combined with stress management does the trick, she says. "And it's well worth the effort. Now I can wear my hair off my face, sometimes pulled straight back. My skin is the best it's ever been—pure peaches and cream."

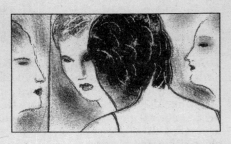

BODY IMAGE

WHAT WE—AND OTHERS—SEE

When you look in the mirror, what do you see? If you're like many women, it's not what's reflected back. Rather, your mind's eye sees your body critically as an intricate, continuously changing collage of past and present experiences, of forgotten praises and remembered insults. Of feeling too fat, too curly, too tall or too hippy, at a time when skinny, straight, petite or narrow hips were the signs of true beauty. Of never fitting in, if it means looking like the models in magazines or the smooth-skinned actresses who bare their perfect bodies on larger-than-life movie screens. Of wondering at times who will love an average, normal human woman like you because you don't look as desirable as society and Madison Avenue make you feel you should.

"Of all the ways people think of themselves, none is so primal as the image of their own bodies," says April Fallon, Ph.D., assistant professor in the Department of Psychiatry at the Medical College of Pennsylvania in Philadelphia. "The way we view our bodies is a reflection of our self-esteem. It is subject to the same psychological distortions as our sense of self and will in turn affect the way we view ourselves.

"Girls and women are generally less satisfied with their bodies, in particular with their weight, than boys and men," continues Dr. Fallon, who has done extensive research on body image. "Even the thinnest girls point to specific areas

that they see as too big—thighs and hips in particular."
Studies conducted by Dr. Fallon have shown that, in general, women think they are heavier than others see them, whereas men have a more accurate assessment of their body shapes. What's more, women's perception of what men consider to be the ideal female figure is significantly thinner than the figure that males actually desire.

HEARING IS BELIEVING, TOO

The development of a negative body image is rooted in childhood, adds Mary Froning, Psy.D., a clinical psychologist practicing in Washington, D.C. Our society focuses too much on physical appearance. Everywhere girls and women turn, ideals of beauty scream out at them—from TV and magazines to the women chosen to be Miss America.

Little girls who grow up outside the "ideal" are often told so in so many words by other children and insensitive adults—a kind of emotional abuse that scars the psyche. It is invisible to the outside world but indelibly etched in the mind of the receiver, says Dr. Froning.

"I grew up thinking I was a hideous monster, a freak," admits Darlene Balin, a successful businesswoman of 41. "I was overweight, tall, and when I hit puberty was graced with an overabundance of body hair. Once when I was standing outside a supermarket waiting for my father to pick me up, a little boy about 5 years old looked up at me and said, 'You're ugly.' Everywhere I went it felt like I was running a gauntlet. Walking by a group of teenage boys was the worst nightmare. It's pretty hard to feel good about yourself when the world is telling you otherwise."

DAMAGED-GOODS SYNDROME

It would be a mistake to underestimate the influence of abuse on how women feel about their bodies, Dr. Froning says. Believe it or not, random surveys of adults have indicated that as many as half of all women report having been sexually abused in some fashion one or more times before age 18. Twenty to 25 percent have experienced childhood sexual abuse. "This kind of abuse creates what is known as the damaged-goods syndrome," she explains. "That is, women often feel that the abuse has somehow damaged their bodies and that everyone will be able to see how hideous they really are. In fact, I've had some truly beautiful women express to me how ugly they think they are. These women often struggle to attain body perfection through excessive dieting or numerous cosmetic surgeries because they believe it's the only way to rid themselves of feeling ugly."

BUILDING ON THE POSITIVE

If it's any consolation, many women grow more accepting of their bodies as they age. Not that they suddenly love their too-broad hips or too-long nose. But their so-called flaws become less important to their total perception of themselves.

You can help yourself achieve a kinder view of your body shape, too, if you haven't quite managed it yet. Here's what the experts advise.

Recognize the problem. Issues of body esteem and body image are a result of a complicated set of cultural pressures, says Dr. Fallon. The fact is, these pressures have influenced your ideas and attitudes about the importance of beauty and physical attractiveness. In other words, you did not become so critical of yourself in a vacuum.

Improve what you can, within reason. A responsible effort to lose weight, and an exercise program to tone muscles and improve cardiovascular fitness, can do wonders to improve body esteem. But beware, says Dr. Fallon, that you don't go overboard in your effort. It's not for nothing that the women who are the most likely to be excessively critical of their bodies are also those most likely to develop disorders such as anorexia nervosa (self-starvation) and bulimia (bingeing and purging)—dieting gone haywire.

It's not unreasonable to consider cosmetic surgery, adds Dr. Froning. "Sometimes a consultation with a plastic surgeon can reassure you that your particular 'flaw' is certainly within normal limits. It's like getting an affirmation from an authority figure, someone who really knows," she says. On the other hand, surgically fixing a bothersome physical characteristic can sometimes initiate a process of emotional healing, Dr. Fallon states—especially in a person who is otherwise realistic about her physical appearance.

Rephrase negative thoughts into positive ones. Dr. Froning teaches women to say something positive about a part of themselves they don't like but can't do anything about. "A woman might say to me, for example, that her breasts are too small," says Dr. Froning. "She can turn that statement around and say instead, 'My breasts are exactly the right size for my body and I feel good about them. They're part of me and I'm satisfied with them.' This is what we call an affirmation, and I'll advise the woman to say this statement ten times a day for 21 days. That's because if you repeat something over and over and over again, it becomes part of your belief system."

Accentuate the positive. Everybody has something— hair, eyes, hands—that they can feel good about. You may be the best friend a person could ask for, or you may be particularly sensitive to others. Whatever it is, if you draw attention to what you like best about yourself, you are directing others' attention there, too.

Develop a sense of humor about yourself. Sandra Gursky, 35, a housewife and mother, recalls a particular event, while on a trip to the British Isles, where her sense of humor came to her rescue. She had met a man, a rugby player as it turned out, in a pub. They began to talk and suddenly he commented to her, "You have a really big, long nose." Sandra started to get upset, but something stopped her. "I looked him square in the face," she says, "and noticed for the first time that he had braces on his teeth—so many that it looked like high-tension wires spanning his mouth. I replied to him with a big grin, 'I may have a big nose, but at least I can go outdoors in a lightning storm.' "

Sandra says that the man burst out laughing and said it was the funniest thing he'd ever heard. "I think that pointing out his flaw somehow made us equal," she says. "It dawned on me then that people pick on another's foibles and flaws because they are so conscious of their own short-comings. I gained a new sense of power that night."

Change your priorities. What's really important to you? How you look or who you are? A person who grew up in a family that emphasized physical attractiveness is likely to place more importance on body image than someone from a family that stressed education and achievement, says Dr. Froning. "The fact is, a woman who feels generally happy with her work or school or family can let physical imperfections go, place less importance on them." The culture may still hound you to be thin and perfectly proportioned, but you will be better able to withstand the pressures and focus on what's really important—your relationships and your behavior.

Learn to erase "old tapes." You are not your nose. You are not your hips—in spite of the distressing messages you remember from your past. Donna Degregorio, sensitive about the size of her hips (which were not outlandishly large), always thought that people saw only that about her. She wondered how she looked to others and sought comparisons. When walking behind a woman, she'd ask her husband, "Is that what *I* look like from behind?" Her husband was always astonished by her choices, for the women she compared herself to were often grossly obese. It turned out that Donna's oldest sister had broad hips, too, and Degregorio grew up hearing her family despair over her big sister's "figure flaw."

"People who focus on negative body images have been given reason to feel this way," Dr. Froning points out. "They carry these messages with them into adulthood, like audiotapes that are programmed to replay at the appropriate signal. You have to go back and erase those abusive messages from your memory. Whenever you feel people are judging you by your particular 'flaw,' immediately recognize the connection to past messages and tell yourself that it is not true, that's not what they are doing, that your body is fine the way it is. Say it over and over, turning a negative thought into a positive affirmation."

Recognize that beauty comes in many forms. Michelle Pfeiffer is beautiful. So are Barbra Streisand, Oprah Winfrey, Sinead O'Connor and Jessica Tandy. The point is that there are many ways to be beautiful. Today, more often than not, an interesting face garners as much attention, if not more, than a classically beautiful one, like Christie Brinkley's. And that's good news for all of us.

See also Self-Esteem

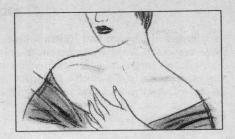

BREAST CARE

WHAT EVERY WOMAN NEEDS TO KNOW

*E*very couple of months or so, sometimes less, I do a half-hearted examination of my breasts," says Marlene Egan, a sales representative for a major computer company. "I know I should be more conscientious about it. After all, I'm 41.

"But I feel all these bumps and ridges in there and I wonder if I'd recognize a dangerous lump even if it should appear. So mostly I rely on my doctor to check me over once a year, and get mammograms when he tells me to," she says.

Marlene's breast-care plan is fairly common. Surveys have shown that most women know about breast self-exam, but only about one-third actually do it. And although more women are likely to get at least one mammogram, the National Institutes of Health report that only 31 percent of women age 40 and older get them as often as recommended by the National Cancer Institute (NCI). Indeed, breast cancer screening is so underutilized in the United States that the NCI believes it could be a major reason why breast cancer death rates have not declined over the past three decades.

KEEPING A CAREFUL WATCH

Although there is no sure way to prevent breast cancer, experts will tell you that your best chance for survival is early detection. And to that end most specialists recommend that every woman past the age of 20 do the following:

- Perform a monthly breast self-examination (see "How to Perform a Breast Self-Exam" on page 45).
- Have a breast examination by a doctor every three years up to the age of 40 and yearly thereafter.
- Have a baseline (first) mammogram between the ages of 35 and 39.
- Have a mammogram every one to two years between the ages of 40 and 49 and once a year thereafter.

Sounds simple enough, doesn't it? Then why aren't most women following this advice?

One reason is that breast self-examination isn't taught very well, says Susan Love, M.D., director of the Faulkner Breast Center in Boston and clinical assistant professor of surgery at Harvard Medical School. "We tell women to look for a change, but then we don't tell them what kind of a change. Nor do we tell them what a cancerous lump feels like."

Like Marlene, most women who try to do a breast self-exam give up or do it only sporadically because they are frightened by what they're feeling. "They lack confidence in their technique or they're afraid they'll find something," says Wende Logan-Young, M.D., director of the Breast Clinic in Rochester, New York, and a consultant to the Roswell Park Cancer Institute in Buffalo. "Either way it creates a great deal of anxiety.

"I've had women say to me, 'Look, I know how to do a self-exam, but if I ever found a lump I would just curl up and die. I couldn't handle it.' They want someone else—their physician—to take the responsibility," she adds.

Even women who have gone through the discovery of a benign lump are reluctant to perform a self-exam. In a study of 655 women, researchers from the University of Michigan School of Public Health in Ann Arbor found that women who discovered a lump that later proved to be benign were three times more likely to *stop* practicing self-exams than women who had never discovered a lump.

It's as if the women who discovered their own lumps were saying that they brought the whole unpleasant experience on themselves because they performed breast self-examination, the researchers speculate. Even though the outcome was clearly favorable, the stress, discomfort and inconvenience that accompanied the event apparently had such a negative impact that self-examinations were discontinued by many. These women in particular, say the researchers, need to be encouraged by their doctors to continue self-care.

Women who are so overwhelmed by anxiety that they just can't do a breast self-exam should simply see their doctor more frequently, perhaps every three or four months, says Dr. Love, who is also the author of *Dr. Susan Love's Breast Book*. "Then they don't have to deal with the anxiety of doing it themselves, but they do get the advantages of relatively early detection of a lump.

"Don't feel like you're some kind of nut if performing a self-exam freaks you out," adds Dr. Love. "We've all got our 'crazy' areas, and you're entitled to some irrational feelings."

EARLY DETECTION CAN SAVE YOUR BREAST

Breast self-examination can mean early detection, and early detection can mean less disfiguring surgery, says Dr. Love. "It may mean the difference between a larger or smaller lumpectomy, or even the difference between a lumpectomy and a mastectomy."

But even though early detection is important, you need to realize that whether you discover a lump this month or next month isn't. "Breast lumps are generally slow-growing," explains Dr. Love. "And some of them are sneaky. They don't become 'feelable' until they're fairly large, because the cancer has to grow big enough for the body to create a reaction—a fibrous, scarlike tissue forms around the cancer—which is actually what you feel." Unfortunately, the notion that you've "missed" a lump is the source of a lot of unnecessary guilt, says Dr. Love. A woman often

HOW TO PERFORM A BREAST SELF-EXAM

Most breast lumps (about 90 percent) are discovered through self-examination. So the better able you are to do a thorough examination, the more likely you will be to discover a problem as soon as it makes its appearance. Before you get started, here's what you will be looking for.

- New lumps
- Puckering of the skin
- Dimpling of the skin
- Thickening or hardening under the skin
- Retraction of the nipple
- Bleeding or discharge from the nipple
- Any other unusual appearance of the skin or nipples

Now here's how to look, according to the American College of Obstetricians and Gynecologists and the Albert Einstein Healthcare Foundation.

In the shower. Raise one arm. With fingers flat, touch every part of each breast, gently feeling for a lump or thickening. Use your right hand to examine your left breast and your left hand for your right breast.

Before a mirror. With arms at your sides, then raised above your head, look carefully for changes in the size, shape and contour of each breast. Look for puckering, dimpling or changes in skin texture. Gently squeeze both nipples and look for a discharge.

Lying flat on your back. This is the most important step because it is the only position in which you can feel all the tissue. Place a folded towel or a pillow under your left shoulder and place your left hand under your head. With your right hand, keeping the fingers flat and together, gently feel your left breast without exerting too much pressure. Use small circular motions with your fingers starting at the outermost top edge of your breast and spiraling in toward the nipple. Examine every part of the breast. Repeat for the right breast. Be sure to examine the area below the armpit, which also contains breast tissue.

feels that she screwed up and missed something obvious when it's simply not true.

PICTURE THIS

If performing breast self-examination has the potential for early detection, consider what a mammogram can do.

"Although mammograms aren't perfect, on the average, a mammogram can pick up a cancer two years before the patient or her doctor can," says Dr. Logan-Young, adding a few words of caution. "It's not perfect. The fact is, if a woman's breast tissue is very dense, the woman or her doctor may feel a lump before it's visible on a mammogram. Still," she insists, "it's amazing what mammograms can pick up. One of the reasons is that half of all cancers contain clusters of calcifications—calcium salts left as cellular debris—which show up as white specks visible even among dense breast tissue."

"If a tumor develops around the edges of the breast or if it doesn't create much fibrous reaction or if the breast is exceptionally dense, a mammogram may not pick it up, either," adds Dr. Love.

Nevertheless, mammogram screening improves the survival rate of women over age 50 with breast cancer by 30 percent.

"That's why I firmly believe in it," says Dr. Love. "And mammograms become more effective the older you get. As you age, your breast tissue becomes less dense and more fatty, making it easier for the mammogram to detect an abnormality."

WAITING-ROOM WILLIES

It's not without some anxiety that women schedule a mammogram. "Whenever you go for a mammogram, you go with fear and trembling," admits Dr. Love. "After all, why are you there if not to look for cancer?"

"When I go for my yearly mammogram, I can't help thinking about the reason I'm there," confirms Samantha Kern, a 52-year-old freelance writer. "This is no ordinary x-ray, after all. This is not the dentist looking for a cavity. I'm here to look for breast cancer, and there's no getting around that fact," she admits. "As I sit in the waiting room, I think about my future and my health. 'What if they find something?' I think to myself. Worse yet, 'What if they *miss* something?' It's a sobering experience that always leaves me feeling vulnerable."

Vulnerable, yes. But—once the results are in—probably relieved as well. Because the truth is that the vast majority of women are sent on their way with a clean bill of health. "For every 200 mammograms we do in our office," says Dr. Logan-Young, "we will find only one cancer. The other 199 are okay."

But what if it's *your* mammogram that's abnormal? Finding an abnormality—whether it turns out to be benign or malignant—causes significant anxiety, doctors agree. In a study conducted by Caryn Lerman, Ph.D., director of behavorial oncology at Fox Chase Cancer Center in Cheltenham, Pennsylvania, and her associates, found that about 40 percent of the women with suspicious mammograms worried frequently about breast cancer from the time of their mammograms to their diagnostic follow-ups. About 25 percent of those said that these worries were so significant that it affected their moods. And 20 percent reported that they had trouble handling daily activities.

Unlike those who discovered a problem through self-exam, however, those with abnormal mammograms were more likely to return for subsequent ones than those whose mammograms were perfectly normal.

EXCUSES, EXCUSES

But what keeps most women from getting routine mammograms isn't always fear or anxiety. It's ignorance.

According to a survey by the Jacobs Institute of Women's Health in Washington, D.C., and the NCI, women are operating under a number of false assumptions that could hurt them.

Thirty-five percent of the women surveyed who had had only one mammogram believed, for example, that if it showed no problem, they did not need to have another, according to Sharyn Sutton, Ph.D., chief of the National Cancer Institute's Information Projects Branch. The survey also indicated that more than 25 percent of the women who had never had a mammogram believed that they were not at risk for breast cancer. And about 40 percent felt that they weren't at risk because no one in their family had a history of breast cancer. They were totally unaware that, as Dr. Sutton points out, "up to 80 percent of breast cancers occur in women who have no family history of the disease."

The survey also showed that those who had never had a mammogram were more likely to believe that mammograms are important only for women who feel a lump or have other symptoms of breast cancer.

If you're waiting for your doctor to recommend that you get a mammogram, however, be prepared to wait a long time. Despite the American Cancer Society's recommended schedule for mammograms, one study found that almost half of the women who had never had a mammogram said that their doctors had never recommended it.

Yet, when a doctor does recommend a mammogram, says Dr. Lerman, the vast majority of women comply. Indeed, one survey sponsored by the American Cancer Society found that 94 percent of women whose physicians had recommended mammograms had had one in the past two years, while only 36 percent of women whose physicians had not made the recommendation had had one.

As one expert puts it, doctors are missing quite an opportunity. If physicians ordered mammograms at the time they performed breast examinations, and if all patients complied, mammography could approximately double nationally. And how do you think *that* would affect breast cancer mortality rates?

WHEN A LUMP IS SUSPICIOUS

It happens. You or your doctor or a mammogram finds something suspicious. It's a scenario dreaded by every woman and met head on by thousands every year.

When Annette Sobel, a 49-year-old teacher, found a

lump in her breast, she says she thought about it off and on for two weeks before deciding what to do. "I had my period when I first noticed it, and so I thought I'd wait to see if it went away after it was over," says Annette. "It didn't. I kept thinking it couldn't be anything—no one in my family has ever had cancer of *any* kind. But it nagged at me, and every time I got undressed I would look at it and feel it and get more nervous. Finally, one night I burst into tears and told my husband what I'd found. The very next day we both went to see my doctor. She said it did indeed feel suspicious, although she tried to reassure me by saying that nobody could tell for sure until a biopsy was done. My stomach went into knots, and a wave of nausea came over me. Tears came later."

"There are as many different reactions to the news of possible breast cancer as there are women," says Dr. Logan-Young. "There are women who go into shock and they aren't able to think at all. They're so overwhelmed by the information that their brain circuits sort of spin. Nothing we tell them locks in. In fact, we've actually had to drive some women home, they were so knocked off their feet by the news."

"Our patients tell us that they go through periods of denial and disbelief, numbness and absolute terror," adds Mary Jane Massie, M.D., an associate attending psychiatrist at Memorial Sloan-Kettering Cancer Center who counsels breast cancer patients. "Some of those emotional reactions may keep people from moving forward for the final diagnosis, but for most it has the opposite effect. They must have an answer immediately."

"But most women are really tough," says Dr. Logan-Young. "They react in a very pragmatic way. They'll say, 'Okay, describe to me what has to be done and I'll do it.' And we write all the instructions down: that they're going to see a surgeon, that the surgeon will make a date for the biopsy, that on the day of the biopsy he'll either put them to sleep or do it under a local anesthetic. And we give them copies of their mammograms and any other diagnostic tests to take along to the surgeon.

"We give patients as much information as we can," she

continues. "We show them their mammogram and the area in question. If they haven't felt the lump yet—because it was found on a mammogram, for instance—we have them feel it. If we think it's highly suspicious, we'll tell them so, and if we think it's likely to be benign, we'll tell them that.

"I also give women my home phone number," says Dr. Logan-Young, "and tell them to call me at any time if they have any questions at all. Women have told me that even though they didn't call, just knowing that they could was a great comfort."

IN LIMBO

The worst time for a woman is that period of time between finding out she has a suspicious lump and the biopsy results. "It's that fear of the unknown," says Dr. Logan-Young. "And even though the odds are in her favor—nationally, only one of every seven biopsied lumps turns out to be cancer—she can't, of course, get it out of her mind that she could be that one."

For Annette, that time in limbo was "the longest week of my life," she says. "I had to get through the long Memorial Day weekend before the biopsy could be done. My husband and I went to the video store and rented more than a dozen movies—thrillers, comedies, adventures, science fictions—anything but tear-jerkers. Believe it or not, I was actually able to laugh during that weekend, and I was able to escape reality for a few hours at a time," says Annette. "But at night, I'd wake up and imagine what my future might hold—illness, pain, disfigurement, maybe death. I didn't want my life and my lifestyle to change. I didn't like being forced to face my own mortality. I wasn't ready."

GETTING THROUGH THE WAIT

"We try to get our patients through the diagnostic workup as quickly as possible," says Dr. Massie, "because there really isn't anything that any wise psychiatrist can say, and there's no magic pill that takes away the horrible fear these women are going through. That's why women need compassionate doctors who truly understand what a terrible time this is for them."

Dr. Logan-Young says she usually sees two different coping strategies among her patients. One group wants to talk to everyone they know about it, the other group wants to read everything they can. "Both help," says Dr. Massie, "but I always encourage verbal communication. This is not the time to spare your family members. You need all the support you can get. For women who prefer the intellectual approach, though, I suggest appropriate books and articles."

Annette told her close friends and her two daughters about the upcoming biopsy and what it could mean. But she didn't tell her mother and sister until she had a diagnosis. "I knew they would just fall to pieces until they knew the outcome," she explains. "I would have wound up comforting them and reassuring them instead of the other way around. Besides, I felt that I had ample support from my husband, children and friends to get me through.

"After the biopsy I called my mother and sister to tell them what I'd been through," she says, "and also to give them the *good* news—that it was a benign fibrocystic change, not a single cancer cell to be found.

"We all cried together, and I had the best summer of my life," adds Annette.

See also Pregnancy

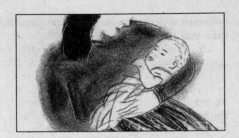

BREASTFEEDING

A SPECIAL KIND OF BOND

*B*efore her first baby was born, Marianne Lupinski thought that breastfeeding was the most natural thing in the world. She soon discovered differently.

When her son, Brian, was born with low blood sugar, he was taken from her to the nursery, where he was given glucose solution to help stabilize him. "When I saw him again the next day," recalls Marianne, "the nurses wheeled him in in a little bassinet that contained several tiny bottles of sugar water and formula. I thought I was supposed to give him this until my milk came in, so I did."

In between bottle feedings, Marianne made her first attempt at breastfeeding. "I figured he'd grab onto the nipple, suck away and that would be that. Well, he treated my breast as if it were coated with poison. Not only did he not latch on, he pushed it out of his mouth with his tongue. I made a few more attempts over the next day or so, with some of the nurses trying to help, but it didn't work. I felt like a total nincompoop. Here I was, a well-educated, highly paid lawyer, and I couldn't do what millions of women in Third World countries do every day. I thought breastfeeding was something that you just did, not something you had to learn to do."

Marianne and Brian did finally settle into a successful nursing routine, but only after Marianne contacted a lactation consultant she found through her local breastfeeding support group. The consultant was able to show her what she and her newborn were doing wrong.

MASTERING A SKILL

"Breastfeeding is an art and a skill," says Marsha Walker, R.N., president of Lactation Associates in Weston, Massachusetts, and an international lactation consultant. "It is something that has to be learned. Both the mother and baby have a set of reflexes and behaviors that allow it to happen, but it needs practice."

For some women and their babies, nursing seems to be second nature. "I breastfed my son right in the delivery room," says Maureen Becker, who nursed both her children into toddlerhood. "I had so much milk I thought I could feed the entire nursery. I felt like a real Earth Mother."

Other women and their babies, like Marianne and Brian, need help. But, like Marianne, many mothers may not anticipate it before they undertake "the most natural thing in the world."

It helps, says Walker, to be prepared. That can mean taking a course in breastfeeding *before* your baby is born. Many hospitals and midwifery centers and most breastfeeding support groups, such as La Leche League International and Nursing Mothers Council, offer sessions for mothers-to-be. "Although there are outstanding books on breastfeeding," says Walker, "it's difficult to understand some of the subtle points by looking at pictures and reading words. Some classes have breastfeeding moms who will demonstrate, so you can see how it's done and can ask questions. Plus, the babies are so cute and the mothers have such wonderful smiles on their faces that most couples see this and say, this is what we want for ourselves. We want to sit there and smile like that."

GETTING PSYCHED

You may need that motivation. The early days of breastfeeding, even if you have a minimum of difficulty, can be trying. Often tired and sore from childbirth, you're getting used to your newborn and getting used to your new role as mother, plus you're practicing a new skill, usually 8 to 12 times a day—and night. "A new mother is *very* vulnerable," says Walker. "You need to believe in yourself and your decision to provide optimal nutrition to your newborn. All this has a payoff not found through formula feeding.

"Breastfeeding gives a baby an edge," she says. "Studies show that breastfed babies are healthier than bottle-fed babies." For one thing, breast milk contains the mother's antibodies to infections and diseases. Studies have shown that breast milk helps protect babies against gastrointestinal distress, allergies and infections. It may also be a baby's first "brain food."

Breast milk contains "long-chain fatty acids whose composition is very much like brain tissue," says Walker. "That's why it's so important to feed a species its own milk, otherwise you may be laying down an entirely different matrix in the brain. Breast milk is exactly the right food physiologically for babies. It also assures contact with the mother, which the baby needs to become socialized."

STRAIGHT TO THE HEART

And that's where the other payoff—the psychological one—comes in. "Nursing mothers say it gives them a great sense of pride and fulfillment to actually give of themselves to their babies," says Walker.

And most mothers who successfully breastfeed their babies say the time investment is worth it once a nursing baby looks into your eyes and smiles. "When Terence was about 6 months old, he would smile at me, touch my face, which is really when I started to feel we had established a strong, loving bond," says Penny Stevens, a 34-year-old mother who also runs her own home sewing business.

Bottle-feeding does offer some advantages—extra sleep and more freedom to go out. But it's not necessarily more convenient. It is also more expensive—up to $1,000 per year. Breast milk doesn't need to be stored at the proper

WHEN TO WEAN

How long should you nurse?

"As long as you want to," says international lactation consultant Marsha Walker, R.N., of Massachusetts. In some societies, babies aren't weaned until they're 3 or 4. "The norm is well into the second year. That's traditional," says Walker.

Weaning, she says, "is appropriate when the baby or mother says it's enough. A lot of times it coincides with a developmental milestone like walking. The baby thinks, 'Do I want to walk more than I want the breast?' They cruise by and take a sip and run off. The mother may get tired of getting up four or five times a night or the baby moves onto other things."

One reason you don't have to wean, says Walker, is because you're going back to work. If you have a flexible situation at work—if you work at home, for instance, or have on-site or near-site day care—you can continue to breastfeed your baby at least part-time. Even mothers employed full-time can express milk and breastfeed at home.

Generally, Walker says, breastfeeding provides the baby with the disease protection mother's milk confers before the baby's immune system begins functioning and thereafter as the baby is exposed to more of the environment. The American Academy of Pediatrics recommends mothers nurse for a year, although no harmful effects have been noted from changing to cow's milk and supplements after six months. "The breast milk still provides nutrients that the pureed foods do not, so they still get benefits in the second half of the first year," says Walker.

She recommends that you wean gradually, stopping one or two feedings every few days and substituting cuddling, attention or playing. This way the baby isn't deprived of the closeness you and he have come to know as well as of the breast. You don't want to deprive yourself of it, either.

temperature, heated, measured or poured. And while nursing mothers may lose a little more sleep than bottle-feeding mothers—which may account for the higher rate or postpartum depression some studies found among nursing mothers in the early months—many mothers avoid that by napping when their babies nap or by rousing themselves only lightly during the night.

AN OUNCE OF PREVENTION

Most nursing problems can be solved or prevented if mother and baby get off to a good start, says Walker. Sometimes that means that you may need to ask for help from a breastfeeding counselor or hire a lactation consultant, as Marianne Lupinski did. "I couldn't imagine what I was doing wrong and, after she took my history and watched me try to feed Brian, she told me I wasn't doing anything wrong. The problem was that Brian had gotten off to a bad start in the hospital with those bottles," Marianne says.

It's important, says Walker, that your baby be put to the breast as soon as possible after birth, preferably in the birthing, delivery or recovery room. A baby who is given a bottle has to configure his mouth and suck in an entirely different way than a child who is nursing from a breast. "I think it also has something to do with imprinting in the baby's mouth," says Walker. "The first objects that go in the mouth are extremely important. They're a major avenue of communication for a baby. Artificial nipples are nothing like a human nipple. Pacifiers and artificial nipples encourage babies to shut their mouths, pull back their tongues and bite. Mothers wind up with sore nipples and babies who do not get any milk. All your efforts have been sabotaged, so you wind up supplementing with a bottle."

Using one of dozens of techniques a skilled lactation consultant knows, Marianne's consultant helped her teach Brian how to suck from a breast. Her problems could have been prevented had she investigated the breastfeeding policies at the hospital where she delivered, says Walker.

Your breastfeeding experience will be off to a smoother start if the hospital or birth center where you deliver encourages breastfeeding by keeping mothers and babies together, rather than isolating the babies in the nursery. "What you need is lots of practice and lots and lots of contact," says Walker.

A study done several years ago found that even some mothers who intended to breastfeed before the birth of their babies were influenced by the practices of the hospital where they delivered. If the hospital formula-fed babies in the nursery or presented new mothers with gift packs containing formula, the mother was more likely to bottle-feed using the brand of formula the hospital used, even though it was costly.

Some mothers reject the idea of rooming in because they feel they won't get enough sleep after delivery, but Walker says there's no evidence you'll get any more if the baby is in the nursery. "You talk to any night nurse and she'll tell you how much sleep mothers get," she says. "Studies show they get about 5 hours of sleep at night whether or not the baby is in the room with them. So there's no purpose in isolating the baby from the mother. You sleep better and the baby sleeps better when it all works according to human physiology."

A LITTLE TENDERNESS

Some of the most common breastfeeding problems can be prevented by a little foreknowlege. Although most women will experience some initial tenderness when they begin nursing, says Walker, breastfeeding shouldn't cause a lot of pain. There's very little that is necessary to prepare your nipples, except for spending time braless to allow your breast to gently rub against your clothing and for air to circulate around them.

After a week or two the tenderness should disappear. If it doesn't, or worsens or hurts during feeding, says Walker, your infant may be positioned incorrectly or sucking improperly, or your breasts may be engorged (too full of milk), which are the usual causes of breast pain during early nursing.

You may need help in positioning your baby or in determining if he or she is sucking properly. To latch on properly, a baby needs to open his mouth wide to take the nipple and ¼ to ½ inch of the areola—the pigmented area around the nipple—into his mouth. You can use your free hand to support the breast and keep it in the baby's mouth. Use your four fingers under the breast and thumb on top. You can hold the baby at your breast by positioning him on his side or his tummy against your tummy, with his mouth at nipple level.

To help the baby get started, express some milk into his mouth to encourage him to open wide, suck and swallow.

PRACTICE MAKES PERFECT

What helps with all of these problems is frequent practice. Frequent nursing—even of short duration—can help prevent sore nipples, engorgement, plugged ducts and mastitis, a breast infection. It will also assure you a good milk supply as your baby grows, says Walker.

Limiting the time your baby spends at the breast—advised by some experts—won't prevent sore nipples, says Walker. Most newborns can feed from a few minutes to 20 minutes per side. A baby should be kept on the first side for as long as he will stay before being switched to the other side. "Since sore nipples are usually caused by positioning or sucking problems, limiting the time isn't going to help and may even cause problems," she says. "These kinds of restrictions can limit the amount of milk a mother will produce further down the line."

Breast milk contains chemicals called suppressor peptides that automatically regulate the amount of breast milk. If milk builds up inside the breasts and they become engorged, the suppressor peptides build up and slow the milk production. As long as you're taking milk out—either by nursing or pumping—the peptides won't build up. "The only thing that limits the amount of milk you can make is the appetite of the baby," says Walker. "That's why mothers can feed twins and triplets."

TAKING YOUR CUE

As a general rule, Walker says, you should be feeding your newborn 8 to 12 times in a 24-hour period. But don't feed by the clock, Walker warns. "When you feed by the clock, you are literally doing that, feeding whether the baby is ready to feed or is overhungry. You're feeding the baby according to some outside influence, like a production line in a factory."

Mothers who "feed on demand" usually consider "demand" to mean when the baby is crying, which experts say isn't always wise. "When they're crying, they're overhungry," says Walker. "Babies don't feed well when they're overhungry. Feeding 'on cue,' which is preferable, would be 20 minutes before they start crying."

To feed on cue means you need to be alert to the baby's subtle signals that mean I'm hungry. Sleeping babies—and many newborns are—will offer some clues when they move from the deep to lighter sleep phase. You'll see rapid eye movements, mouthing and increased restlessness, says Walker. Awake babies will also be more restless and may begin moving their mouth in instinctive sucking. Keeping an infant in a front pack or sling is very helpful in learning to read a new baby's cues, because, cuddled so near the breast, the baby will probably begin rooting toward the smell of the milk and the feel of the breasts, says Walker.

Another sign you want to look for is whether your baby, who is sucking away like mad, is actually swallowing milk. "Babies at the breast normally do some nonnutritive sucking," says Walker. "They'll be sitting there gumming away, hanging out, little jaws going a mile a minute, but there's no swallowing of milk. Generally, newborns suck one to three times and then you need to watch and listen for swallowing. Unless some mothers are made aware of this, they will happily put their babies to the breast for 15 minutes on a side like the books say and walk in at the two-week checkup with a baby who has not gained any weight or who has lost weight."

CHAPTER 10

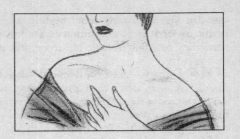

BREAST SURGERY

TRAUMA, FEAR AND DECISIONS

$\mathcal{F}$inding a lump in her breast was nothing new for Kerry McGinn, a 48-year-old registered nurse from San Francisco.

"My breasts were cyst farms, and I always had abnormal mammograms, so I routinely saw a breast surgeon every six months," explains Kerry. "This tiny lump showed up right before my regular checkup, and I wasn't concerned about it at first. Neither was my surgeon, and he planned to see me again in six months. The next month it was still there, and I just got a gut feeling about it.

"The mammogram didn't show anything, and after a second exam, the surgeon still insisted it was nothing," says Kerry. But Kerry was so persistent that he agreed to do a needle aspiration—a relatively painless procedure in which a few cells are drawn out through a needle and examined under a microscope—if it was still there in another month.

"I agreed to wait," she says, "and a month later I was back in his office. He did the needle aspiration, and 20 minutes later I had one shook-up surgeon on my hands."

The lump had felt so different from others she'd discovered that Kerry said she wasn't surprised by the news: breast cancer. "I was surprised at just how quickly I got the news," she says. "I thought I'd have to have a biopsy and wait several days for the results. Instead, I knew immediately. 'Oh, God,' I said to myself, realizing instantly what I was in for. But at first I found myself consoling the surgeon because he was so upset that he had missed it."

THE CHILL OF DISCOVERY

Ronnie Kaye, a Los Angeles psychotherapist in private practice, also had been plagued with numerous "false alarms"— breast lumps that had turned out to be nothing. But at one particular routine exam, she knew something was wrong when she heard her doctor sigh. "Ronnie," he said as he carefully felt the lump, "this has to come out right away. Do you have a surgeon?"

In her book *Spinning Straw into Gold*, Ronnie describes her immediate reaction. "I remember feeling terribly cold. The nurse brought blankets, and they piled them on top of me as I lay there shivering. It was quite a while before they could stand me up on my feet. I was overcome with shock and a sense of unreality. 'This cannot be happening to me,' I thought. But it could and it was."

Ronnie was on an operating table for a biopsy of the suspicious lump less than 24 hours later, but somewhere inside herself she felt sure that a reprieve would be forthcoming. She was wrong. At 37, she was diagnosed with breast cancer. "I didn't know it then," she says, "but that was the beginning of the most incredible journey of my life."

OPTIONS AND OUTCOMES

An estimated 175,000 women in the United States embark on that same journey each year, and nearly 25 percent of them die, according to National Institutes of Health statistics.

Nevertheless, treatment options and outcomes have never been more promising. Gone are the days when the breast, the surrounding chest muscle and lymph nodes were automatically removed—sometimes before you even knew whether or not your lump was cancerous. Kerry McGinn says that back when she had her first biopsy—some 25 years ago—she had to sign a consent form allowing the surgeon to perform a mastectomy if her lump should prove to be cancerous. "When they put me to sleep," she says, "I didn't know if I'd wake up with or without a breast."

Today, doctors know that removing more tissue does not necessarily improve survival rates or increase longevity. Indeed, 17 years of study have shown that lumpectomy—removing the cancerous lump while leaving the breast virtually intact—provides survival rates equivalent to those of total mastectomy—removing the entire breast and sometimes part of the chest muscles.

So why choose a mastectomy when a lumpectomy is an option? Well, a mastectomy is an option for anyone with breast cancer, explains Jeanne A. Petrek, M.D., an attending surgeon at Memorial Sloan-Kettering Cancer Center in New York City. But you must meet certain criteria to have a lumpectomy.

For one thing, your diagnosis must indicate that you have a stage I or II breast cancer. "Stage I is a cancer that's less than 2 centimeters in diameter—about the size of a nickel—that has not spread to the lymph nodes," says Dr. Petrek. "Stage II means that the cancer is larger than 2 centimeters even with nodes, or that the cancer is larger than 2 centimeters but less than 5 centimeters with noncancerous lymph nodes." Fortunately, 75 percent to 80 percent of breast cancers are classified as stages I or II.

There are other considerations as well, adds Dr. Petrek. "The breast has to be large enough so that removing the lump with about a centimeter of visually normal tissue around it will not leave the breast distorted or deformed. And the cancerous cells have to be the kind that are sensitive to radiation therapy—the next step after lumpectomy."

LOADING THE DICE IN YOUR FAVOR

Actually, your doctor will probably recommend chemotherapy and/or hormone therapy after surgery and radiation, says Susan Love, M.D., director of the Faulkner Breast

Center in Boston and clinical assistant professor of surgery at Harvard Medical School. That's because breast cancer is systemic—it can spread throughout your body. Cancer cells start cruising your bloodstream two or three years after cancer originally begins to grow at a specific site, says Dr. Love. And cancer can be in the breast ten years before it is detected by a physical exam. "In some lucky women, the body's immune system will identify the circulating cancer cells and knock them off. In other women it won't."

Doctors don't know whose immune system will zap the cancer and whose won't, adds Dr. Love. So virtually everyone with breast cancer, whether they choose a lumpectomy or a mastectomy, now gets a course of chemotherapy—mostly given to premenopausal women—or hormone therapy—more commonly given to postmenopausal women.

"What we try to do with surgery, radiation and chemotherapy or hormone therapy is to reduce the total number of cancer cells so that your immune system can take care of the rest," says Dr. Love. In effect, your immune system is the major weapon against breast cancer. The treatments provided by your doctor just give it a helping hand.

A diagnosis of breast cancer is commonly followed by days and weeks of consulting other specialists, gathering information and making treatment decisions, says Mary Jane Massie, M.D., an associate attending psychiatrist at Memorial Sloan-Kettering Cancer Center who counsels breast cancer patients.

The time between initial diagnosis and surgery is very hard. "You're always thinking, 'Am I making the right decision?' and, 'What are the consequences of the decision I make?' " says Dr. Massie.

It's also a time of such soul-freezing fear that women are frequently afraid "to let go." Kerry McGinn says that at first she was so busy seeing cancer specialists, seeing another surgeon for a second opinion and having blood tests, bone scans and chest x-rays that she didn't take time to cry.

"I felt that I couldn't afford to relax and let myself go," she says. "Not until I was sure I knew what I was going to do."

TAKING YOUR TIME

Despite the deadly nature of breast cancer, its slow growth means that you don't have to rush into making a decision. You have time to think, decide, reconsider and decide again before you begin treatment.

It takes about 100 days for a single cancer cell to double itself, explains Dr. Love. And it takes 100 billion cells to grow a centimeter's worth of cancer.

That's why "most doctors believe that it would be entirely safe to have treatment within three weeks after the biopsy," adds Dr. Petrek. "And if you need to wait a little longer, that would probably be okay, too." After all, most cancers have been around eight years before they were spotted on a mammogram—ten years before they were felt as a lump.

MAKING THE RIGHT CHOICE

Although you have several weeks in which to make up your mind, deciding which cancer treatment will give you the best chance of survival is probably one of the toughest decisions you'll ever have to make.

Kerry was leaning toward having a lumpectomy until she saw the radiation specialist. "He went on and on about how wonderful lumpectomy was and that it was equally as effective as mastectomy," Kerry says. "Then he felt my breasts and said, 'Have you thought about having a mastectomy of the other breast? You'd be better off if you did.'

"That radiation therapist told me there was no way of finding anything in my breasts because they were so lumpy to start with and had large amounts of scar tissue from previous biopsies.

"I knew he was right," says Kerry. "So I had a double mastectomy. I didn't want to lose my breasts, but I realized that was the best alternative for me. With a strong family history of breast cancer, I had a major chance of other breast cancers cropping up. I could have lived with that if I had a reliable way of detecting any problem early. But I didn't. My mammograms had always been a radiologist's

nightmare, and everyone agreed that my breasts were extremely difficult to examine. I was seeing myself as a member of the biopsy-of-the-month club."

Ronnie opted for a lumpectomy, which was a relatively
new procedure at the time she had it. "I had to look very
closely to see any difference between the way I looked
before and after surgery," she says. "There was no blatant
physical reminder that I had had cancer, which helped me
get out of a marriage that really needed to end. Had I been
unable to choose this procedure, had I lost my breast, I
seriously doubt that I would have had the courage to leave
the relative safety of my marriage. The social world of the
single woman would have seemed totally inaccessible, and I
would have been terrified that no man would ever want me."

Three-and-a-half years later, however, Ronnie had a recurrence of the cancer and had to have a mastectomy after
all. "I felt the fear, the terrible anticipation of a surgery
that might save my life but leave me disfigured in a way I
didn't know I could accept," she says. "I felt the dread of
a disease that might kill me and a flood of feelings so
complex that I was totally overwhelmed."

WOMEN OF STRENGTH

The initial numbness, denial and shock that follow breast
surgery, particularly mastectomy, actually only lasts a couple of weeks, says Dr. Massie. "Then there are a few more
weeks of anxiety and difficulty in concentrating. But generally—and I must point out that these times vary greatly
among individuals—after a few months women start to get
themselves back in order. Their families are running again,
their jobs are being handled, the marriage has settled down
and life is moving along smoothly once again."

When you see someone you know going through something like breast surgery, you think that you could never
handle it, adds Dr. Massie. But the fact is that when you're
faced with a life-threatening illness, you do.

"Women are so strong and adaptable," she continues.
"The remarkable courage and staying power that women

CONFRONTING THE REALITY OF BREAST CANCER

"The first thing that anyone thinks of when diagnosed with breast cancer is 'Will I die?' " says Susan Love, M.D., of the Faulkner Center in Boston. "This is quickly followed by 'Will I have to lose my breast?' "

With these kinds of questions tumbling through your mind, it's clear that confronting the reality of breast cancer will have a major psychological impact.

"You're shocked that your body could do this to you," explains Dr. Love. "And you're particularly shocked because you don't have any symptoms. It's hard to believe that you can have a life-threatening disease going on in your body when you feel fine."

Kerry McGinn recalls those feelings well. Especially the numbness. "Mostly, my husband and I just held each other and talked," she recalls. "I was trying to get some sense of control over what was happening—the initial diagnosis leaves you feeling very *out* of control—but I felt confused.

Often when women are faced with breast cancer, they want the quickest way out of the situation. "In fact," says Dr. Love, "during the first 24 hours or so, women are likely to say, 'Just cut it off.' It's a sort of naive view that if you cut off the breast, the cancer will be gone and you can forget about it. Forget about the fact that cancer is a disease that spreads throughout your body. It's as if you think you can trade your breast for your life.

"While this is a perfectly understandable emotional response at the time," says Dr. Love, "it's not one that you should act on. Getting your breast cut off will not make your life go back to normal. Your life has been changed. And you need to realize that it will never be the same again."

have never ceases to amaze me. Most people find reasons to become optimistic. They make relationships with their doctors and nurses. They agree to a course of treatment and adhere to it. And they are able to pull themselves out of their fears and slumps and move ahead."

A FEELING OF BEING LESS THAN WHOLE

Women who have been able to have a lumpectomy often have an advantage when it comes to emotional healing.

Research studies have shown that women who choose lumpectomy have a much better body image and a greater sense of sexual desirability than women who choose mastectomy, scientists report. And at least one study has found that half of the mastectomy patients it studied regretted not having chosen lumpectomy.

"On the whole, lumpectomy patients fare better because they are more able to forget about it," explains Dr. Petrek. "When they take a shower, for example, they're not always being reminded of the event."

On the other hand, a woman who has had a mastectomy may feel disfigured by the procedure, says Jimmie Holland, M.D., chief of psychiatry services at Memorial Sloan-Kettering Cancer Center. She may feel she is no longer human, no longer the person she was, no longer attractive to her husband. That feeling, which also leads to the fear that her husband might abandon her, adds to the emotional turmoil surrounding the operation and knocks her self-esteem to the ground.

Although the emotional impact of mastectomy can be reduced when a woman undergoes reconstructive surgery, the problem of poor self-esteem is frequently compounded by the woman's husband, adds Dr. Holland. Most men are reluctant to initiate sex after such a major operation because they don't want to "bother" their wives. Ironically, their loving concern strikes a staggering blow at their wives' self-esteem because women interpret their husbands' reluctance as "proof" that they're no longer sexually appealing.

Do husbands feel that a woman who's had breast surgery is unattractive? "No," emphatically states Joanne Cipollini, R.N., a cancer clinical nurse specialist at the Montgomery Cancer Center of the Fox Chase Cancer Center network in Norristown, Pennsylvania. "I have *never* heard someone's husband say, 'She is no longer attractive to me.' "

THE YEARS AHEAD

Although the fear of being unattractive will eventually be laid to rest, nothing can apparently diminish the fear that breast cancer will recur.

"Not that it's foremost in a woman's mind," stresses Dr. Massie. "But women tell me that whether they are coming in for checkups three times a year, twice a year or once a year that their degree of anxiety, restlessness, sleeplessness, fear or terror right before a checkup is just as horrible as it was around the time of their diagnosis."

That's one of the reasons that belonging to a support group is so important, says Dr. Massie. Women who have had breast surgery need to know that what they're feeling is exactly what every other woman is feeling after surgery. They need to know that it's normal and not at all outrageous.

Besides, adds Dr. Massie, "a shared burden is a burden that's easier to handle."

Kerry McGinn agrees. "Everyone in my group was going through treatment at the same time," she says. "Some women had had lumpectomies, some mastectomies, some had had reconstruction. We laughed, we cried and we became as close as any sisters."

The group also helped her realize that the experience of having breast cancer was not without its positive side. "I'm not going to be a Pollyanna and say I'm glad I had cancer," says Kerry. "But I gained a lot of respect for myself. I think I handled the whole ordeal with reasonable courage. I learned to prioritize, to take better care of myself. I like the changes I've made, the person I've become."

Ronnie Kaye had a similar realization. "I searched within, looking to connect with my core self, to reestablish feelings of self-worth, to question and redefine femininity, sexuality, acceptability and beauty and to come to terms with my own mortality," she says.

"In the process, I learned more about myself than I had in years of therapy. I changed and grew in unexpected and very gratifying ways. I became more assertive, more self-assured, more open about my feelings, better able to ask for and accept comfort. I'm a very different person today than I was at the time of my mastectomy," she says. "And I like the changes that have taken place. In a strange way, breast cancer has been one of the most valuable experiences in my entire life."

See also Cancer

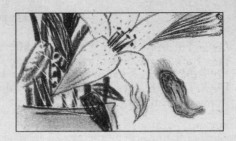

CANCER

COPING, HOPING AND HEALING TECHNIQUES

*J*udith Martindale, a certified financial planner from San Luis Obispo, California, was 41 when she learned that she had cancer.

"I've been fired twice in my life, my husband came to me and said he was in love with another woman, and I've had a doctor tell me I have cancer," says Judith. "All of those things were emotionally excruciating, but nothing was equal to being told about the cancer."

In fact, there may be no other disease that has the power to terrify like cancer, an insidious disease characterized by abnormal, runaway cell growth that kills 242,000 women (and 272,000 men) every year. That's 700 women every day, or about one death from cancer every 2 minutes.

Although heart disease is still the number one killer of Americans, most people fear cancer more, says Barrie Cassileth, Ph.D., former director of psychological programs at the University of Pennsylvania Cancer Center and currently professor of medicine at Duke University in Durham and the University of North Carolina.

GOOD NEWS OBSCURED

In reality, any illness that confronts us with our own mortality has the power to terrify. But the horror associated with cancer is so deeply embedded in our psyche that it persists despite the fact that survival rates for cancer have improved over the past 30 years. "Cancer is no longer an automatic death sentence," says Jeanne A. Petrek, M.D., a breast surgeon at Memorial Sloan-Kettering Cancer Center in New York City and author of *A Woman's Guide to the Prevention, Detection and Treatment of Cancer*. New advances in cancer treatment—whether that treatment involves surgery, radiation, chemotherapy or experimental therapy—means that about half of all those diagnosed with cancer will be alive five years later.

Despite these advances, the realization that you have cancer leads to a period of serious emotional turmoil, says Jimmie Holland, M.D., chief of psychiatry services at Memorial Sloan-Kettering Cancer Center. "But once you develop a treatment plan, you begin to get more hopeful. You think, 'I can do this, this, and this, and the doctor says I'm not going to die tomorrow the way I figured.'

"For most people, getting into treatment makes them feel they're back in control," adds Dr. Holland. And no matter how arduous the treatment, at least they're doing something that makes them feel hopeful and optimistic again."

YOU COPE AS YOU ARE

Of course, anything that sounds that easy isn't. Cancer is a life-threatening illness, a major life trauma. And how you deal with it is going to depend largely on your psychological makeup, on how you've dealt with other major events in your life.

"People don't change just because they have cancer," says Dr. Cassileth. "They are who they were before. If they're the kind of people who can roll with the punches, then they're going to do that. If they're the kind of people who fall apart when problems strike, they'll do the same in response to the diagnosis of cancer."

Women who discover that they have cancer are likely to run the gamut of emotions detailed in the work of death expert Elisabeth Kubler-Ross, Ph.D.: denial, fear, anger, despair, depression, hope, acceptance. But each woman will feel them in her own order, her own way. And no one should expect it to happen "by the book," cautions Dr. Holland.

"Everyone goes through it," says Joanne Cipollini, R.N., a cancer clinical nurse specialist at the Montgomery Cancer Center of the Fox Chase Cancer Center in Norristown, Pennsylvania. "The difference is some people do it in 5 minutes, some every 5 minutes."

Judith Martindale says her first reaction was, "Why me?"

"I didn't have any risk factors for breast cancer," she says. "I kept thinking, I've always been such a good person, how could this happen? I had always eaten well and exercised. Getting cancer never entered my mind."

Although she spent some time living in fear and self-pity, she says, her own personality gradually surfaced. "My history has always been, 'I can do it myself.' I realized that I didn't have an answer to the question 'Why me?', but I did have some choices: What doctor I was going to see, what kind of treatment I was going to have, where I was going to have it. It gave me some power back over my life in an area where I didn't have any."

EMOTIONAL TURMOIL

Not everyone bounces back the way Judith did, of course. About one-quarter to one-half of all cancer patients can suffer from depression serious enough to warrant the use of antidepressants or psychiatric therapy. Others go through a bout of mild depression that may require some counseling

CAN YOU CURE CANCER WITH YOUR MIND?

Confronting cancer patients these days is a controversial theory that their physical illness has psychological roots. The theory is based on studies that suggest that people who repress their emotions or who are depressed may be at higher risk for cancer. The idea is that people allow their emotions to eat away at them.

Some studies have also found a link between attitude and cancer survival. Notably, studies of women with breast cancer conducted at the Royal Marsden Hospital in Surrey, England, found that those who exhibited a fighting spirit or denied the seriousness of their diagnosis were more likely to be alive within five to ten years than those who felt helpless or hopeless.

Frances Weaver is a woman who believes in developing that fighting spirit. The 69-year-old former decorator and grandmother of four learned in June 1991 that she had ovarian cancer. Doctors removed her ovaries and she underwent chemotherapy. And, like the patients in the Royal Marsden Hospital study, she practices denial. "I know I have a 50 to 80 percent chance of surviving this," she says. "But I don't read about my disease. I don't want to know about it. I don't think it will help me. I feel real upbeat about it. I feel great. I feel that I'm going to get better. I try to maintain that attitude. To think otherwise is too depressing."

But doctors warn that a positive attitude may complement, but should not replace, medical treatment. Duke University professor Barrie Cassileth, Ph.D., conducted two studies of women with cancer in advanced or intermediate stages and found that psychological profiles—whether they felt helpless or exhibited a fighting spirit—had no effect on survival rates. She says that often cancer patients, lured by the notion that they can "think their cancer away," abandon traditional therapies for alternative and often controversial treatments.

"It would be wonderful if we could wish cancer away," adds Dr. Cassileth. "But if that were possible, everyone would get better. As we know, they do not." Studies may have shown that psychological factors can alter the immune system, but those changes are not necessarily going to cure a disease.

However, most experts, including Dr. Cassileth, agree that attitude can be of the utmost importance in cancer treatment—not because it enhances your immune system, but because a good mental attitude helps women adhere to arduous treatment regimens. It also helps women and their families cope with the disease. In fact, adds Jimmie Holland, M.D., of Memorial Sloan-Kettering Cancer Center, an attitude of "positive" denial can be "a very healthy mechanism" in illness.

or may lift all by itself once the initial shock of diagnosis wears off and treatment begins.

The depression is understandable. "For most people the cancer diagnosis means first of all, 'I may die,'" says Dr. Holland. "Then they think, 'I may be disabled, dependent on other people, disfigured. I won't look the same. People won't be able to love me the same. I'll be isolated and will lose those around me because they won't be able to tolerate me with a disease like this.'

"For a woman, there's an added meaning. 'I'll lose some of my attractiveness. I may be less feminine. I may lose my hair. I may lose my sexual organs, my sexual attractiveness, my sexual responsiveness, therefore I'll lose my opportunity for intimate relationships.' And if it's a young woman, it's, 'I'll lose my chance to have a home and children.' All of those losses are profound and may lead to anticipatory grieving," says Dr. Holland.

COMBATING PAIN

But of all the fears that accompany a cancer diagnosis, studies have shown that what women with cancer fear most is pain. "Most people say they're more afraid of dying in pain than they are of dying," says Cipollini.

According to a number of clinical studies, about half of all cancer patients undergoing treatment suffer from pain caused by the cancer itself or by the treatment. Seventy percent of those with advanced cancer are in severe pain. But through a variety of means, pain can be controlled satisfactorily in more than 90 percent of all cancer patients.

Behavioral and relaxation techniques normally used to treat anxiety and depression can be very helpful for moderate pain and discomfort from both the cancer and its treatment and as a nonchemical booster to drug treatment. They are particularly effective when a woman with cancer is anxious or depressed, says Kathleen Foley, M.D., chief of the Pain Service at Memorial Sloan-Kettering Cancer Center. Although these emotions don't cause physical pain, they can make it worse, she says.

Some techniques include progressive muscle relaxation, an approach in which patients tense and relax muscles one by one; meditation, an approach involving the mental repetition of a word that draws attention away from distressing thoughts; and distraction, an approach in which you do something engrossing—calculating an arithmetic problem or mentally reciting a poem, for example—to divert attention from the pain or the procedure. Other techniques include biofeedback, which uses electronic sensors to detect changes in body temperature and muscle tension; hypnosis and even music therapy.

PHOBIC RESPONSES

Relaxation is a behavioral technique that is particularly helpful for women who become fearful about procedures or uncomfortable side effects. For some women, nausea and vomiting associated with treatment can elicit anxiety and conditioned reactions—that is, thinking about the treatment can bring on the symptoms. In one reported case, a woman who had been successfully treated for cancer ten years earlier became nauseated every time she drove by the hospital where she had received her chemotherapy.

To help women overcome this kind of anxiety, a skilled therapist helps them achieve a relaxed state and, while in that peaceful mood, visualize a peaceful scene. If they do it often enough, many women will find that when they're undergoing treatment, their anxiety—and its attendant discomfort—has diminished.

Drugs such as morphine can also be very useful in controlling cancer pain, doctors agree. Unfortunately, many women—and some clinicians—worry about addiction. As a result, some cancer patients are "undertreated"—they either are not given morphine or receive amounts of the drug inadequate to dim their pain.

Yet morphine is not reserved for people who are lying on their deathbeds, says Dr. Cassileth. It's an effective way to reduce severe pain if it occurs during the course of disease. And addiction is simply not a problem for women with cancer.

Fortunately, doctors now have an arsenal of preventive measures that can diminish and even eliminate the side effects of treatment. Nausea, for example, which is a common side effect of chemotherapy, can be lessened by taking antacids, adding high-potassium foods to the diet, resting after meals or eating smaller, more frequent meals.

QUESTIONING SEXUALITY

One side effect that's difficult to treat is the damage done to a woman's sexuality. Even when a woman with cancer doesn't have disfiguring surgery, she may feel her sexuality has been destroyed by her disease, explains Cipollini. "In the support groups we run, many women have said they feel that their sexuality isn't an active part of them anymore. While they're undergoing treatment, they have strangers touching and looking at their bodies all the time. When that happens, you may feel it's not yours anymore. You don't have any control over what happens to you on the inside or the outside."

With some gynecological cancers, surgery—which may involve removing sexual organs or even the vagina itself— may physically reduce or eliminate sexual responsiveness or make intercourse no longer possible. Many women with cancer may need therapy to help them cope with what, for some, is a fundamental change in the way they express themselves.

Unfortunately, although sexuality is a major issue for cancer patients, "it's also one of the hardest for the patient and staff to talk about," says Cipollini.

"Patients don't want to ask and doctors don't want to ask," says Dr. Holland, whose department has one of the few programs in the country in which staff are trained to handle sexual dysfunctions among cancer patients. Staff members broach the subject with patients and discuss new ways to express their sexuality.

LOOKING GOOD, FEELING BETTER

When cancer treatments change how a woman looks, there are usually a number of ways she can look and feel attractive once again.

Breast reconstruction, for example, is frequently done at the same time as or shortly after mastectomy. That's what Judith Martindale had done. "I went home with a little roundness, which was just right for me, because it felt so future-oriented."

Temporary hair loss can also change your looks. Fortunately, your doctor should be able to predict whether or not it will happen so you can prepare for it. "At Penn, we had a young woman with very long hair that was her pride and joy," says Dr. Cassileth. "When she was diagnosed with cancer, she knew she would lose it. I sent her to a hairdresser who cut her hair into an attractive short hairdo, and then made a beautiful wig out of her own hair.

"If you don't have long hair," she adds, "you can get wigs today that look wonderful. You can even have fun with it, getting all different kinds of lengths and colors."

Several years ago, the American Cancer Society, in cooperation with the Cosmetic, Toiletry and Fragrance Association Foundation, developed a program called Look Good . . . Feel Better to help women with cancer feel better about themselves and their looks. Today volunteer cosmetologists and beauty advisers help women learn to take care of their skin and hair, apply makeup and choose wigs or turbans. Makeover videos and instructional pamphlets are provided to various support groups as well as complimentary makeup kits for each participating woman.

The premise of the program is that if a woman who has undergone cancer treatment looks good, she'll feel better and the quality of her life will improve. It's based on the Lipstick Theory, an observation by medical professionals that once a woman battling cancer starts to put on lipstick, she is on the road to recovery or, at the very least, restored self-esteem.

YOUR CANCER-PREVENTION PROGRAM

What's the best thing you, as a woman, can do to avoid dying of cancer?

"Stop smoking," says Jeanne A. Petrek, M.D., a surgeon at Memorial Sloan-Kettering Cancer Center. Smoking is the only known risk factor for lung cancer—the number one killer of American women.

Although breast cancer occurs in higher numbers, more women are likely to be cured, says Dr. Petrek. Very few survive lung cancer. Unfortunately, many women are unaware they are at high risk of contracting and dying from both lung and colorectal cancers. The perception is that these are men's cancers, although they are the first and third leading causes of cancer death in women. Breast cancer ranks number two. They are followed by pancreatic and ovarian cancer, both silent, insidious cancers that are lethal largely because they are rarely detected in early, curable stages.

Here are the American Cancer Society's recommendations for helping to prevent cancer.

Stop smoking. Tobacco use has been implicated in lung cancer as well as cancers of the mouth, tongue and throat. Seventy-five percent of all women who develop lung cancer smoke.

Eat a high-fiber, low-fat diet. A number of studies indicate that a high-fiber diet, rich in fruits and vegetables containing vitamins A and C as well as betacarotene, may protect against a number of cancers, including colon cancer. Studies also show that low-fat diets may exert a protective effect against some cancers.

Limit alcohol use. Alcohol, in conjunction with smoking, may increase your risk of developing cancers of the mouth, larynx, throat, esophagus and liver.

Limit smoked or cured foods. In areas of the world where salt-cured and smoked foods are eaten frequently, there is a higher incidence of cancer of the esophagus and stomach.

Avoid obesity. People who are 40 percent or more over their ideal weight increase their risk of colon, breast, gallbladder, ovarian and uterine cancer.

Wear sunscreen. Exposure to the sun is believed to be the leading cause of skin cancer.

Have regular cancer screenings. From the time a woman

is sexually active, or at least by the age of 18, she should begin to have regular screenings for cancer. These are the recommended guidelines for early detection of cancer, according to age.

Ages 20 to 39
- A cancer-related checkup every three years, which includes examination of the oral cavity, thyroid, skin, lymph nodes and ovaries.
- A breast self-exam should be performed on a monthly basis; a clinical breast exam should be done every three years, although some doctors recommend yearly exams.
- A Pap test and pelvic examination should be done every year, or less frequently if the exam has been negative for three consecutive years.
- A baseline mammogram should be scheduled sometime between the ages of 35 and 39.

Ages 40 to 49
- A cancer-related checkup every three years, which includes examination of the oral cavity, thyroid, skin, lymph nodes and ovaries.
- A breast self-exam should be performed on a monthly basis; a clinical breast exam should be done every year.
- A yearly Pap test, pelvic examination and digital rectal examination.
- A stool blood test, barium enema with sigmoidoscopy or total colonoscopy every three to five years in women with a family history of colorectal cancer.
- Mammogram every one to two years, and at menopause, an examination of endometrial tissue in women whose doctors have said that they are at risk for endometrial cancer.

Age 50 and Older
- A cancer-related checkup every year, which includes examination of the oral cavity, thyroid, skin, lymph nodes and ovaries.
- A breast self-exam should be performed on a monthly basis; a clinical breast exam should be done every year.
- A yearly Pap test, pelvic examination, digital rectal exam, stool blood test and mammogram.
- A sigmoidoscopy every three to five years.

BE WHO YOU ARE

One of the most important things a cancer patient can do for herself is to keep on living the way she did before her diagnosis. Although the temptation is to feel your life has stopped, says Dr. Cassileth, you simply can't give in to it.

One woman, for example, says that she stopped flossing her teeth while she waited for the results of a biopsy. "I figured, if I'm going to die, who cares if I have nice teeth?" she confesses.

"That's a phase that many women go through," says Dr. Cassileth. "But then they'll realize that they'll probably have to live with this for a while. So you start reevaluating what's important, integrate your illness into your life and readjust your goals." Beware, however, of taking on a new identity as "a cancer patient."

"The worst thing that can happen to a patient is that she becomes her illness," says Dr. Cassileth. "You want to keep the illness in its place and make sure you continue all of the other roles that have been important: wife, mother, friend, career person. It's very, very important for your mental health and for the quality of your life to keep the other areas of yourself alive." You can't allow the cancer to dominate your life.

FRIENDS AS MEDICINE

One of the most therapeutic things you can do for yourself is to reach out to others, either through a formal or informal support group. The American Cancer Society sponsors a number of educational programs such as I Can Cope, and many hospitals and cancer centers have their own groups, some for specific cancers.

Joanne Cipollini runs several cancer support groups, including one for women with breast cancer. "For our patients, a support group offers both education and camaraderie," she says. "It's a safe place to say what your feelings are, feelings you may not be able to say to your family and friends. As one woman put it during one of our groups, 'The people who don't have cancer don't know how we're feeling. You do know what I'm going through and you don't think I'm crazy.' "

There's even some evidence that support groups may prolong as well as improve the quality of your life. Researchers at Stanford University, who were examining the effect of support on the quality of the lives of women with terminal breast cancer, were "amazed" to find that the women who regularly attended support groups were living twice as long as the women who didn't. It was a finding they hadn't anticipated.

"Social support works for everything," says Dr. Holland. "There's good evidence that people who are part of a group, either as part of a couple or who have friends who are there for them, find it easier to tolerate a chronic illness such as cancer. And it's clear from a number of studies that if you perceive yourself as isolated and alone, there's a higher mortality from *all* diseases."

PERMANENT CHANGES

A cancer diagnosis will likely make an indelible mark on your life. Even those who survive it find that their lives are never the same. This has, however, both positive and negative aspects.

"Probably the cardinal problem of cancer survivors is that heightened fear, which they never lose, that the cancer might come back," says Dr. Holland. "You will find people, even ten years later, who are still afraid. When they have to come in for a physical exam, they'll become anxious. They'll ask, 'Could it have come back? I know it hasn't, but I won't feel all right until I get the report.'

"This goes with the territory," says Dr. Holland. "You learn to live with it. You learn to count to 10 and remind yourself that the ache in your big toe doesn't mean that the cancer has returned."

Although it will sound incomprehensible at first, cancer may be, as Judith Martindale found, something that changes your life for the better. Like the people facing death in the Stanford study, Judith has become "an expert in living."

"It reorders your priorities," she says. "I don't sweat the small stuff any more. I take time to enjoy people. I'm much more aware of taking care of my body and where I spend my energy. And it certainly helps with procrastination," she adds with a laugh. "I have a sense of urgency running me that I can trace back to cancer. It's changed my life more positively than anything else."

See also Breast Surgery

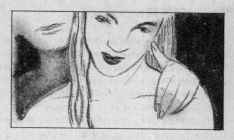

THE NEW CELIBACY

BUT IT'S THE SAME OLD SONG

No one's quite sure how it started, although some speculate it was a logical extension of yuppie life. Devotion to work and climbing the corporate ladder, perfecting the body inside and out, renovating an old home, acquiring the "right" belongings to grace rooms and fill closets. It's a lifestyle that leaves precious little time—or energy—for a sexual relationship.

No wonder some people are turning celibate—there is no *time* for sex!

Kidding aside, is there really a new trend toward a chaste lifestyle? Sort of, but not quite, say the experts. The "new celibacy" is really a misnomer, says sex therapist Lonnie Barbach, Ph.D., author of *For Yourself: The Fulfillment of Female Sexuality*. There really isn't anything new about it. People who are celibate today are celibate for the same reasons people were celibate ten years ago and ten years before that. Possibly what's new is that people are more willing to talk about it.

"Many women go through periods when they're not sexually active," says Dr. Barbach, who is also on the clinical faculty of the University of California at San Francisco Medical School. "Sometimes their careers or other aspects of their lives simply take priority for a while."

This is especially true for single, career-oriented women who put all their energy into their work, she says. It's hard enough to meet someone—but it's impossible to meet someone when you're too busy and too tired to even go out and look. Some women are celibate because they don't have any other choice! They're also a little too smart for indiscriminate sex; chancing diseases such as herpes and AIDS just isn't worth it. If there's a new celibacy, *this* kind of thinking is what it is all about.

But there *are* a lot of celibate women out there, says Dr. Barbach, and they're not all overworked and stressed out. For many of them, celibacy is a soul-searching conscious decision, often emerged from an experience that's been happening to women since the beginning of time: getting dumped.

REJECTION PROTECTION

"If you've had enough bad relationships, you become wary of giving your heart away one more time," says Judith Sills, Ph.D., a clinical psychologist practicing in Philadelphia. "You get sick of giving yourself emotionally to someone who doesn't give you anything in return. It makes a woman feel used, so she starts to hold back as a form of self-protection."

Margaret Kelsey, a 35-year-old high school teacher, says her year of celibacy followed what she refers to as her "year of living dangerously. I had been dumped by a man I thought I wanted to spend the rest of my life with, and I tried to replace him as quickly as I could. I dated heavily and slept with 11 men in one year in a desperate search for companionship, friendship and love. None of these relationships went anywhere and I was left feeling worse than ever."

So she decided that she needed to take stock of her life. She wanted to get back her self-esteem; the best way to start was to get men out of her emotional life.

Kathryn Webster, a 40-year-old bank executive, has been celibate for ten years for the same reason. "I think I really want a relationship now, but I don't even go out. I'll show interest in someone, but when he asks me out, I chicken out. I just don't want to get tied up in that knot again." It's not really sex that she's looking for, she says.

It's a relationship. "But where are you going to get one without the other?"

For women like this, celibacy is a shield. "The goal of being celibate is to avoid dating and hoping," Dr. Sills points out. "Getting involved sexually makes you vulnerable. Celibacy is a way of avoiding vulnerability."

BACK IN THE SADDLE AGAIN

Celibacy can be a positive experience if it serves to heal rather than make wounds, say therapists. It was for Margaret. "I'd describe my year of celibacy as very peaceful," she says. "I did things I wanted to do and went where I wanted to go. Going through a year without any emotional upheavals was wonderful."

Celibacy normally is not a permanent condition. "Women come back to the sexual life when they find a reason to," says Dr. Barbach. "When they feel they are able to take control of their lives and relationships. When they know they can't be buffeted about by other people who use and discard them. When they feel capable of deciding what they want from a relationship and when they want it."

Margaret knew she didn't want to get involved with anyone on an intimate sexual level until she was involved with him on an intimate friendship level first. "I didn't want the illusion of intimacy, which is what I had before. I wanted the real thing." And she got it. Two years later she was married. She now has two children.

CHAPTER 13

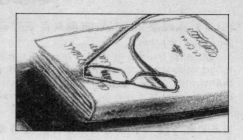

CELLULITE

THE FACTS ABOUT THIS STUBBORN FAT

*T*echnically, it doesn't even exist. You won't find it in a medical dictionary or anatomy book. But it's a word in the mind of every woman past the age of 20 when she looks at her own body in the mirror.

Cellulite may be a concept hyped by magazines and beauty consultants, but what it signifies is very real. Any woman who's looked in the mirror at dimply, bumpy lumps of fat poised defiantly upon her thighs or bottom knows what cellulite is and what it means to have it: It means never having to say good-bye. Because no matter how much you diet, how much you exercise or how much weight you lose or muscle you build, this stubborn and unwanted sign of aging is there to stay.

Most women (but not men!) eventually end up with some amount of cellulite, says Diane Gerber, M.D., a plastic surgeon in Chicago. What makes women the unlucky bearers? "Women have a tendency to put fat onto their thighs and hips partly because of their hormonal makeup."

The other factor is the *way* women pack fat. "The dimpling is caused by fibrous cords that connect the skin to the underlying tissue," explains Dr. Gerber. "These cords tether the skin to the deeper structures, with the fat lying between the layers. As fat cells accumulate, they push up against the skin, bulging out around the long, tough cords." Sort of like the buttons on an overstuffed sofa.

JUST ANOTHER WORD FOR FAT

The word *cellulite* was coined back in 1975 when a best-selling book hit the market, making women aware that there was just one more thing—cottage cheese–like thighs and fannies—contributing to their less-than-perfect bodies. Since then, the word has been blasted from magazines, newspapers, books and advertisements, and women have responded by spending millions of dollars each year trying to rid themselves of their cellulite.

"I tried it all," admits Vera Hoffman, a 46-year-old writer saddled with her own lumps of cellulite. "It used to make me crazy when I'd look in the mirror and see my cottage-cheese butt. It's not even fat, just lumpy."

Cellulite is perfect fodder for the "miracle cure" because you'll never find anyone who likes it or thinks it's attractive, notes Dr. Gerber. But it's not a disease. It's not even abnormal. It just *is*. Nevertheless, many women attack it with a vengeance. They try to massage it away, loofah it off, wrap it, pound it and make it disappear with lotions and oils. But the truth is, notes Dr. Gerber, none of these methods work.

Getting rid of cellulite, however, is not a totally hopeless cause.

DIMINISHING RETURNS

Just like other problems related to fat, some cellulite (but not all) can be lost through diet and exercise. Fat-burning exercise means the aerobic variety—jogging, swimming, biking, fast walking. But you have to keep it up at a good pace for 20 minutes or more to actually burn fat. It's true that you can't turn fat into muscle, but firm, toned muscles may help smooth out the skin and reduce the appearance of cellulite.

You can also help get rid of excess fat and keep down the amount of fat you accumulate through a low-fat diet. Eat more fruits, vegetables and fish and less meat, dairy products and butter, which contain saturated fats.

Doctors agree that these measures will get you some results. Yet some women still opt to go a more drastic route. For a few thousand dollars you can have the fat in your thighs removed through liposuction, a surgical procedure in which the fat is literally siphoned out. But does it work?

"It helps a little," says Dr. Gerber, "but it really doesn't get rid of the dimple. Liposuction just evens the surface slightly by getting rid of the fat that produces the mountains and valleys."

But there's a newer procedure that some claim can even help get rid of the dimpling, she says. Here's how it works. The doctor first aspirates the fat through standard liposuction. Then a special instrument with a cutting edge is inserted and moved back and forth. This catches and severs the fibers that are causing the dimpled skin. The doctor then reinjects fat to smooth the area further.

This technique is still considered controversial, says Victoria Vitale-Lewis, M.D., a plastic surgeon with Plastic and Reconstructive Surgery Associates in Melbourne, Florida. "I know of one doctor from Brazil whose results do look impressive, but we know from experience with fat injections that they are not lasting. So far, there have been no good studies that show this procedure works over the long term."

FACING FAT

Is it possible—or even realistic—to go through middle age with smooth skin below the waist? Probably not. Your chances of avoiding the problem are better if you *never* get overweight and *always* stay in good shape, say medical experts. But you can still get cellulite, despite good diet and exercise habits. It really is a question of genetic makeup.

"I used to go crazy comparing me and my flaws to photos of models with perfect bodies," says Vera Hoffman. "Sometimes it still bothers me. I have to keep telling myself that that's how they got their jobs. Their bodies *are* unusual. I tell myself 'real' women are supposed to have hips and thighs."

As one doctor put it: "It's okay to decide that it's okay to be less than perfect."

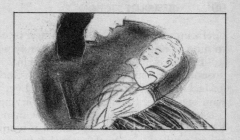

CESAREAN SECTION

WHAT THE STATISTICS ARE SHOWING

One out of four women who enter a hospital to have a baby will have a cesarean section, and for many of them it will be the unkindest cut of all.

According to a study of C-section rates in 41 states, 475,000 women who could have had a vaginal birth were given C-sections—exposing them to a maternal death rate that may be two to four times higher than for a routine delivery. Every year, unnecessary C-sections cause about 25,000 serious infections, mean an extra 1.1 million days in the hospital and cost more than $1 billion. The study also showed that in states with high C-section rates, there has not been a corresponding lower rate of newborn deaths. Yet, Japan, which has one of the lowest infant and newborn mortality rates in the world, also has a very low C-section rate.

What these sobering statistics don't reveal is the profound and, to many women, bewildering psychological trauma that accompanies the physical pain of a cesarean.

FEELINGS OF FAILURE

Her own experience with a cesarean caused Esther Zorn of Syracuse, New York, to found the International Cesarean Awareness Network, formerly the Cesarean Prevention Movement, in 1982. Esther was in labor for 36 hours when her doctors made the decision to operate. "I went into that operating room full of Demerol and thinking I was going to die and hoping that at least the baby was going to make it," Esther recalls. "Afterward, I was in a lot of pain. I went around for six months thinking, 'My God, I've been hit by a Mack truck.' I'll never be the same. Even after the physical pain was gone, I just couldn't stop crying."

Studies have shown that some women who have C-sections tend to feel they have "failed as women" because they were unable to give birth naturally. In one Canadian study, women who had C-sections said they were angry with themselves and felt guilty because they were so dissatisfied and unhappy with their childbirth experience despite having had healthy babies.

For many women, like Esther, a cesarean represents a "loss of expectation." A woman who becomes pregnant today usually goes through many hours of childbirth preparation—for a vaginal birth. Her fears and her fantasies revolve around a picture of "normal" childbirth that, more and more, comes from viewing a video rather than from hearing other mothers' stories. Deprived of what is essentially the fulfillment of a dream, some women may feel that they are less than a woman. While most women who give birth feel euphoric, even victorious, many mothers who have had C-sections feel defeated or disappointed.

As one mother put it: "Cesarean is a gyp."

Some women also initially have trouble caring for their new babies. The women in the Canadian study, like most cesarean mothers, were separated from their babies for several hours after birth. Most said they were unable to "mother" as they wanted to because they were in so much pain, fatigued or simply unmotivated, all common complaints among cesarean mothers.

OF HUMAN BONDING

A woman who is separated from her baby at birth—or who may not have seen the birth because she was given general anesthesia—is deprived of an important time of bonding to her infant. "With my first child," says mother-of-two Peggy Hathaway, "I was able to hold her and nurse her right away. With Jimmy, I didn't see him for 18 hours. It took me a long time to feel close to him."

It's not hard to understand a woman's mixed emotions after a cesarean. It's considered major abdominal surgery—equivalent to having an appendix or gallbladder removed—and C-section recovery can be long and painful. Unfortunately, it also coincides with the demanding and fatiguing first months of motherhood. The surgery just makes the demanding job of caring for a newborn that much harder.

For some women, looking at the new baby may trigger memories of a stressful and traumatic childbirth. "For months after the operation," says one C-section mother, "I couldn't bear to even talk about babies or pregnancy. Seeing a pregnant woman would make me start to shake. Of course, I also felt guilty because I wasn't 'in love' with my baby the way other women were. Then, I was reading an article about the psychological problems of Vietnam veterans and I realized I was suffering from post-traumatic stress disorder. It was like I had come back from a war, too."

But not all women who have cesareans suffer psychological trauma. A woman who needs an operation to save her or her child's life—or who believes she does—is more likely to view the operation positively. "Usually, these women have had some warning, usually even a sixth sense that told them something was wrong," says Esther. "They integrate it into their lives and accept it. They may have some postpartum blues, but nothing compared to the woman who was not ready for it and more important, doesn't believe it needed to happen."

PREVENTION AS CURE

The 41-state study discovered that the greatest single reason for a cesarean is a previous cesarean. The main argument against vaginal birth after cesarean has been the risk of uterine rupture. About one in three C-sections is a repeat.

In 1988, the American College of Obstetricians and Gynecologists announced its thinking on repeat cesarean—the universally followed rule, "Once a cesarean, always a

MAKING THE MOST OF IT

If you need to have a C-section, you don't necessarily have to feel cheated out of a satisfying childbirth experience. Suzanne Pope, Ph.D., director of the Colorado Institute for Marriage and the Family in Boulder, had her first child, Sophie, by scheduled cesarean, and recalls it as a wonderful experience.

"I learned that just because you can't have natural childbirth doesn't mean you can't have it the way you want it," she says. In fact, she says, you need to insist on having it your way.

Her advice: Decide what you want and ask for it.

Do you want your husband and a family member or friend with you? Do you want soft music playing? Do you want to nurse immediately after the delivery? Do you want your delivery filmed? You can probably have it all if you talk to your obstetrician and pediatrician in advance.

For example, Dr. Pope says, she decided she wanted to make the birth experience as comfortable for her daughter as possible. So she questioned a number of standard hospital procedures that she felt would upset Sophie—the drops they would place in her eyes to prevent infection (usually only a problem in vaginal deliveries), the vitamin K shot, the heel-prick blood test.

"My doctors and I reviewed them and we decided that some things like the eyedrops weren't really necessary," she says. "Some of the procedures they do are simple convenience—for them—and others are done for good medical reasons. Once you talk to the doctor, you begin to learn which is which. Also, they don't all have to be done right away. Some can be done an hour later, after you've nursed.

"Don't be afraid to say, 'Let's not do everything by the manual,'" suggests Dr. Pope.

Another negotiable item: Who is in the delivery room with you. Dr. Pope got the hospital to agree to allow both her husband and her mother to attend the birth and to permit her mother to videotape it. Be insistent, she advises, but don't be combative or aggressive. Use the best negotiation skills you can muster, realizing the medical professionals may try to scare you and "won't roll over easily."

Find an advocate, "someone who is on your side or who has been through it, someone who will help you challenge things,'' she says. ''You need someone who has the knowledge to help you question some of the procedures.''

Read as much as you can and talk to other mothers who have been through the procedure. You'll pick up a lot of useful information that way, she says.

Perhaps the most important thing you can do is stay involved in the process, says Dr. Pope. ''I think a lot of women have problems because they play a passive role in their own childbirth. I realized that all the work I was putting into this birth was part of stepping in to be Sophie's mother. I was fulfilling my job as a parent, deciding what was correct for her and me. It was all part of becoming a mother.''

---

cesarean.'' It now advises its members to encourage women who have had cesareans to attempt a subsequent vaginal birth. In studies of women who had low transverse uterine incisions—a horizontal incision as opposed to a vertical incision—half to 80 percent were able to deliver vaginally in a subsequent pregnancy. Seventy percent of women who had had cesareans because their labors were long or difficult were able to deliver their next child vaginally. Most important, the mortality rates for mothers and babies were lower than for repeat cesareans.

Other reasons that account for the explosion of C-sections include dystocia, the medical term for prolonged, difficult labor, fetal distress and breech deliveries, in which the baby is pointing feet- or buttocks-first rather than head-first toward the birth canal. Ironically, among many C-section experts, those are rarely considered mandatory reasons for a C-section.

BE A CHILDBIRTH CONSUMER

Perhaps the best thing a woman can do to avoid an unnecessary C-section is to become an informed consumer. Only two states—Massachusetts and New York—have laws requiring hospitals to provide women with their cesarean rates and the number of vaginal deliveries after C-sections they perform. "But you can certainly ask them yourself," says Esther Zorn.

You may want to ask your caregiver his or her position on fetal monitoring and the criteria used to determine when a labor is failing to progress. If you have previously had a cesarean, you may also want to know your caregiver's views on trying for a vaginal delivery. If you want to avoid a repeat cesarean, you will need a caregiver who will be sympathetic and supportive and not contribute to your doubts and fears.

One of the reasons many women feel psychologically traumatized after a cesarean is that they feel childbirth was out of their control. "You have to be making some of the decisions yourself," says Esther. "You can't put all your faith, especially blind faith, in your caregiver. It's not fair to them or to you."

While gathering statistics can help you choose a good caregiver, Esther recommends a final test. "You need to be able to look in a person's eyes, with your clothes on, and say, 'I trust this person. I know this person is going to value my opinion and values the information I have gathered and cares to ask me what it is that I would like.' If you can't do that, then you need to go somewhere else."

See also Childbirth

CHAPTER
15

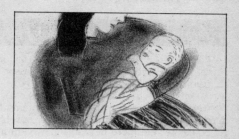

CHILDBIRTH

A UNIQUE EXPERIENCE—EVERY TIME

*F*or a woman, there is no more intense or unforgettable experience in life than childbirth.

"I think that a woman going through birth is probably equivalent to a man who is going through a war," says Deborah Gowen, a certified nurse-midwife at WomenCare at Malden Hospital and Brigham and Women's Hospital in Boston. "When soldiers come back from a war, they feel that no one could know what it was like except someone else who has been through it. Even if each war story is different, it was for them a rite of passage. It's the same with childbirth. When I visit nursing homes, I meet 80-year-old women who don't remember their own lives, but they can tell me their birth stories."

But if childbirth is like a war, it's one without a Geneva Convention. There are no rules, no fixed standard by which a woman can measure or predict her own experience. No two childbirth experiences are the same, not even for the same woman.

There are easy births and difficult ones, although no one has a painless birth. Some women experience more and some less pain, for both physical and psychological reasons. Although studies have shown that anxiety may affect the course of labor, even make it more painful, there's no guarantee that the woman who goes into it brimming with confidence will have a better experience than the woman

5 MEASURES OF PAIN

Researchers have found that these five factors—some physical, some psychological—are often associated with how painful women report their labors to be.

MENSTRUAL SYMPTOMS. Generally, women who have severe cramping and other symptoms during their periods report more pain during labor, possibly because their bodies secrete more prostaglandins, a group of chemicals that stimulates uterine contractions and is associated with pain.

SOCIOECONOMIC LEVELS. Women in higher income brackets and with more education tend to report less pain, largely, researchers say, because they are more likely to have learned and use pain-control techniques (such as Lamaze breathing) and have supportive mates, which help reduce their apprehension.

AGE. Older women report having less labor pain than younger women, possibly because they feel more in control of their lives—a factor which reduces stress—and have more support than younger women who are more tense during childbirth.

ANXIETY LEVELS. Researchers have found that anxiety at 32 weeks was the best predictor of drug use for labor pain in first-time mothers.

PARITY. First-time mothers feel more pain than women who have already had children, possibly because the first-time mothers have unrealistic expectations of labor pain. Second-time mothers know what to expect and so worry less and are less tense than first-timers.

who arrives at the hospital or birthing center biting her lip and wringing her hands.

Yet as individual as the *experience* may be, the physical process is basically the same for every woman. At some point in a pregnancy, the body and the fetus signal the uterus to begin contracting, and irrevocably, birth begins. Although doctors can temporarily stop it or speed it up, it is a process with the power of a juggernaut.

Pain, fear, loss of control—these are the facts of childbirth. How each woman deals with them are as individual as her fingerprints. Like pregnancy, childbirth is a psychological crisis. Your past history may be the best predictor of how you will handle its challenges.

"Generally, a woman labors as she lives," says Christiane Northrup, M.D., a gynecologist in private practice in Yarmouth, Maine, who is also co-president of the American Holistic Medical Association.

THE REIGN OF PAIN

How painful is labor? One research study put it quite succinctly: When surveyed, 115 laboring women tended to rank it "distressing" in its earliest stage, "horrible" in active labor and "excruciating" during transition—the last stage of labor.

Of course, some women do have relatively easy labors. In *The Motherhood Report*, authors Eva Margolies and Louis Genevie, Ph.D., found that 8 percent of the 1,100 women they surveyed reported having had easy, fairly painless labors. But pain-free or not, 6 out of 10 of all the women surveyed recalled childbirth as a peak *positive* experience in their lives. Pain seems to be a matter of attitude as well as a physical reality.

Becky Stern, a 32-year-old mother of two, had heard more than a few horror stories before the birth of her first child and was pleasantly surprised by her own experience. "For some people it really is genuinely very, very painful. But it wasn't for me," she says. "I mean it was more painful than anything I've experienced in my life, but the thing about the pain of labor is that it comes and goes. It's not like someone dangles you by your hair and leaves you there for 35 hours."

One reason the pain of childbirth, while unforgettable, may be viewed in a more benign way than, say, a broken arm, is that unlike the pain of injury or illness, it's not threatening. In fact, it serves a positive purpose. One pain expert says that pain that isn't perceived as harmful may be barely felt.

PICKING A CAREGIVER

Clearly, reducing anxiety is key to improving your chances of having a shorter, more manageable labor. But how do you reduce anxiety when you are facing what for most women is the worst pain they have ever experienced?

Perhaps the most important thing you can do is choose the best caregiver for you. You need to pick a caregiver—obstetrician or midwife—with whom you feel secure and comfortable, who will be there when you give birth and who is willing to consider and meet your needs. Not only will you feel less anxious when the big day arrives, studies show you improve your chances of having a good experience, a healthy baby and fewer medical interventions and complications if your caregiver is sensitive, patient and supportive.

"It sounds like such a little thing," says Kathy Scott, the mother of two preschoolers, "but with my first child, my doctor pulled some strings and made arrangements for me to have a private room because she knew I was so nervous. Her sensitivity made the real difference for me. I was still nervous, but I felt *safe*. Her attitude wasn't, 'I've done this a million times.' It was, 'This is the first time *you've* done this.' "

Kathy was fortunate. She found a caring, supportive doctor who not only met her needs but sensed them. Finding that kind of person is often easier said than done. Since childbirth moved from the home to the hospital, it has been, in the words of one expert, "medicalized."

"*You* need to take control," says Dr. Northrup. "The experience of a beautiful delivery with a delayed cord clamping so the baby can rest on your abdomen in the dim light is nice, but depending on where you have your baby, you may have to fight for it. What needs to happen for childbirth to change is for women to begin trusting themselves—and for their caregivers to begin trusting them, too."

Unfortunately, what often happens is that the woman is surrounded by her caregivers, who are all urging her to push, to not push, to breathe, to not breathe. In short, running the birth as if it were scripted instead of assisting her to give birth in her own time and way. Add to this such restrictive, dehumanizing and stressful medical protocols as frequent vaginal exams, fetal monitoring and depriving the pregnant woman of food and drink, and you have "a crisis atmosphere," says Dr. Northrup, which can only serve to increase a woman's anxiety and may even affect the process and the outcome of her delivery.

In a study done at the University of Colorado Health Sciences Center School of Medicine in 1989, researchers watched and analyzed videotapes of the labor and delivery process and found that the kind of feedback mothers get from their caregivers can affect the quality of the baby's health after delivery. Joyce Roberts, Ph.D., a certified nurse-midwife, and her colleagues discovered that both the mother and her baby were healthier after delivery if her caregivers were "responsive"—allowing the mother to choose her delivery position and to push when she felt the urge—rather than "regulatory," which Dr. Roberts defined as attempting to speed up the birth process by telling the mother what to do, including pushing when she didn't feel ready.

NO GAME PLANS

When *you* are in labor, it's clear the last thing you need is a coach with a game plan. What you really need, says nurse-midwife Gowen, is a supportive person you know is there to meet, not dictate, your needs. Even if you've never given birth before, says Gowen, you instinctively may know best, even when what you want to do flies in the face of hospital protocol, what you learned in your birthing classes, even your own everyday character.

"In our practice," says Gowen, "we follow the woman's lead. If she needs to sleep, then we need to let her sleep. If she wants to walk, then she gets to walk. If she wants to be nice or bitchy, then that's what she does. She can cry like a baby, say she wants to go home or close herself in a dark bathroom and not talk to anyone, and that's fine.

This is the one time in her life she gets to say and do and be anything she wants with impunity."

A woman who is allowed to labor as she wills with the help of a supportive companion may also reduce her need for painkilling drugs, says Gowen. In fact, several studies have shown that women who are supported in their labor by companions—not necessarily medical personnel—have an easier time all around. They may have shorter labors and fewer medical interventions, including cesarean sections, and they and their babies may experience fewer health complications. Researchers speculate that the presence of a companion may help reduce the woman's anxiety, which in turn—in as-yet-unknown ways—has a positive effect on both her childbirth experience and the outcome.

GO WITH THE FLOW

Female birthing experts say you'll also reduce your labor anxiety if you follow two pieces of seemingly conflicting advice: Be prepared and expect the unexpected.

Many studies have shown that taking childbirth preparation classes can reduce your anxiety and dread and give you more positive feelings about labor and delivery. For one thing, you eliminate part of your fear of the unknown. Although you may not have experienced childbirth, the classes, offered by most hospitals, give you the opportunity to ask others—from childbirth educators and nurses to experienced mothers—what it's really like.

Talking to other mothers can be quite helpful, says Gowen, if you talk to enough of them. There's a danger, of course, that in any group of women sharing childbirth stories you'll hear your share of horrors. "But I think that if women had heard birth stories from the time they were children, then it wouldn't be as frightening because they would have heard a variety of stories," Gowen says. "Occasionally women have easy labors. But 98 percent of the women who go through difficult labors find out the next day that they're walking and talking and living, and they'll tell you that there's a sense of achievement in going through that and coming out okay."

UNNATURAL CHILDBIRTH

Childbirth experiences vary widely, even for the same woman. "A bad first experience does not a second one make," says Gowen. And a good first experience doesn't predict the next either. Lois Bjornsgaard had a short, nearly pain-free delivery with her first child. With her second, she expected the same. "Only shorter, since I heard the second one is faster," she says. To her surprise, her son, Luke, "took his own sweet time in arriving, and I was in excruciating pain. So much for the old wives' tales," she says with a laugh.

Studies have also shown that a totally intervention-free birth is rare. At the bare minimum, you'll leave the hospital or birthing center with an episiotomy, an incision in the pelvic floor and vagina made to prevent tearing during birth. Nine out of ten American women do. Even with all your childbirth preparations, your caregiver may decide at the last minute, because of circumstances, that your labor needs to be helped along with drugs or that you need a cesarean. You need to be flexible enough to recognize that like all best-laid plans, this one can go awry. You need to find a way to work with your caregiver to make a good experience out of a medically assisted childbirth, recognizing that your safety and the safety of your baby must take first priority.

And even some of the proponents of natural childbirth agree that drugs—especially epidural anesthesia—are the best way for some women to have a good childbirth experience. When given by an experienced person—nurse-midwife or doctor—medications can make the difference between a terrible experience and a joyous one, with little or no ill effects on you or your baby.

Pain-control techniques, while very effective for many women and highly recommended, aren't a panacea. And they're likely to fail you if you expect them to guarantee you a painless labor and delivery. The breathing exercises taught in most childbirth classes are really a relaxation technique, a way to help you cope with but not eliminate pain, although they may do that to some degree. "I never tell women the breathing is going to reduce pain," says Diane Courney, R.N., a clinical specialist in childbirth education and assessing problem pregnancies at the University of Texas Health Science Center in San Antonio. "I try to make it clear up front that it's going to control how they feel about the pain, how they respond to the pain. I tell the women, 'At some point in labor, maybe even more than once, you're going to say this is not working, and you're going to give up doing your breathing. But you're going to

TRAINING FOR LABOR

You can get yourself in good physical shape for labor, and you don't need a gym membership to do it. There are a number of simple exercises that can help you learn to relax during extreme discomfort and prepare you for some of the sensations you may feel during childbirth. They may also help you avoid lacerations during delivery and may benefit you in other ways after your baby is born.

Your doctor or midwife will probably counsel you to do what are known as Kegel exercises. Every day, as often as you can, contract and relax the muscles of the pelvic floor. You can do this sitting, standing, lying down or in your bedroom, the car or the supermarket. Simply contract the muscles of your anus and urethra. It will feel as if you are controlling the flow of urine and a bowel movement. Hold for a few moments, then release.

What this exercise does is help you learn to relax the muscles used in childbirth, which helps reduce your risk of tearing. If you have a hard time isolating a muscle, try it with your arm first, suggests nurse-midwife Deborah Gowen of Boston's Brigham and Women's Hospital. Tighten a specific muscle, then relax it. Some experts recommend you do this same exercise with all of your extremities because it will help you to relax during the tense times of your labor. A class in yoga may also help you learn to tighten and relax specific muscles and to accomplish overall relaxation.

After you have your baby, the Kegel exercises will help you keep the pelvic floor muscles toned to prevent bladder problems.

realize very quickly that that's the best thing you had going, so you're going to go right back to it.' "

But you're not a failure if you ask for medication. Expecting to go through childbirth stoically is setting yourself up for disappointment. Mimi Cohen chose to have her first baby at a birth center staffed by midwives because she wanted to experience "natural" childbirth, which for her meant no drugs of any kind. Fearing she wouldn't live up to everyone's expectations, including her own, Mimi toughed out a difficult labor and birth and, in retrospect, regrets she didn't ask for some kind of medication. When she talks about the birth of her daughter, she sounds bitter. "My experience was horrendous and now, two years later, I still don't think I could ever do it again. I was left thinking that all that breathing was basically a plot by people who have to be there while you're giving birth to give you something to do besides scream. I'd just as soon scream. And I'd just as soon you get out of the room if you can't take it."

Carol Tucker, on the other hand, had a "blissful" childbirth. "Unnatural, of course," she says cheerily. "They gave me an epidural, I went into the delivery room, they told me when to push, and in 15 minutes my daughter squirted out. It was fast and easy and my hair didn't even get messed up. I watched her being born in the mirror and it was like someone else was having a baby. There was no pain. It was wonderful."

THE RIGHT ATTITUDE

Most childbirth experts agree your best bet for getting through labor is to forget what you've heard it's "supposed to be like." Instead, prepare to "go with the flow," recognizing that once your uterus takes over, anything can happen. "We have to learn to fly by the seat of our pants," says Dr. Northrup.

Some women dread the idea that they may "lost control" during labor, screaming, cursing, even defecating—all things that can and do happen. This can lead a woman to be very fearful, even panicky. "I had heard that sometimes women go to the bathroom right on the delivery table and I thought, 'Oh, my gosh, if that happens, I'll just die,' " recalls Kathy Scott, who admits she was unusually nervous about her delivery. "I was even too afraid to ask my doctor about it, and I was so happy when it didn't happen."

For some women, to "lose control" is a blow to their self-esteem, especially for many professional women who are used to controlling nearly every aspect of their lives, says Dr. Northrup, who speaks from personal experience. With her first child, she says, she expected to go through natural childbirth virtually without breaking a sweat. But instead of "going" with her labor, she says, "I fought it.

"I was shocked at how much it hurt. I had watched hundreds of labors, I had been up all night every third night for four years delivering babies, and wouldn't you have thought that I might have gotten the idea that maybe this was uncomfortable? But you see, I knew it was—for *them*. But I was Superwoman. It wouldn't happen to me. This is the time where your body takes over, so you really need to let go big time. Most women today, especially those in their thirties who are control freaks, have a hard time doing that," she says.

She's convinced her attitude affected her labor, which "got stuck at 6 centimeters," was very painful and for some time was nonproductive.

That's why she recommends women get involved in a physical activity—yoga, massage, exercise—that helps them get in tune with how their bodies work. (See "Training for Labor" on page 102.) "You need the chance to tune in, to learn to trust your own body wisdom," she says. "There is an old axiom among obstetricians that the people with the most detailed birth plans—'this will happen to me, this won't happen to me, do this, don't do that'—are the most apt to get into trouble. They have no faith in themselves and they want everything planned beforehand. Well, there are some things you can't plan, and this is one of them. This is the biggie."

CHAPTER
16

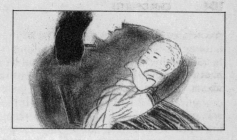

CHILD CARE

THE GUILT COMES NATURALLY

*I*n 1986, a leading expert in day care research struck terror into the hearts of millions of working women whose infants were in day care. That year, developmental psychologist Jay Belsky, Ph.D., announced that his studies had found that infants who spent more than 20 hours a week in day care were at risk of not developing a secure attachment to their mothers and of having behavior problems by the time they reached school age.

"Boy, did that push my guilt button," says LeeAnn D'Andrea, whose 7-year-old daughter had been in day care 40 hours a week since she was 4 months old. "I began to watch my daughter for signs that she wasn't attached to me, but it didn't happen. But the whole Belsky thing left a nagging doubt in my mind. Even today I wonder if some horrible 'Bad Seed' kind of thing is suddenly going to happen just because I left my daughter in day care all those years."

Day care and guilt. For many mothers, the two go hand in hand. Although many experts disagreed with—and poked holes in—Dr. Belsky's findings, and other studies have shown that good day care is far from harmful and can even be beneficial, many parents approach the whole concept of leaving their children in the care of others with uneasiness.

That was abundantly clear in a survey of 4,050 people—2,009 of them parents—conducted by Louis Harris and

Associates. More than 95 percent of the parents said that having a relative care for their children at home would be in the child's best interest and would provide them with peace of mind, but only slightly more than half said that was a realistic option, and only 39 percent were actually doing it. Only 8 percent said they felt the child care system was working "very well," and 38 percent said it was working "not very well at all." Only 25 percent of the total number of people surveyed, including the nonparents, said they believed children received quality care while their parents were working.

PLEADING GUILTY

Guilt appears to be universal among working mothers. In a readers' survey conducted by *Working Mother* magazine, most of the 3,000 respondents said they occasionally had pangs of guilt—"like the throbbing of a bad knee on a cloudy day," according to survey consultant Carin Rubenstein, Ph.D.—and most said it was self-inflicted. What makes them feel guilty? Forty-four percent—the largest consensus—said it was not spending enough time with their children. In fairness, their now-and-then bouts with guilt seemed to be offset by the pride and self-esteem they gained by working and providing for their families.

But guilt isn't necessarily always a bad thing. It does serve as a signal to do some soul-searching, says child care expert Ellen Galinsky, co-president of the Families and Work Institute in New York and coauthor of *The Preschool Years* and a number of other books on child care and child development. "Guilt is a signal that we're not living up to an expectation," she says. "What we need to do in that situation is ask, 'Is our expectation realistic or not?' "

Women who work do so because they either want to or have to—and sometimes both. In today's society, the working woman is the norm. Of women who return to work within a year of the birth of their first child, most do so within three months. But many also grew up with the expectation that, like their mothers, they should stay home with their children. Some women find they're constantly waging the battle of "shoulds": I should be working because we need the money. I should be working because my job makes me feel fulfilled. I should be at home because children should be raised by their parents.

SELF-FULFILLING PROPHECY

One of the few ways to avoid feeling guilty is to be convinced that you're doing the right thing. Otherwise, says Galinsky, your guilt can become "a self-fulfilling prophecy." A study done by Ellen Hock, Ph.D., professor of family relations and human development at Ohio State University, found that a mother's attitude toward leaving her child influences how the child reacts to separation. Guilt may also prompt you to act in ways that are detrimental to your child.

"You think you're damaging your child, therefore you may begin to act as if your child is damaged," says Galinsky. "You may begin to feel like you have to 'make it up' to your child because you work."

What often happens is that, out of guilt, parents indulge their children, acquiescing to the constant "gimmes" and allowing kids to stay up late at night, ostensibly to spend more time with them. Others attempt to be Supermom and burn themselves out in the process. The result can be confused or mixed-up kids who "know what you're doing is not quite right," says Galinsky.

Rather than handle it that way, she says, "face the guilt squarely in the eyes and say, 'Am I going to work or am I not?' And if you are, then come to some sort of terms with it. Don't let it seep into the relationship because the thing parents fear worse can happen. You can damage your child."

Investigate ways in which you can spend more time with your children. If your company offers it, take advantage of flex-time, or work part-time if it's a viable option. Take a look at your priorities. Are you working to keep food on the table or to keep up the payments on the time-share condo? If you can live comfortably if not luxuriously on one income and would like to stay home—at least until your children are older—then consider a new career as a stay-at-home mom.

PICK THE RIGHT CARE

But if you need to or want to work, it will help to be convinced that you've picked the right day care situation for your child, says Galinsky, who has done several studies on what makes parents happy or unhappy with their child care arrangements.

While you need to pay attention to your "gut feelings" when interviewing nannies or investigating family child care homes or day care centers, there are some other important specifics to look for.

Ask if you're permitted to drop into the home or center at any time. Your child care provider shouldn't be concerned about keeping any secrets from you. You want to be able to see the center or home at its worst as well as its best. You want to know where your child is going to be all day long, and what she's going to be doing. "There should be an open-door policy. Otherwise, go someplace else," advises Nancy Balaban, Ed.D., author of *Learning to Say Goodbye: Starting School and Early Childhood Separations* and director of the Infant and Parent Development Program at New York City's Bank Street College Graduate School of Education.

Find out the ratio of adults to children. Some states that license child care providers have their own guidelines, but the American Academy of Pediatrics recommends a child care facility have one adult for every three or four infants, four or five toddlers and six to nine preschoolers. Parents often prefer to have in-home care for infants, to assure the child will get sufficient attention, but that is scarce and unaffordable for many. Family child care may be a good alternative, because care is usually provided by another mother in her own home, and if she is licensed, is restricted in the number of infants she can care for, says Dr. Balaban.

What kind of training do the child care workers have? Is the area safe? What special activities does the caregiver or center offer? How are meals, discipline or illnesses handled?

LEARNING TO SAY GOOD-BYE

Walking out on a wailing child left in the care of a babysitter, teacher, child care worker or even a relative can cause high anxiety—for you as well as your child.

Children go through several predictable phases of separation anxiety, although some temperamentally find it hard to say good-bye, says New York child care expert Nancy Balaban, Ed.D. Generally, however, somewhere between 7 and 10 months, most children will raise a fuss if you leave them, even if it's to go into another room. "At this age, it's really clear to them that you are somebody special and they're going to put up a fuss when you leave them," Dr. Balaban says.

Most babies get over their anxiety in time, only to have it recur somewhere between 14 and 15 months and 2½ years. "These kids feel it even more intensely," says Dr. Balaban. "They know how vulnerable they are, how much they need you."

You need to acknowledge their feelings—"I know you feel sad because Mommy is leaving"—and give them a little extra TLC, says Dr. Balaban. "Never reject them or shove them away if they get clingy."

Just make a graceful exit, smiling after a hug and a kiss. Even if you're feeling separation anxiety, too—mothers do—try not to communicate it to your child. One tearful person per parting scene is enough. "And never, ever sneak out," cautions Ellen Galinsky, of the Families and Work Institute in New York City. "It might work the first time, but you pay for it the second and the third because you're not trusted."

She recommends that you leave something of yours with the child "like a symbolic gesture of your return—a transitional object that allows the child to keep 'home' with him until you return."

What's the turnover rate? When and how often does the center close? Does the family child care provider have backup for illnesses or vacation? These are some of the factors that can spell the difference between a good child care situation and a nightmare, yet many parents fail to place the importance on them they deserve. Galinsky says that her research found that most predictive of parents' satisfaction was a warm, caring relationship between their child and the child care provider. Research confirms parents' understanding that this relationship is, in fact, the most critical component of quality. "But research also shows a warm and caring relationship is much more likely to happen when the teachers are trained, the adult/child ratio is right, there isn't a high turnover and so on," says Galinsky. That makes these vital questions for every parent to ask.

EXTENDED FAMILY

It's also important that the staff or caregiver truly be caring to your child and supportive of you. What you are looking for is "family-centered" child care, says Galinsky. First, you want to know that your caregiver wants to help you in the challenges you face in balancing family life.

"In one study, we found that teachers were less supportive of parents when they didn't believe mothers should work," she says. "That seems like an oxymoron, but about a quarter of the staff at a representative sample of centers where we did our study strongly did not believe that mothers should work. Because we asked, we found out that most parents were unaware of the teachers' negative feelings about their working. Those parents whose children were cared for by staff who didn't believe mothers should work reported a lot less support from the staff. So, it would be very important to ask, 'Would you put your child in this program? Do you believe that mothers should work?' If the caregiver doesn't believe in child care, then, from my point of view, it's not a good program."

This is an especially important question to ask a family child care provider, because many are mothers of young children who have chosen to supplement the family income by providing child care to other children so they don't have to work outside the home.

There's another important sign to look for that signals a good "family-centered" child care situation. "When you walk in," says Galinsky, "are the parents kidding around with the staff in the morning? Do they act like they have a good time together? If you ask a staff member about a child's family and they say snide and awful things, they might say that about you, too. Sometimes a program will be just child-centered. If the staff is child-centered, you may get the impression they feel 'I'm going to save this child.' They think of themselves as the repository of all wisdom and think they know more about children than the parents. They really do care about the children, which is good, but it can breed some negative feelings between the parents and the staff."

What if you can't find a family-centered child care provider? Will a child-centered one do? "Well," says Galinsky, "if I had to trade off a good environment for me versus a good environment for my child and that was the only choice I had, I would pick out an environment for my child and figure as an adult, I could cope with it. But family-centered is really better for everyone."

See also Motherhood versus Career

CHAPTER 17

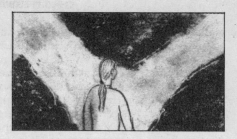

CHILD-FREE BY CHOICE

AN ALTERNATIVE LIFESTYLE

Thirty, even 20 years ago, a woman who decided to forgo motherhood would have been viewed at best as a curiosity, at worst a social outcast. She would have been "committing a taboo," in the words of one researcher. In fact, back then, the social pressure to have children probably forced many women who were dubious about their own maternal feelings to become reluctant, unhappy mothers.

Today, though not gone, that pressure is slowly easing. With motherhood increasingly regarded as a choice rather than a destiny, the few women who do choose childlessness—by one estimate, about 3 to 6 percent of all married women—find their decision is more accepted, and in many cases, supported. In fact, the negative appellation "childless" is rapidly being replaced by "child-free," which more accurately describes the way women without children see themselves.

Fading, too, are the assumptions about child-free women: that they're selfish, immature, maladjusted, unhappy and view kids with indifference at best.

CONFLICTING INTERESTS

Psychologist Mardy Ireland, Ph.D., who conducted indepth interviews with 100 child-free women, found that the majority of women who don't want to be mothers actually like children, but they place a higher value on other aspects of their lives, such as their careers or their relationships.

"I actually expected to find more women who didn't like kids, but they were a minority," says Dr. Ireland, adjunct faculty member at Santa Clara University in Berkeley, California, who is herself child-free. "Rather, these were women who valued the egalitarian nature of their primary relationship and were concerned that becoming a parent would change that. They also valued their personal freedom and their spontaneous lifestyle and had strong creative work interests that made them feel they couldn't do both to the degree of success that they wanted to."

Some of the women in Dr. Ireland's study even tested their feelings by deliberately spending time with the children of friends or relatives. "This was a way for them to find out how much they wanted to be involved with children. Obviously they decided, 'Not this much,'" she says.

Other studies have found that women who don't want children tend to be well-educated, high-achieving women with fulfilling jobs who don't think motherhood offers the same rewards. Many believe that demanding careers and children don't mix. They may sense that even in an "egalitarian" marriage, child care tends to be woman's work.

Elsa Harrow, a 34-year-old research scientist, says she's sure children would be a source of conflict in her ten-year, happy marriage. "Ed's a psychologist who sees people until 9 at night, so I would be the one doing everything, and I know I would get aggravated at that. I know I would start resenting him for working late, and I'd start feeling like a single parent."

A SOUL-SEARCHING DECISION

The crucial test of the wisdom of forgoing children comes in a woman's later years, when not having children could be a disadvantage. Gisela Booth, Ph.D., a clinical psychologist and assistant clinical professor at Northwestern University in Chicago, says she has seen a number of older women in her practice "who felt unconnected and isolated" when facing old age without children.

That may be true in some cases, particularly for those women whose husbands have died and who may have retired from their careers. But when studies focus on older women, the picture of the desiccated, unhappy childless woman simply doesn't emerge. In one study of women between the ages of 60 and 75, the childless women saw more advantages—personal freedom, privacy, less stress, a better marriage—than disadvantages to their lifestyles.

Having and being able to make friends—child-free or otherwise—serve as a buffer against loneliness. Unless you're a loner at heart, your friends can be as good as or better than children and grandchildren as you get older.

But the decision to give up parenthood is not one you should make lightly, especially if you are planning to take the virtually irreversible step of sterilization. You need to be sure you're doing it for the right reasons, and be aware of the pressures you're going to face as part of a very small minority in this society.

Most engaged couples feel each other out about children, and with good reason. When one wants kids and the other doesn't, it doesn't bode well for the relationship. "This is a fundamental conflict with only one solution: Someone has to change their mind," says Dr. Ireland. "Otherwise, the relationship won't last."

EXAMINE YOUR SUBCONSCIOUS

Jacqueline Fawcett, R.N., Ph.D., a researcher in maternity nursing at the University of Pennsylvania School of Nursing, knew from a very early age that she wanted a career and didn't want to be a mother. Nevertheless, she says, "I went into therapy because I wanted to make sure I wasn't specializing in maternity nursing for the wrong reasons."

Therapy might help you make a clear and balanced decision, especially if you have some unresolved conflicts from your past or some misconceptions about what it's like to be a mother. Some women may have a distorted view of parenthood—as all give and no get, for instance. Others may fear childbirth. Others may be what one psychologist calls parental children, who cared for siblings or acted as caretaker for dysfunctional parents in their childhood and are now "exhausted" by the parenting role.

"The sad thing is that if your choice is rooted in an emotional wound, you can go through life continuing to pay prices for that original wound," says Suzanne Pope, Ph.D., director of the Colorado Institute for Marriage and the Family in Boulder. "If you're not conscious of it, it can color everything you do."

Women who were parental children, says Dr. Pope, were robbed of their childhood. "Now, in their adulthood, they're robbed of being parents." It's a cycle that needs to be broken.

"It's more of a reactive choice," says Dr. Ireland, "or in some cases an active choice but not a very conscious one. Therapy can help you work through those conflicts. You still might make the same decision, but it will be a clearer one."

WAIT 'TIL YOU'RE THIRTYSOMETHING

You may want to put off sterilization until you're in your thirties to determine whether your feelings about parenthood change, suggests Dr. Ireland. They can and do. Decisions you make in your twenties might not work for the person you'll become later on.

"I couldn't have cared less about having kids until I was in my midthirties," says Bernadette Grundy, a marketing researcher who eventually did have a child when she was almost 40. "I was wrapped up in my career and my social life. Then, some of my friends started having babies and motherhood started to look appealing. I sneaked one in under the wire, and I'm glad I did."

"It's hard not to get a deviant feeling when you spend so much time with women who are mothers," says Dr. Ireland. Since most women are, you run the risk of feeling very isolated, unless you have child-free friends.

"It's like when you are single and everyone else is married," says Dr. Booth. "You may be perfectly comfortable being single and may even have chosen to be single, but you feel somewhat different."

EVERYBODY'S BUSINESS

And not only will you feel different, you really will *be* different. Which means you can expect social pressure. And expect it from your families first.

"Most parents want grandchildren," says Dr. Booth. "They feel deprived on a narcissistic level by not being offered grandchildren. They want to see some kind of family continuance."

Dr. Fawcett's mother-in-law pressured her and her husband to have children. "The pressure from my mother-in-law was because my husband is an only child," she says. "I became annoyed about constant references to other people's children. After several years, I asked my husband to tell his parents that it was a mutual decision, not just his wife depriving them of grandchildren. So he wrote his parents a letter."

But even if you successfully defuse the pressure from your family, don't be surprised if friends—even total strangers—offer their opinion. "The longer Ed and I have been married, the more people think it's their business," says Elsa Harrow. "One of my good friends has three kids and one day she said, 'Well, it's probably none of my business'—and I'm thinking, oh, boy, here it comes—'but how come you and Ed don't have kids?' I was floored. I would never dream of asking her why she has kids, which is as legitimate a question."

One thing that may help you get through this eventuality is to prepare for it. Have an explanation ready for parents and others who ask about your childlessness. "You can say, I just didn't want to have any children, I'm busy enough now or not everybody is meant to be a parent," suggests Matti Gershenfeld, Ph.D., director of the Couples Learning Center in Jenkintown, Pennsylvania. "Prepare yourself a line. You can count on the fact that people are going to ask you."

By remaining child-free you are choosing an alternative lifestyle, but you're not abnormal. Not every woman—nor, for that matter, every man—is cut out to be a parent. "We tend to forget that there is a vast spectrum of maternal instinct among women, even women who have children," says Dr. Booth. "There are some women who really wouldn't make good mothers, and maybe they know it. There is nothing that says women are supposed to have children just because they are women."

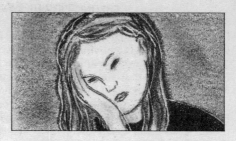

CHRONIC FATIGUE SYNDROME

TIREDNESS THAT WON'T GO AWAY

*I*t's been called the yuppie flu and Raggedy Ann syndrome. It's also been called bunk. But don't let that put you off—it's for real. Chronic fatigue syndrome (CFS) is an illness characterized by continual dog-tiredness, achy muscles, fever, drowsiness and the blahs that last for months—sometimes even for years.

"Although anyone can get chronic fatigue syndrome, the typical patient is most likely to be a woman between 20 and 50 years old and often highly successful, educated and articulate," says Dedra Buchwald, M.D., assistant professor of medicine at the University of Washington and director of the Chronic Fatigue Syndrome Clinic at Harborview Medical Center in Seattle.

The typical patient is also likely to have difficulty finding someone to take her symptoms seriously.

Just ask 30-year-old Roberta Holland. "I told each doctor that I went to that I had a headache for three months and my joints and muscles were so achy that even lying down could hurt," she says. "I told them I couldn't think straight, I couldn't remember. I even had a hard time spelling. I told them I was exhausted all the time, yet I'd lie awake all night." But Roberta had a hard time finding someone who would take her symptoms seriously.

A medical librarian, Roberta looked for the answer on

her own. Her best educated guess: CFS. But her research did nothing to help convince the doctors.

She says she must have gone to a half-dozen specialists before she found one who was sympathetic to her problem. "A psychiatrist told me that I didn't have CFS, I had depression," she remembers. "An internist said it couldn't be CFS because my lymph glands weren't swollen and I didn't have a low-grade fever, even though it followed a flulike illness. One doctor finally admitted to me that he didn't believe that CFS existed. No wonder he couldn't diagnose it!"

THE PROCESS OF ELIMINATION

Dr. Buchwald admits that there are some doctors who are reluctant to recognize or diagnose CFS, although this is not as common now as it was a few years ago. And she also admits that *true* CFS may be difficult to diagnose. One reason is that doctors frequently hear about excessive fatigue from their patients. But only a minority actually fit the criteria for CFS, devised by more than a dozen experts along with the Centers for Disease Control in Atlanta.

According to these criteria, people who truly have CFS are those who have suffered debilitating fatigue (or easy fatigability) that has lasted at least six months and who have reduced their daily activity level by at least one-half. They also must have ruled out (with the help of their doctor) any psychiatric diseases such as depression that may mimic CFS symptoms, physical problems such as various infectious diseases, hormonal disorders such as thyroid disease, drug abuse and exposure to toxic agents. They must also have at least 8 of the following 11 symptoms recurring or persisting for six months or longer.

- Chills or mild fever
- Sore throat
- Painful or swollen lymph glands
- Unexplained general muscle weakness
- Muscle discomfort

- Fatigue for a least 24 hours after previously tolerated exercise
- Headache unlike any previous pain
- Joint pain without joint swelling or redness
- Forgetfulness, excessive irritability, confusion, inability to concentrate or depression
- Disturbed sleep
- Quick onset of symptoms within a few hours or days

Patients also may meet the Centers for Disease Control criteria by reporting six of these symptoms and having two of the following three physical examination findings: a low-grade fever, an inflamed throat and palpable or tender nodes in the neck or under the arms.

THE CFS MYSTERY

But exactly what is chronic fatigue syndrome? And why was there a problem recognizing it as a disease?

"This could be the $64,000 question. Doctors, researchers and patients have been scrambling for the past few years looking for the answer," says Dr. Buchwald. "Right now there are only theories. CFS may be caused by the immune system or a chronic viral infection, and *several* viruses may be capable of producing the syndrome."

Indeed, most CFS sufferers say that their fatigue started abruptly following an infection, such as the flu. They may even be able to name the exact day they became ill.

"The syndrome often begins during a stressful time, when unusual demands are being made upon the patient," says Dr. Buchwald, "such as during a divorce, career change or a death in the family.

"Laboratory tests of CFS patients may show abnormal white blood cell counts, slight abnormalities in liver function, elevated antibody levels to various tissues or viruses or a mild increase or decrease in total antibody levels. The patterns are not clear-cut, though. There are some immunologic factors that are suppressed and some that are overactivated. Whatever this is, it's a very diffuse process."

It's also one that is still being studied and slow to be diagnosed.

"It's true that patients get very frustrated when they can't find someone who knows anything about chronic fatigue syndrome or who will listen to them," says Dr. Buchwald. "Many patients are told their symptoms are all in their heads, and that they should just snap out of it and get back to work. By the time patients get to me—which is usually at the end of the line—they are deep in despair."

Even with treatment, chronic fatigue syndrome can be long-lasting. It can last months or it can last years.

"During the worst part of the illness, I couldn't work or read at all," says Roberta Holland. "It's been a year, and I still can't read anything too complicated. And I still have trouble organizing my thoughts. I have days now when my energy level feels almost normal. But then suddenly, I won't feel so great. It seems to change from hour to hour or day to day, and I sometimes despair that I'll never be completely well. Although overall, I've improved tremendously over the past year or two, I know the disease can last for years and be chronic forever, and this knowledge haunts me."

MEDICATIONS CAN HELP

With this kind of struggle to face, how can you pull through? While there's no proven cure yet for CFS, there are a number of treatments that often help reduce the symptoms.

Doctors have tried various drugs to help boost the immune system or to attack specific viruses. "There are no medications approved specifically for chronic fatigue syndrome," says Dr. Buchwald. "The choice of drugs used is based on clinical experience. And all have varying degrees of success.

"A variety of antidepressants has helped many. Not only do these drugs increase energy and improve mood, they may help patients get a good night's sleep, which in turn

GIVE YOURSELF A LIFT

Although you need to enlist the help of a doctor to fight the energy-depleting symptoms of chronic fatigue syndrome (CFS), there are several things you can do for yourself. Here's what experts say you should try to do, even if you don't feel up to it.

Eat right. CFS is not thought to be associated with vitamin or mineral deficiencies, but eating meals with adequate amounts of nutrients (including calories) does make a difference in how some CFS sufferers feel. Some report feeling better when the diet is low in sugar and fat.

Exercise every day. Even a little bit, such as simple stretching, can help. Chronic overexertion tends to worsen symptoms and may prolong the course of the disease. Most experts do not believe people will get better faster if they stay in bed for long periods of time. This can be psychologically and physically devastating.

Prioritize your activities. Be ruthless, says Dedra Buchwald, M.D., director of the Chronic Fatigue Syndrome Clinic at Seattle's Harborview Medical Center. Eliminate those things that are least important. "This involves learning to say no to tasks that can be put off," she says, "so you can carefully parcel out your available energy among those things that have to get done."

Spare your family and friends. Pouring every detail of your illness out to close relatives can backfire. "Family members and friends are not equipped to deal with the devastating nature of CFS over the long haul," explains Dr. Buchwald. "It's okay to educate those close to you about it, but be careful to monitor the amount of personal details you burden them with. You don't want to drive your most important network of social support away."

Get help. Patient support groups can be a great source of comfort for many on how to deal emotionally and functionally with the disease. Others have found counseling and physical therapy to be beneficial.

Continue living. If you can't walk a mile, walk a block. If you can't work full-time, try to do it part-time, says Dr. Buchwald. In other words, try to do the same things you used to do, even if you can only handle a fraction of the activity.

Maintain a positive attitude. Those who do seem to cope the best.

helps reduce fatigue. Most people don't realize that antidepressants have multiple uses." People with CFS usually require much smaller doses of these medications than are prescribed to treat depression. Doctors have also tried antiviral agents, gammaglobulin, vitamin B_{12} shots, opiate and histamine blockers and more, she says.

Whatever treatment you try, CFS experts recommend being cautious of unproven therapies promoted as sure cures. It's not necessary to fly across the country to find a doctor. You can find quality care at home. Try looking for a CFS specialist affiliated with a teaching hospital or university. Or ask a local support group to recommend a helpful doctor. And until a cure is found, focus on safe, doctor-approved treatments, say the experts.

See also Fatigue

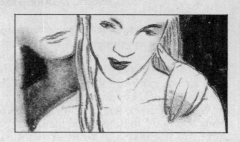

CONTRACEPTION

MAKE IT *YOUR* BUSINESS

*T*he rise in sexually transmitted diseases—AIDS, herpes, precancerous genital warts and the like—has forced women to realize that the purpose of contraception is more than just preventing babies. It's protecting their health and well-being.

And that—plus the fact that women are more vulnerable to sexually transmitted diseases than their partners—is why many experts feel that women should take charge when it comes to birth control.

Just one unprotected sexual liaison with a man infected with gonorrhea means you have a 50 percent chance of getting the disease yourself, according to statistics. For chlamydia, herpes or syphilis, the chances are 30 to 40 percent.

How likely is it that anyone you make love to has any of these diseases? Pretty likely. Scientists report that 1 in 25 American men has herpes, and 1 in 60 carries chlamydia.

Yet, despite the risk, experts say that most women tend to choose their birth control method based more on what they've heard or the scary and often contradictory headlines they've read in a newspaper rather than on factual information intended to protect their health. As a result, some women are apparently so confused about what to use that they place themselves in harm's way by using nothing at all.

SOME THINGS TO THINK ABOUT

Surveys show that about one in ten sexually active women who are at risk of becoming pregnant uses no birth control at all, says Jacqueline Darroch Forrest, Ph.D., vice-president of research of the Alan Guttmacher Institute in New York City, a nonprofit organization that does research in reproductive studies. And these women account for over half of all the unintended pregnancies in the United States.

Heaven knows, choosing a contraceptive method isn't easy. The particular method that each woman selects depends upon her goals, lifestyle, health, financial status and relationships at any given moment.

A sexually active woman who has not yet settled into a monogamous relationship, for example, might want the protection of a birth control pill and a condom, while a woman who is in a mutually monogamous relationship may turn to the diaphragm. Ten years later—and still fertile as a turtle—these women may very well exchange places and methods of contraception.

The point is that every woman who values her health must take the time to sit down and evaluate her options and needs. Often this means finding the method that—for her—confers the greatest degree of protection from pregnancy *and* sexually transmitted diseases, says Dr. Forrest. When it comes to smart sexual practices today, say the experts, women must consider barrier methods. And leading the list is the condom.

YOUR BEST BET

Condoms can be an effective birth control method for any woman, but given the 12 million new cases of sexually transmitted diseases (STDs) each year, they're de rigueur for a woman with more than one sex partner—or for a woman whose sex partner is having sex with others as well. They're also ideal for people who aren't having sex on a regular basis.

Condoms can be nearly as effective as oral contraceptives and the IUD. Failures—typically around 10 to 15 percent—are generally blamed on the users rather than the condoms. Unfortunately, it's easy to make some dangerous mistakes with male condoms. Unrolling the condom before putting it on, for example, can lead to tears or breaks. Putting the condom on during intercourse rather than before allows unprotected contact that can lead to both pregnancy and disease. Or exposing condoms to excessive heat, light and humidity can also affect their effectiveness, as can oily lubricants.

If you do need additional lubrication, doctors say, stick to water-based lubricants such as glycerin and K-Y Jelly. Or use spermicidal jellies and foams with the condom. In fact, some condoms already come with a spermicide; the failure rate for spermicide-coated condoms is generally lower.

As far as your health is concerned, the condom has a lot going for it. When used properly and consistently, studies show that it can reduce the transmission of bacterial STDs and viral diseases such as AIDS, herpes and warts. Because they help prevent STDs, condoms also protect against pelvic inflammatory disease—a disease that can result in infertility—and ectopic pregnancy. And since doctors now believe that cervical cancer can be caused by certain strains of the human papilloma virus, a sexually transmitted disease, a condom can prevent that as well.

Condoms can help prevent both pregnancy and sexually transmitted diseases because sperm and other organisms cannot pass through the latex rubber sheath. STD experts, however, warn against using "lambskin" condoms because infectious organisms, including those that cause AIDS, can pass through, making it ineffective for disease prevention.

CONDOM SENSE

The biggest problem with condoms is compliance, says Dr. Forrest. Unlike other contraceptives, the condom is used by your partner, so his cooperation is unavoidable. Yet some men object to the condom because they say it reduces sensitivity. And both men and women complain that condoms are messy and bothersome and interfere with the passion and spontaneity of the moment.

If you're single and otherwise unattached, however, your biggest problem may be condom etiquette. Studies show that women like condoms more than men like to use them, says psychologist Linda J. Beckman, Ph.D., director of research at the California School of Professional Psychology in Alhambra, so it may not be easy to convince a partner that it's in his best interest to wear the colorful, ribbed condom you just happen to have with you. Women must be able to do it, however, because roughly 40 percent of condom buyers *are* women.

How do you ask a man to wear a rubber? "A lot of women think that such a question might be construed as an insult," says Dr. Beckman, also an adjunct professor in the Department of Psychology at University of California, Los Angeles. They're afraid that it might be construed as a lack of trust.

But trust is not the issue, she points out. You're not trying to protect yourself because you suspect that he's withholding pertinent information but because he may not even know if he's been exposed to an STD. The AIDS virus, for example, can lie dormant for years, producing no symptoms.

The bottom line? Condoms are effective, cheap and readily available in drugstores and restroom vending machines. They come in a variety of sizes, colors and textures and are now the third most popular contraceptive among American women.

With the alarming rise in STDs, however, most experts hope that they will soon be number one.

THE FEMALE CONDOM

For those who want to avoid the sometimes treacherous negotiations with condom-resistant males, female condoms may provide an alternative.

The first to hit the market is Reality, a 7-inch-long, prelubricated, polyurethane pouch that is inserted like a tampon.

BEFORE-YOU-HIT-THE-PILLOW TALK

The most important thing to remember when you begin a sexual relationship is that you're not crawling into bed with *one* man, says Jacqueline Darroch Forrest, Ph.D., of the Alan Guttmacher Institute in New York City. You're also sharing space with all the people *he* had sex with—*and* all the people *they* had sex with!

"Our biggest problem is not contraceptive technology—the hardware, so to speak—but the software of our own behavior and how we deal with our relationships with one another," says Dr. Forrest. It's often a lot easier to have sex than it is to talk about it.

But talk you must. And the International Planned Parenthood Federation offers these suggested responses for women negotiating over condom use.

HE: I know I don't have any disease. I haven't had sex for a long time.

YOU: As far as I know, I don't have any disease either. But I still want us to use a condom since either of us could have an infection and not know about it.

Or:

HE: What an insult! You think I'm the sort of person who gets AIDS?

YOU: I didn't say that. Anyone can get an infection. I want to use a condom to protect us both.

Or:

HE: I love you. Would I give you an infection?

YOU: Not deliberately. But most people don't know they are infected. That's why this is best for both of us.

Other suggestions:

- Discuss condom use before you're physically close, when you still control your feelings.
- Rehearse what you want to say to your partner. Have a close friend role-play with you.
- Bring up the subject by mentioning a news item or TV program you've seen about condoms.

- If your partner doesn't have a condom, pull one (make sure you have one at all times) out of your handbag and say something simple and clear such as "Let's use this condom for protection."
- Be assertive. Be clear; don't get drawn into an argument. It's your life and health at stake.

The Reality female condom is designed for women to use to help prevent AIDS, other sexually transmitted diseases (STDs) and unintended pregnancy. The device, which is *under the control of the woman*, is comfortable and easy to use. Reality covers the cervix and lines the vaginal canal, preventing skin touching skin. The sole purpose of this device is to reduce the risk of transfer of virus, bacteria and sperm between sexual partners.

Reality is made of polyurethane, a thin but strong material which is very resistant to rips and tears during use. The disposable barrier device consists of a soft sheath that is open on one end and closed at the other. It has two flexible rings: one is used to insert the device and hold it in place over the cervix; the other remains outside the vagina after insertion. Reality covers the woman's labia and the base of the penis during intercourse. It comes prelubricated in its package, is disposable and is to be used for only one sex act.

Although women who have tried the device generally find it comfortable, some did not like the visibility of the outer rim.

Laboratory tests indicate that the condom will provide equal protection against all STDs. During typical use, it is about as effective as the diaphram, sponge and cervical cap in preventing pregnancy. Ongoing clinical studies are looking at how effective it is in protecting against STDs during actual use. The Reality female condom is available over the counter at drug stores and other retail outlets wherever condoms for men and other family planning products are sold. It also can be found at many public health and family planning clinics.

ANOTHER ALTERNATIVE

A barrier method that's totally dependent on the woman is the diaphragm, a soft, dome-shaped rubber cap with a flexible rim that fits in the vagina and covers the cervix. It prevents conception in the same general way a condom does—by preventing sperm from entering the cervix and heading for an egg. It is normally used with a spermicide, which can help kill any sperm that manage to get around the rim.

The diaphragm can be inserted up to 6 hours before intercourse so you don't have to worry about "spoiling the moment," but you need to have planned for it. It should never be left in for more than 12 hours. But taking it out too soon may increase your risk of pregnancy. Check with your doctor.

When used with a spermicide, diaphragms decrease the possibility of transmitting STDs and pelvic inflammatory disease. They also protect against cervical neoplasia, an often precancerous condition that has been linked to cervical cancer.

The diaphragm can be nearly as effective as birth control pills, but only if used properly and consistently. In one study, for example, older married women who had been using a diaphragm for more than five years had a failure rate—in this case, pregnancy rate—of only 1.1 percent. When a group of younger married and unmarried women was studied, however, the pregnancy rate was 21 percent the first year and 37 percent the second.

Clearly, depending on the motivation of the woman using it, the diaphragm is either nearly foolproof—or a disaster.

GETTING RISKIER

Other barrier methods are somewhat less effective. But given your options, they are better than nothing at all. These include spermicides and sponges.

A spermicide is a chemical that immobilizes or kills sperm. It comes in various forms, including foams, jellies, suppositories, creams and films that dissolve in the vagina. The active ingredient in most spermicides is nonoxynol-9, a chemical that can reduce sexually transmitted diseases, both bacterial and viral.

Pregnancy rates for spermicides can be as high as 28 percent, studies reveal, although the typical failure rate is around 13 percent. It is most effective when used in conjunction with another barrier method such as the diaphragm, sponge or condom.

The sponge is a pillow-shaped, polyurethane device that contains nonoxynol-9, so it is technically both a barrier method and a spermicide. The sponge itself traps sperm, while the spermicide kills them. It fits in the upper vagina with its concave side covering the cervix so it's less likely to be dislodged. It has a loop for easy removal, comes in one size and is available over-the-counter. It offers protection for up to 24 hours, no matter how many times you have intercourse, after which it must be discarded.

The sponge has a 17 to 25 percent failure rate, studies reveal, and because of the spermicide, it can help reduce the risk of sexually transmitted diseases, both bacterial and viral.

Unfortunately, the sponge may cause allergic reactions and vaginal irritations such as vaginal dryness, itching, stinging, a foul odor and vaginal discharge. There may also be an increased risk of yeast infections and toxic shock syndrome, although toxic shock is rare.

The sponge is not the right choice for a woman for whom effectiveness is a priority. For the highly motivated woman, however, the sponge has some pluses: It's inexpensive, easy to use, doesn't require a doctor's visit and protects against disease.

So which contraceptive is right for you?

Take your choice and discuss it with your doctor. But remember that deciding which contraceptive to use is only half of what you need to do to protect your body. *Using* it is the other half.

See also Birth Control Pills, Sexually Transmitted Diseases

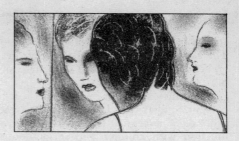

COSMETIC SURGERY

APPEARANCE AND SELF-ESTEEM GET A LIFT

*E*ver see a book with before and after pictures of cosmetic surgery patients? You probably spent more time gazing at the photos than a kid with a toy store catalog. And why not? There, laid out before you, was visible evidence of the magic that could be yours. Bumpy noses turned straight. Lumpy thighs turned smooth. Sagging faces turned fresh. Small breasts turned full. Tummies turned tighter. It's the ultimate wish book, isn't it? What *you* could become—if you had the money and the nerve.

Well, it takes a lot less nerve than it used to (although the cost is still pretty steep). "There has been so much social change in the last ten years that cosmetic plastic surgery has reached a level of acceptability never thought possible before," according to Caroline Cline, M.D., Ph.D., a San Franciscan trained as both a plastic surgeon and a psychologist.

"People are getting in shape in every way," adds Diane Gerber, M.D., a plastic surgeon practicing in Chicago. "They go to health clubs, jog or walk regularly and are careful about what they eat. Cosmetic surgery is an extension of wanting to look your best."

HEALTHY, YOUTHFUL MOTIVES

"What people see when they look in the mirror has a big impact on their self-esteem," notes Dr. Cline. "Can you imagine what it would be like if someone made you a dress that was the wrong size or shape and then made you wear it for the rest of your life?"

That's how Melita Koch felt about her stomach. "I've been a physically active person all my life," says the 56-year-old registered nurse. "But after four pregnancies, my stomach got in the way of the activities I liked most of all—volleyball, bike riding and jogging. When pedaling my racing bike, my knees kept hitting my stomach. And I always looked three months pregnant, even though I was not overweight."

When Melita inherited some money a few years ago, she decided it was time to do something about her belly. "I didn't decide to have a tummy tuck with the idea of looking more beautiful or for approval from anyone else, including my husband," she insists. "I did it for my own comfort."

Like Melita, people want to look as young, vibrant and attractive on the outside as they feel on the inside, adds Victoria Vitale-Lewis, M.D., a plastic surgeon with Plastic and Reconstructive Surgery Associates in Melbourne, Florida. Or they feel that they have one body part that's inconsistent with their idea of themselves. That was particularly true of Michelle Fitzgerald, a 24-year-old secretary. "I think it was the wedding video that finally convinced me to get my nose fixed," she says. "All I could see was my nose sticking out of my veil. It's a long nose, which I actually didn't mind, but it had a big bump on the top which simply ruined my profile. My aim was to get the bump removed, that's all. I didn't want to look different, only better," she says.

Fixing a troublesome body part helps people get on with their lives, to put painful memories behind them, says Dr. Vitale-Lewis. Barbara Aston remembers being called "monkey ears" as a child. "The insult stung because I knew it was true," says the 28-year-old newspaper reporter. "From the time I was a child, I always wore my hair long so it would cover my ears. When I went swimming (which I loved), the first thing I would do when I came up to the surface was quickly pull my hair over my ears. I never wore my hair in a ponytail no matter how hot the weather.

Getting my ears fixed meant that I could forget about them. They're just ears now, completely indistinctive and unremarkable. Nobody notices them anymore, not even me."

UNREALISTIC EXPECTATIONS

Cosmetic surgery will not save a failing marriage. It will not magically shave 20 years off your appearance. It will not necessarily give you a better chance of attracting a new boyfriend. It will not secure that promotion you've been aiming for. In fact, even if you're counting on surgery to deliver great or rested looks, you may be disappointed, says plastic surgeon Elizabeth Morgan, M.D., in her book *The Complete Book of Cosmetic Surgery*. "Surgery can only *help*. Successful surgery may not deliver such specific goals as looking good in certain clothes or hairstyles. To want to be able to 'see the change in the mirror' is realistic; to have exactly a 28-inch waist may not be." Unless your hopes are compatible with what surgery can realistically deliver, she says, you may not be happy with the results.

Doctors say, however, that it can be healthy for you to participate in planning your surgery by indicating which looks you like and which you don't—up to a point. Dr. Cline recalls a 28-year-old patient who pointed to a photo of her older sister, saying, "I want a nose just like hers." Upon further probing, it became apparent that the patient's sister was a professional model who was perceived as hogging all the limelight in the family. The woman secretly believed that if she had her sister's nose, she would have her lifestyle, too. Dr. Cline advised against surgery and encouraged her to seek psychological counseling.

Even if your motives are healthy and your expectations realistic, cosmetic surgery still may be inappropriate. A good surgeon will tell you, for example, if she thinks enough improvement can be achieved to outweigh the costs and discomforts of the procedure you want. Patricia Christman says she was satisfied with her looks in general but felt that her aging face needed improvement. "Looking older seemed to come upon me too suddenly," explains the 48-year-old personnel manager. "I thought having a face-lift would improve my self-confidence and make me feel younger." Patricia went to see two plastic surgeons and both told her that it was too soon to operate. "They felt that the improvement would hardly be noticeable. In other words, why go through all that discomfort and expense for such minimal results?"

But Patricia didn't listen. Instead she searched for a doctor who could give her the kind of results she was after, and she found one. "I should have listened to the advice of the first two doctors," she concedes. "I spent $6,000, suffered some severe complications and when I look in the mirror, I can barely see an improvement. Nobody would ever believe that I had my face lifted just a year ago."

FEARS CAN COME TRUE

Cosmetic surgery is not like a trip to the beauty parlor, reminds Dr. Gerber. It's surgery, and it's not without pain, discomfort and some risks, although severe complications occur only rarely. It's normal, in fact, expected, to feel anxious about having cosmetic surgery, adds Dr. Vitale-Lewis. You're putting yourself under the knife, and in some cases, under general anesthesia for what many perceive as vanity, not a medical condition.

A good surgeon will explain the operation in full to you, including how much bruising, swelling and pain might be expected. She should also discuss the possibility of minor or major complications, how frequently they occur and how they can be corrected. The fact is, postsurgical bleeding, blood clots, unsatisfactory scarring, nerve damage and infection can happen. No wonder anxiety is a part of the equation!

Patricia says the surgeon who agreed to do her face-lift de-emphasized her concerns about severe complications. Patricia was particularly worried about facial paralysis—a serious complication that occurs when a nerve is damaged—because it happened to a friend. Although rare, it can leave half your face "frozen" for more than a year.

"When the bandages came off, the doctor asked me to close my eyes," she recalls. "Although I had the sensation

LIPOSUCTION: FAT DEPOSITS WITHDRAWN

It's probably the hottest cosmetic surgical technique to come along in years. In fact, since its introduction into this country in the early 1980s, liposuction has become the most commonly performed cosmetic surgery procedure, with more than 109,000 done in 1990, the most recent year for which statistics are available.

Liposuction is a procedure intended to permanently remove deposits of excess fat that are resistant to diet and exercise—like "saddlebags" and "love handles." To perform liposuction, a doctor inserts a blunt-ended metal tube, called a cannula, through a small incision in the skin, then tunnels repeatedly under the skin in a radiating pattern to dislodge and remove fatty tissue. The cannula is connected by a plastic hose to a vacuum aspirator that suctions out the fat, which is mingled with blood and body fluids.

The procedure, which takes from 30 to 90 minutes, can be done under local or general anesthesia. Afterward, you must wear a support garment, such as a girdle or chin strap, depending on the liposuction site, for a few weeks. This helps prevent dimpling by smoothing out the fat that remains under your skin. If your thighs, buttocks or hips are suctioned, you may not be able to walk or sit comfortably for a few days. Bruising, swelling and some pain may linger for up to three months.

The people who can expect the best results are those who maintain good health, are at their ideal weight, are age 40 or younger and have excellent skin tone. Liposuction can still be successful if you are between 40 and 60 if you have somewhat resilient skin, are in good health and weigh no more than 10 pounds more than your ideal weight.

that both eyes were blinking, in fact, only one was. I also couldn't curl back the left side of my upper lip. And when I smiled, only one side of my face turned up. I had suffered the one complication I feared the most."

Patricia says that at first she was frantic. Not only did she look grotesque, she wondered how she could face people at work. But her friends and colleagues were extremely supportive, she reports. Just as the doctors predicted, the damaged nerve slowly recovered, although it took more than a year.

Complications aside, it's not unusual for patients to be fearful of the outcome, says Dr. Vitale-Lewis. The fears are all the same: How long will it take for me to feel well? Will I be able to handle the pain? Will the results live up to my expectations? Will I like the new look that's been created? "I try to alleviate any fears patients may have by being completely honest about what they can expect," states Dr. Vitale-Lewis. "Sometimes I show them pictures of other patients, but only if I can find some that are very close to what I'm trying to achieve for them."

THE STORM BEFORE THE CALM

No matter how happy people are with the final results (and they almost always are, by the way), there's a healing process to get through first. Pain, bruising and swelling can be quite unpleasant for the first few days or weeks after surgery, depending on the procedure you had done. Yet, patients happy with their new or revised features seem to put the pain aside rather quickly. Perhaps it's like having a baby. You don't dwell on the discomfort you went through because you're so pleased with the final reward.

Melita Koch says that the first two days after her tummy tuck surgery were the worst. "There were drainage tubes coming out of my abdomen. My stomach felt so tight that I had to sit and walk bent over," she recalls. "And I had to sleep on my back with pillows under my knees so the stitches wouldn't pull. Even my breathing felt different. Before the surgery my stomach kind of flopped south when I breathed in and out. Afterward it was held firm."

According to Barbara Aston, the bruising and swelling from her ear surgery were far worse than she had expected. "There was some bleeding the day after the surgery and quite a bit of pain," she says, "and so my mother took me back to see the doctor. When he took the bandages off, the look on my mother's face said it all. Even the doctor admitted there was more swelling and bruising than usual. Still, aspirin dulled the pain, and in a few days I felt much better."

Barbara says the bruising lasted several weeks and spread down and around her neck, leaving a mark that looked like someone had tried to strangle her.

For Michelle Fitzgerald, the discomfort she felt after her nose surgery was relatively minor. "When I touched my face it felt swollen out to there. I was uncomfortable for the first 24 hours. My head felt heavy and there was a fair amount of bleeding, but there was no pain."

A TOUCH OF THE BLUES

During recovery, it's not uncommon to go through some emotional flip-flops, says Dr. Gerber. Everybody wants the results to be immediate, but the reality is that right after surgery, you'll have to go through several weeks of swelling, bruising and discomfort. "That's especially true of face-lift surgery," she says. "You're swollen, cooped up at home and your head may be bandaged so you can't even wash your hair. Patients often start feeling a bit depressed."

A study of those who underwent plastic surgery of the nose (rhinoplasty) showed that 20 percent experienced some dissatisfaction and depression during the first 30 days after the operation. The feelings lasted up to six months.

There are a couple of reasons why some patients may be prone to some temporary blue feelings after rhinoplasty, says Marcia Kraft Goin, M.D., clinical professor of psychiatry at the University of Southern California, Los Angeles, and author of the study. "First, it can take some time before the swelling and bruising disappear and the patient can see the true results of the surgery. And second, rhinoplasty is somewhat like breast reduction because it changes the body shape a person basically 'grew up' with," explains Dr. Goin. "Unlike a face-lift, which returns your features to the way they've always been, a rhinoplasty creates a whole new shape you've never had before. And no matter how much you wanted that change, it can be a shock at first."

Dr. Goin also found in her research that the patients most likely to experience temporary feelings of depression and dissatisfaction were also the ones who reported higher-than-normal levels of anxiety before surgery. A doctor who is sensitive to her patients' moods, she says, may be able to anticipate which ones are most at risk of having postoperative blues and offer extra support and reassurance.

A LITTLE LESS CHEST

"It's me, only better," is the theme echoed by those whose expectations were met or exceeded, no matter what the new look may be. But according to the experts, perhaps the happiest patients of all are those who have had breast reduction surgery. These are the women whose whole lives have often been dominated by the size of their breasts. Sure, there were the catcalls. But there was other pain as well. Most of these women experienced severe back problems and constant physical aggravations from deep indentations of their bra straps caused by the sheer weight of their breasts. Almost unanimously, these women wish they had had the operation years earlier.

Esther Goldman, a 56-year-old wife and mother, marvels over her new size 34C—down from a very full 36D. "It may not sound like that much of a difference, but let me assure you it most certainly is," she says. "Immediately after the surgery I felt younger, lighter. If my bra rubbed against the stitches I thought nothing of just slipping it off and going without it! I had never been able to do that in my life," she crows. "Suddenly I could wear clothes I never had before—a strapless bathing suit, a little tank top. And my back problems completely disappeared."

A HAPPY NEW ME

Most people are happy with the results of their surgery, no matter what the procedure, says Dr. Gerber. And that's probably because today's plastic surgeons are extremely careful to choose patients with realistic expectations. Although most praise is word-of-mouth, there have been some scientific studies to support those opinions. Dr. Goin's survey of 120 rhinoplasty patients, for example, showed that 90 percent felt that the surgery had been worthwhile.

If you've undergone a substantial change—a very large

THE HIGH COST OF LOOKING GOOD

Cosmetic surgery isn't cheap, and it generally isn't covered by insurance policies. The table below will give you an idea of the number of surgeries performed each year and the costs for various procedures. These numbers are based on 1990 statistics from the American Society of Plastic and Reconstructive Surgeons. Fees could vary significantly depending on the geographic location and complexity of the particular operation. These fees are for the doctor only and do not include hospital charges.

Procedure	Estimated Number (per yr.)	Fee Range ($)
Breast augmentation	89,400	1,000–2,400
Breast lift	14,300	1,000–2,890
Breast reduction	40,300	1,500–4,400
Chin augmentation	13,300	300–1,580
Liposuction	109,100	500–1,480
Rhinoplasty	68,300	300–2,590
Tummy tuck	20,200	1,200–3,430

nose into a smaller one, or a breast reduction, for example—there's a period of adjustment until you appreciate the new you, Dr. Gerber says. For subtler changes—a face-lift or an eyelid lift—the adaption may be practically immediate. "People can get so used to their new looks, in fact, that they stop seeing the difference. I often have to bring out their original photos to remind them how much of a change was really made," she says.

"I think I didn't fully appreciate my new ears for many months," says Barbara Aston. "One day I was leaning over my desk doing some close work. My hair fell into my face and without a second thought I tucked it behind my ears. I remember smiling to myself," she says, "realizing that I had finally gotten over my old habit of pulling my hair down *over* my ears."

"Believe it or not, I can get into clothes that I wore in high school," says Melita Koch, who had the tummy tuck.

"In fact, I was so pleased with the results that I went back to the same doctor and had a breast reduction a few years later. I feel so good about myself now. I can be as athletic as I want, and no more stomach or breasts flopping around."

Michelle Fitzgerald says her nose doesn't look any different from the front, which is just the way she wanted it. "It was the bump that had bothered me. The doctor took that away and so now I have this great profile. I'd like to go through life walking sideways," she quips. Michelle says she does a lot more with her hairstyle now, too. "I bought all kinds of hair accessories—clips and bows—and now I often wear my hair up and off my face to show off my profile."

KEEP 'EM GUESSING

The question of secrecy has more to do with personal style than anything else, says Dr. Vitale-Lewis. "There's one group of people who like to keep things to themselves. They don't want anyone to know they had cosmetic surgery." One woman who had excess fat removed from her thighs through liposuction (see "Liposuction: Fat Deposits Withdrawn" on page 136) took great pleasure in keeping her aerobics classmates guessing. Even though several commented on how great she'd been looking, she never let on to anyone that her new appearance was due to anything but diligent exercise.

"Then there's the other group who can't keep quiet. They'll be out there in the waiting room lifting up their shirts to show everyone their new breasts, whether they were made smaller or larger," says Dr. Vitale-Lewis.

More often than not, other people will not know that you've had something fixed, adds Dr. Gerber. "Even if you've made a drastic change—a new nose, a face-lift, an eyelift—something right in the middle of your face, people will miss it entirely. They may ask you if you had your hair cut or are wearing new makeup. They may say, 'You look so rested, have you been on vacation?' "

Michelle says she only told a few of her coworkers about her nose. "They were amazed at how much it looked the

CHOOSE A SURGEON WISELY

You have only one face, so if you're considering plastic surgery, you should choose a surgeon carefully.

Look for recommendations from other doctors and nurses you may know. Friends who have had cosmetic surgery can often offer good advice, too, if they're willing to be candid. What's more, at least in some cases, you can see with your own eyes if you like the outcome of their surgery.

A few words of caution: Watch out for a surgeon who is overly enthusiastic, makes unrealistic promises or tries to sell you on more surgery than you really want. Secretary Michelle Fitzgerald says that one surgeon she consulted about a nose reconstruction wanted to do cheek implants, too. He also showed her before and after pictures of his work and everyone had the same nose after surgery—men and women alike.

Make sure, also, that your surgeon discusses the potential risks and complications that can arise with your type of surgery. Even though severe complications are rare, you want to know your surgeon can take the appropriate actions if they should be needed.

Make sure the doctor you select is certified by the American Board of Plastic Surgery. How will you know? Look for his name in your library's *Directory of Medical Specialists*. Your county medical society can also give you the names, addresses and qualifications of several board-certified plastic surgeons in your area.

You can also call the nationwide toll-free Plastic Surgery Referral Service, which provides consumers with the names of board-certified plastic surgeons in their geographic areas. If you're interested specifically in cosmetic plastic surgeons, you can request referral to the American Society for Aesthetic Plastic Surgery.

If you're particularly interested in facial plastic surgery— such as nose reshaping, a face-lift, eyelid lift or chin implant—you can call the Facial Plastic Surgery Information Service in Washington, D.C. They will supply you with a list of board-certified facial plastic surgeons by state and information brochures about the facial plastic surgery in which you are interested.

same and yet different, too. Nobody else noticed or made any comments about it," she says.

If you're the kind of person who would rather publish your bank account than reveal the fact that you had cosmetic surgery, you'll need a plan to field potential nosybodies, says Dr. Morgan in her book. Remember, though, that you have nothing to be ashamed of or defensive about. Try this strategy.

Ignore the question. Add an icy stare if you don't mind offending the person offending you.

Answer a question with a question. If you're asked, "Didn't you just have a face-lift?" Answer, "Where did you hear that?" or "Why do you want to know?"

Use humor. "It's less likely to lead to ruffled feathers— if you care to avoid them," says Dr. Morgan. If someone should ask if you've had a nose job, for example, you could respond, "Are you kidding? Why mess with a work of art?"

Be evasive, and use vague terminology. Say you were "treated" for a condition. Don't use the words "surgery" or "operation," says Dr. Morgan. Breast surgery can be referred to as "a glandular condition." If you had a face-lift, say you were treated for a "muscular weakness."

CHAPTER 21

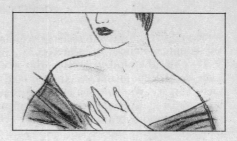

CYSTITIS

HOW TO STOP STUBBORN BLADDER INFECTIONS

*W*hen Lisa Jacobson was in graduate school, she picked up more than an education. It was also her first introduction to cystitis, a urinary tract infection (UTI) all too well known to women.

The symptoms came on fast and furious, says the now 40-year-old photographer, with fierce pain and stinging every time she urinated. "And always there was that uncomfortable feeling that I needed to urinate again," she says, "even if I had just done so minutes before."

Lisa's doctor immediately prescribed an antibiotic to kill the bacteria in her bladder. She recovered quickly and thought that that was the end of it. But soon the symptoms returned, and she needed to be treated again. Her recurrent bouts of cystitis lasted for more than two years, until finally a urologist put her on a longer course of antibiotics, which seemed to do the trick—or so she thought. "A few years later," says Lisa, "my bladder symptoms returned. And they were as stubborn as ever. They hurt so bad when I got them that they interfered with my love life."

COMMON AS A COLD

Lisa is among literally legions of women plagued by this ubiquitous nuisance. In fact, urinary tract infections are so common that it's the rare woman who has never had one.

"They're second only to colds in prevalence," says Kristene E. Whitmore, M.D., clinical associate professor of urology at the University of Pennsylvania and chief of the Department of Urology at Graduate Hospital in Philadelphia.

"Twenty percent of women will have at least one infection a year, prompting about five million visits to the doctor," says Dr. Whitmore, who is also the coauthor of *Overcoming Bladder Disorders*. "Men can get bladder infections, too, but women get them 25 times more often."

And if you've had just one infection, you stand a 15 percent chance of having a recurrent problem. Dr. Whitmore classifies recurrent as more than two within six months or more than three in a year.

AN ANATOMY LESSON

Women are the natural target of this infection by nature of their anatomy. It's a short trip for wandering bacteria from the rectum to the vagina and urethra (the opening that leads to the bladder). As long as they stay where they belong—on the outside of the body—there's usually no problem. But once these normally harmless germs (the most common is *E. coli*) go up the urethra and into the bladder, they turn ornery. What's worse, they settle in and breed.

With the subtlety of a steamroller, the symptoms appear—burning and pain as urine is released and an urgent need to urinate frequently. In fact, your urine may even be tinged with blood, and you could experience soreness in your lower abdomen, back or sides.

If you've ever had one, you know the symptoms are too uncomfortable to be ignored. And they shouldn't be. Left untreated, a urinary tract infection can even travel into the kidneys, where it can cause serious complications.

GERM WARFARE

Fortunately for the vast majority of women, a urinary tract infection is easy to diagnose and easy to treat. The routine treatment is antibiotics, such as amoxicillin.

"For as many as 80 to 90 percent of those with UTIs, a single dose of an antibiotic—just one to four pills at a time—can wipe out the infection and the symptoms, especially for first-time or sporadic cases," says Dr. Whitmore. "Most doctors, though, give a three- to five-day course of treatment to be on the safe side. This is far less than we used to prescribe, and so the likelihood of complications—typically stomach upset and vaginal yeast infections—is greatly reduced.

"If an infection occurs during pregnancy, it still must be treated, but only with certain antibiotics that are known to be safe for the growing fetus," stresses Dr. Whitmore. "If it's not treated, there's a 40 percent chance that the woman will develop a kidney infection during the third trimester."

REPEAT OFFENDERS

If you're one of the lucky ones, a short course of antibiotics should do the trick. For some women, however, bladder infections come back again and again with frustrating regularity, sometimes only days or weeks apart. Why?

Bacteria get in the bladder all the time, explains Dr. Whitmore, but it doesn't automatically mean infection. The germs are simply flushed out by normal voiding—the bladder's most important defense mechanism.

In some women, though, there's a breakdown in the bladder's natural defenses. One theory is that those susceptible to recurrent UTIs have bladder walls that allow bacteria to "stick," making it more difficult for urination to wash them out. In fact, doctors are currently experimenting on ways to prevent bacterial attachment.

THE SEX CONNECTION

When antibiotics fail to stop the recurrences, your doctor may decide to do more extensive testing to check bladder function and also rule out other problems, such as diabetes, tumors, kidney stones or obstructions.

But often the cause of repeat infections is never found.

Even so, there's still a great deal that can be done. For example, some women have found a pattern between UTIs and frequency of sex.

"For women who have a known history of UTIs after sexual relations, we now recommend taking one antibiotic tablet just before or after intercourse," says Dr. Whitmore. "If the problem seems to stem from diaphragm and spermicide use, we suggest trying another form of birth control, such as a cervical cap. Often that's all that's needed to end or greatly curtail the problem."

If this approach is unsuccessful and infections continue to disrupt your life, then a long-term prevention program is often advised, called low-dose suppressive therapy. Doctors have found that one antibiotic pill every other night can often keep women completely free from infection, with a minimum of side effects.

For women who get repeated attacks at random, doctors advise self-medication. You'll be taught about the drugs and then given a supply to keep at home. At the first sign of infection, you can begin a short course of medication. That eliminates calling the physician, waiting until she calls back, going to the office, then getting the prescription filled, which is all so time-consuming and expensive. You *know* when an infection is starting, and this way you can begin medication that much sooner. You'll need to keep a medical diary and know what signs or symptoms still require a visit to the doctor.

If you're past menopause, relief may be as simple as starting estrogen replacement therapy. Sometimes just a topical application of a prescription estrogen cream to the vaginal area is all that's needed, says Dr. Whitmore.

WHERE'S THE GERM?

The symptoms are all there. You know them like the back of your hand. You go to the doctor, and she sends a sample of your urine to the lab for culturing. But this time when the results come back, your doctor calls you and says, "There are no bacteria in your urine." Now what?

First of all, don't be too quick to rule out a bacterial

TAKE THE BLADDER TEST

If you're plagued by recurrent cystitis, the answers to these questions may help you and your doctor find the cause of the problem.

Do you wait too long to urinate? Holding urine in too long before voiding causes the bladder to overfill. When this practice is repeated over and over again, it gradually weakens the bladder, which is a muscle, so that it can't contract with enough force to expel all the urine it's collected. If your bladder is not emptied completely each time you void, then any lingering germs are more likely to take up permanent residence, increasing your risk of infection.

Do you get infections after sexual intercourse? During intercourse, bacteria from the surrounding areas can be pushed into the urethra by the back-and-forth motion of the penis. Some women get an infection almost every time they have sex. One 24-year-old woman found that if she had sex at 10:00 p.m., she could be certain of an infection by 3:00 a.m. In fact, the infection's link to lovemaking is how it got the moniker "honeymoon cystitis."

Do you use a diaphragm and/or spermicidal jelly? Studies have shown that women who use a diaphragm are two to four times more prone to infection than those who don't, says Kristene E. Whitmore, M.D., chief of urology at Graduate Hospital in Philadelphia. "The spring rim of the diaphragm can compress the bladder neck, causing some bruising and swelling, possibly obstructing the free flow of urine, a situation known to promote infection."

Studies also show that the spermicidal jelly used with a diaphragm can upset the vaginal defense mechanism so that unfriendly bacteria can more easily grow and spread.

Are you past menopause? The decreased level of estrogen after menopause can affect the functioning of the bladder and urethra. The tissue becomes thinner and more vulnerable to infection when the ovaries shut down. "What's more," says Dr. Whitmore, "the aging bladder loses elasticity and doesn't contract as efficiently. The result is decreased bladder emptying."

infection. Studies now show that the criteria used to determine a "positive" urine culture are not sensitive enough. About one-third of women with acute UTIs have bacterial counts *below* the level used to define an infection by laboratory standards. Dr. Whitmore says your doctor can request a lab report noting *any* bacteria present.

Sometimes, though, there really are no bacteria present and the diagnosis is still cystitis. And finding the cause isn't always that easy. "There are a number of possible explanations for this condition, but the most common one is, 'We don't know,' " admits Linda Brubaker, M.D., director of the Section of Urogynecology at Rush Presbyterian–St. Luke's Medical Center in Chicago. "The discomfort is real enough, though, so we go ahead and treat the symptoms as best we can while we look for a possible cause."

Dr. Brubaker says she usually spends the first two or three visits reeducating women and proving to them that they do not have an infection. "They find it so hard to believe that those symptoms could be present without germs, even though they are persistently culture negative," she says. "Then we start to look at the things in their lives that could be exacerbating their symptoms. And this is really just trial and error. We don't have any scientific evidence that anything makes a difference."

"We begin by asking questions," says Dr. Brubaker. "Have you started to use a new bath oil? Are you past menopause? Describe your diet. How much stress are you under? We're looking for anything that might cause the bladder to become irritated, and work from there. If it's menopause, we might start them on estrogen replacement therapy. A new bath oil would be discontinued immediately."

DIET AND STRESS CONNECTION

What you eat may be one of the biggest contributors of all, according to the latest opinions from the medical community. For years, women have drowned their bladders in cranberry juice at the first sign of symptoms, believing that acidifying their urine was the key to a healthy bladder. Not

SELF-HELP FOR INFECTIONS

What you do for yourself and the way you treat your body can go a long way in avoiding bladder infections—whether you're plagued by them or have yet to go through the experience.

Here's what experts say you should do.

- Flush bacteria out of your bladder. This is your best defense against infection. You can encourage elimination by drinking six to eight glasses of water a day.

- Empty your bladder completely. When you think you're finished urinating, bend over and push forward over your bladder area. Then stand up, sit down and repeat the maneuver.

- Practice timed toileting. Holding urine too long or trying to void too frequently can both cause problems. Ideally, you should urinate every 3 to 4 hours.

- Urinate before and after sex. Drink water before sex so you'll have something to void afterward. This helps flush out any bacteria that may have entered during lovemaking.

- Use a hand-held shower after sex. This is the best way to wash germs away from your vaginal area.

- Always wipe from front to rear after a bowel movement. And take along personal wipes for those occasions when you need to clean yourself away from home.

- Wear cotton-crotch underwear and avoid tight-fitting clothes. Cotton underwear can help keep the genital area dry; tight clothing, on the other hand, can trap moisture there.

- Change sanitary napkins and tampons frequently. This is basic for good hygiene and infection prevention during menstruation.

- Don't use bubble bath or harsh soaps. They can irritate your urethra and make you prone to infection.

- Stop using a diaphragm and spermicides. Some women are also allergic to the latex in condoms and may need to discontinue their use as well.

- Neutralize your urine with a low-acid diet. Antacids such as Tums or Rolaids can help relieve the burning during a flare-up. So can eating watermelon or drinking a glass of water mixed with a teaspoon of baking soda two times a day. (Note, though, that baking soda can cause fluid retention in certain people. Avoid it if it has this effect on you.)

necessarily so, say the experts, who now believe that acidic foods like cranberry juice may contribute to nonbacterial bladder inflammation. Indeed, some liken it to pouring salt on a wound.

"I probably get about a 60 percent improvement rate taking patients off of all acidic foods," says Dr. Brubaker. Actually, there's no scientific evidence that acidifying the urine helps patients. "On the contrary," she says. "I find that patients who have persisted in that practice can develop this chronic inflammatory bladder disorder." In addition, eating a low-acid diet is one of the safest ways to treat this condition.

Stress, too, can be an instigator. While for some, stress manifests itself as ulcers, migraines or stomach cramps, for others it's bladder symptoms.

"The bottom line is that these bladder problems are probably going to wax and wane over time," says Dr. Brubaker. "And while you may not be able to cure it, you can get some control over your symptoms, whether your condition is infectious in nature or bacteria-free."

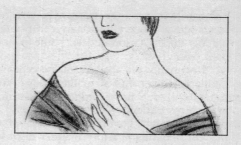

D AND C

THE MOST LIKELY SURGERY

D and C is such a common and routine gynecological procedure that many women quip it's a "Dusting and Cleaning."

"When I was little, I remember my mother telling me that she was going in the hospital for a dusting and cleaning and thought it was kind of funny," says Monica D'Angelo, a 38-year-old beauty salon owner. "Then when I grew up, my doctor told me I needed to have a D and C. When he described what he was doing, I figured the nickname fit perfectly. But it did nothing for my unease about what I was about to go through. I didn't have to go to the hospital like my mother did, though. My doctor actually did the procedure in the office. And it was surprisingly easy and pain-free for me."

D and C actually stands for dilation of the cervix and curettage of the uterus, a procedure in which the uterus is dilated and the inner surface cleansed with an instrument called a curette. Although it isn't performed as much today as in our mother's generation, it is *still* the most prevalent surgical procedure among women. About 1 out of every 200 women undergoes a D and C each year in the United States, according to the National Center for Health Statistics in Washington, D.C.—that's more than half a million procedures.

THE ABCS OF D AND C

Most D and Cs are done to diagnose and/or treat abnormal uterine bleeding, says Dorothy Barbo, M.D., professor of obstetrics and gynecology at the University of New Mexico School of Medicine and medical director of the university's Center for Women's Health in Albuquerque.

"It could be bleeding between periods, excessively heavy periods or bleeding after menopause. Anything that is out of the realm of the normal for a woman," explains Dr. Barbo. "It's also done to remove polyps, which are small growths on the lining of the uterus that can cause abnormal bleeding."

And because abnormal bleeding can be a sign of uterine cancer, a D and C is often performed to rule out cancer. "This is the real bottom line and the one women worry most about," says Dr. Barbo.

D and C is also the procedure of choice to treat incomplete miscarriage and for removal of any remaining fragments of placenta. It is usually done in the hospital under general anesthesia, although it is sometimes done in the doctor's office with a local, as in Monica's situation.

"For most women it's simply too painful to undergo a D and C without first being put to sleep, because dilating the cervix feels like labor pain," says Dr. Barbo. The cervix—the tiny opening to the uterus at the back of the vagina—is extremely sensitive, but with anesthesia, all pain is eliminated.

Once the cervix is dilated, the doctor inserts the spoon-shaped curette and scrapes the lining of the uterus. All the tissue that is removed is carefully collected so that it can be examined microscopically.

"Afterward, it's necessary to abstain from sex for two weeks," advises Dr. Barbo. "And you need to give yourself a day or two to get over the effects of the anesthesia. Otherwise, you're free to resume your normal activities."

Although complications are rare, it is possible to develop an infection following a D and C or to develop heavy bleeding if the walls of the uterus were injured or punctured during scraping. So call your doctor immediately if you develop fever, persistent abdominal pain or cramps, heavy bleeding, faintness or dizziness or an abnormal or foul-smelling vaginal discharge.

ALTERNATIVE PROCEDURES

Although doctors still do D and Cs on a regular basis, fewer women are having them now than in the past. Not that there's anything wrong with the procedure. In many cases—incomplete miscarriage, for example—it's the only one that will do.

But when treating abnormal bleeding today, some doctors are more inclined to do an endometrial biopsy rather than a full D and C. This procedure involves taking a small sample of the uterine lining—the endometrium—to determine whether any abnormal tissue is present. "It's a much simpler, less-invasive procedure that can be done in the office," says Dr. Barbo. "Consequently, it doesn't require anesthesia or the use of an operating room, so it's much more cost-effective. And if you don't get the answer, you can always go ahead and do a D and C later."

Whether you have a D and C or endometrial biopsy, though, it's important to understand that neither can provide absolute assurance that uterine cancer is not present. A small area of abnormal tissue could be missed. If bleeding problems persist after an initial D and C, you may need to have a further evaluation to determine the source of your symptoms.

CHAPTER 23

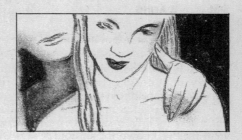

DATING

A GUIDE FOR THE '90S

*H*ere's a scene that could possibly be playing right now in your very neighborhood.

BOY: Wanna go out again tomorrow night?
GIRL: Gee, we were out last night, now again tonight.
BOY: Aw, come on.
GIRL: Well, okay.
BOY: Can I kiss you goodnight?

AIDS, maybe more than anything else, has changed the picture of dating in the 1990s, says Judith Sills, Ph.D., a clinical psychologist practicing in Philadelphia. "It sets sex back about four dates."

Back in the days when sex was free and easy and AIDS was known only as a diet lozenge, a woman felt free to get sexually involved in the first hour of a date, if she so desired. "Before AIDS and herpes, women could get involved sexually on the first date or two," says Dr. Sills. "Today, most women are more likely to take their time and not go to bed with a man until the end of a month or six weeks of dating. The effect is that you have sex with fewer people, because there are fewer people that you have six dates with."

Sexually transmitted disease is literally scaring the pants *on* people. Dating in the 1990s, is getting, well, more refined.

ONLY FOOLS RUSH IN

Putting off sex for a couple of dates is a commendable try but, aside from possibly limiting the number of men you sleep with, it doesn't really reduce your risk of contracting a sexually transmitted disease.

"Women think that sleeping with a man they've known for a few months or a year is safer than sleeping with a man they've known for an hour," says Dr. Sills. "It might be, but it's not necessarily true. It's the sexual contact that puts you at risk."

What, then, is wrong with trying this tack?

GIRL: Before, we, ah, er, you know . . . Ah, do you have any disease I should, like, maybe know about?

BOY: Me!? Heavens, no. Of course not.

"You can't trust him," answers Dr. Sills. And apparently she knows what she's talking about. According to a study of dating practices among 18- to 25-year-old college students, two California researchers found that men, much more than women, will tell a lie to have sex. The survey revealed that 20 percent of men, but only 4 percent of women, admitted they lied about having a negative HIV-antibody test to detect AIDS. And a third of the men, but only a quarter of the women, lied about being sexually involved with more than one person.

PILLOW TALK

This, of course, doesn't mean you shouldn't ask, says Dr. Sills. "If you're not sure how to bring it up, just saying you don't know how to bring it up opens the door. Or start with, 'Well, I guess it's time to have the disease conversation.'"

But the conversation shouldn't end there. If you want to really play it safe, says Dr. Sills, you have to have safe sex. "And make it perfectly clear at the outset that it's the only kind of sex you're interested in having.

"I've also recommended saying, 'Even if you've never

had any disease whatsoever, we're still using a condom.'
And you might add, 'I totally understand that it may interfere with your sexual pleasure. I totally understand why
you may not think it's necessary. But you're not going to
make love to me without a condom. If that's not okay,
please find another woman.' "

Ginny Strickland, a 31-year-old x-ray technician, says
she had gotten "practically paranoid" about checking out
her dates for diseases. "Maybe it's because I'm a health
care worker and I see what carelessness can do," she says.
"But I actually ask any prospective sex partner for a note
from his doctor—in other words, a clean bill of health—
before I'll go to bed with him. One man refused to do it
and I went to bed with him anyway, because I was so
attracted to him and he seemed so nice. Later I came down
with a chlamydia infection."

THE GOOD OLD DAYS

Back in the days *before* sex was free and easy, you may
have known someone for two years and become engaged,
maybe even married, before you had sex.

"When you put sex early in a relationship, you make
courtship and dating a much more vulnerable process,"
says Dr. Sills. "Most women tell me that they become emotionally attached when they take a lover. Emotional attachment makes you vulnerable."

And that attachment to love is what makes the dating
woman of the nineties no different than women who were
looking for love a generation ago. Women go for an emotional roller-coaster ride when dating someone they like.
The anticipation, the anxiety, the waiting, the thrill are all
there.

"In this respect dating hasn't changed at all over the
past 10 to 20 years," Dr. Sills says. "What has changed is
that people have sex at a younger age now and sooner in
the relationship. And that changes everything, especially
for women."

Sex doesn't give men an automatic emotional attachment, says Dr. Sills. "A woman, on the other hand, who may be unsure of her feelings will feel attached once they've had sex. It may come as a shock when she finds out the bond is not shared."

DUTCH LUNCH

What's wrong with this scenerio?

BOY: Waiter, the check.
GIRL: Let's split it.
BOY: But, but . . .
GIRL: I insist.

Absolutely nothing, says Dr. Sills. It's an assertive gesture that easily drives a point. "Splitting the bill conveys something platonic," she says. "A woman likes to split the check when she doesn't want to be sexually involved."

It's a scene, however, that's played out less than you may think. "For many women it's very hard to totally let go of the view that someone's going to come along and pay the bills," says Dr. Sills. "And believe it or not, I hear this more today than five years ago."

See also Contraception

CHAPTER 24

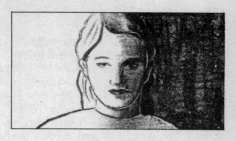

DEPENDENCIES

WOMEN WITH A "MEN'S DISEASE"

*P*atricia Lane is a 33-year-old chemical dependency counselor studying for her master's degree. A woman with a purpose. A woman with a satisfying career. A success story. But until the age of 25, she had a different story to tell. She was out of control, existing in an alcoholic haze, living on frozen lasagna and more than a gallon of wine every time she drank, which was every other night.

"It took years to reach the bottom," says Patricia. "At the age of 12, I was already drinking bottles of cough medicine, which were loaded with alcohol back in those days. By 13, I gave up on that and starting drinking the real stuff. At 18, I knew for sure that I was an alcoholic. I started having blackouts, and I recognized that I had a craving that other people didn't have. After two drinks my friends would say, 'I don't want another because I'm starting to feel it.' And my question would be, 'Well then why don't you want more?'"

Patricia's downward spiral continued until she was in her midtwenties. "My life revolved around drinking. I sought out jobs where drinking was an accepted part of the position. I didn't go places where you couldn't drink. I didn't see a movie for years, for example, because it wasn't a drinking activity. I was an obnoxious drunk, too. I went to bars and drank and then got into fistfights. Sometimes I'd wake up in the park, covered with dirt and grass stains, not knowing how I got there. I drove all the time when I was drunk. It's a miracle that I didn't get myself killed or kill someone else during those years."

By the time Patricia went for help she was in a dire state. "My life was a living hell. I was in such emotional pain that I didn't think I could possibly draw breath *without* alcohol to help me," she recalls. "When I saw myself as I really was—holed up in my bedroom, curtains drawn, with the TV, the telephone and my five liters of wine to keep me company—I knew I had to get out or I was going to die."

But Patricia not only didn't die, she survived and blossomed. "I made a commitment to participate in life, with all its ups and downs and without the 'aid' of alcohol," she says. It was a particularly stunning turnaround by any measure—especially for someone as close to self-destruction as she was.

OUT OF THE CLOSET

Betty Ford, Liza Minnelli, Kitty Dukakis, Elizabeth Taylor—the list of those addicted to alcohol or drugs could go on and on, filled with the famous and the infamous, the rich and the poor, the beautiful and the plain. Yet it wasn't long ago that women impaired by chemical dependency escaped public attention. In fact, they still do far more often than men.

"Before the early 1960s and the emergence of the women's movement, female chemical dependency was regarded as a rare manifestation of an essentially 'male' disease," according to Kathleen Bell Unger, M.D., an assistant clinical professor in the Department of Psychiatry at the University of California, San Francisco. Consequently, women's addictions were often "ignored, underreported, underdiagnosed and most certainly undertreated."

The fact is, 40 percent of all adults who abuse alcohol and drugs are women, and with younger people it's closer to 50-50, adds Jane Gaunt, a certified addictions counselor and clinical supervisor of the women's unit at the Betty Ford Center in Rancho Mirage, California. "At our center about 70 percent of the women are here for alcohol addiction. Prescription tranquilizers and pain medications come in second and cocaine addictions third." But many women are dually addicted as well.

Women are at particular risk for multiple addictions, adds Sherri Matteo, Ph.D., the associate director at the Institute for Research on Women and Gender at Stanford University. They're more likely than men to hide their alcoholism, so when they do see their doctors, they complain of fatigue, depression, anxiety or stress, which is usually related to family, school or job. "All are symptoms that are likely to be treated with the use of sedatives, minor tranquilizers or other psychotropic drugs," Dr. Matteo points out, "without extended questioning that might illuminate a drinking problem." It may not be a total coincidence, adds Gaunt, that two-thirds of all such prescription drugs are prescribed to women.

ADDICTION'S DOUBLE STANDARD

Women are also more likely to hide an addiction because of the way society perceives inebriated women.

"Throughout history, a double standard has existed that allows us to tolerate a drunken man but abhor a drunken woman, labeling her sexually dangerous, promiscuous and generally out of control," notes Dr. Matteo.

"Addiction itself is not something that takes away from a man's masculinity," adds Gaunt. "For women, their femininity is in question. Women are supposed to be pure, the standard for morality."

Dr. Matteo agrees. "The reaction of disgust and repulsion with which an alcoholic woman must contend may well reinforce her reluctance to admit to a drinking problem," she says. Patricia says that if friends brought up the subject of her drinking, she immediately cut them out of her life. "I suppose I knew I had a severe problem, but I tried very hard not to think about it," she explains. "If they questioned me about it, they became a threat to me, a threat to my disease, and so I never saw them again."

So great is the stigma associated with chemical dependence that about 25 percent of addicted women's families actually oppose their seeking treatment for fear of exposure, says Gaunt. That's simply not true for men. "To complicate the issue, women addicts are more often divorced, and consequently, they are more often single heads of families. They have more financial concerns, they have more difficulty paying for treatment and they worry that their children will be taken away. No wonder they try to hide their addictions much longer and come in for treatment less frequently than men do.

"What's more," she continues, "even if a woman does come in for treatment, she will, of necessity, be a participant in a program designed primarily on the male model, since most of our knowledge about addiction and treatment has been based on studies that were conducted almost entirely on male subjects. Of course, that's still better than no treatment."

THE PRISON OF ADDICTION

An addiction is analogous to being in prison, says Angela Burke, Ph.D., a clinical psychologist and director of the Psychology Clinic at the North Texas State University in Denton. "The addiction literally rules your life. It dictates your behavior, your emotions and your goals. Nothing else matters except satisfying that need."

More than likely, you are also creating constant chaos in your family and burdening them financially, says Gaunt. "You will probably be verbally and physically abusive at some point. So you start to figure that the best scenario is to check out from the family, just not be present while you're using." Even then, addiction is still likely to shatter their lives, your life and your self-esteem. "You can't rely on yourself to perform the simplest functions," says Gaunt. "You often lose boyfriends or husbands and alienate friends and family. Your world becomes increasingly isolated and small. If you're younger and single, you're often engaged in a lot of promiscuity, further eroding your self-esteem. It's just emotionally devastating."

WHO BECOMES ADDICTED?

Chemically dependent women are not like everyone else, notes Dr. Unger, not even like chemically dependent men. Women believe that they are "worse" than addicted men, and the men they know usually agree. They lack hope about their lives and feel guilty and responsible for their circumstances. "They are more likely to have come from disturbed families marked by drug or alcohol dependency, mental illness, suicide, family violence and personal physical or sexual abuse," she points out. "In fact," says Gaunt, "about 70 percent of women who are addicted have also been subjected to some sort of childhood or adult abuse."

Patricia says that both her mother and sister are addicted to drugs and that she was sexually abused during childhood and both raped and gang-raped as an adult. "My first memories of sexual abuse were at age 3," she says, "but my doctors believe it began before I was 2. I was in a lot of emotional pain for most of my life. Alcohol was my way of coping, of dulling the pain. I used to rationalize my drinking by saying, 'If you had the life I had, you'd drink, too.' "

Chemically dependent women usually don't recognize that drugs or alcohol are also the cause of problems, according to Dr. Unger. They see such use as a way of coping with losses, with family problems or a bad or violent relationship. "They see their drug or alcohol use as part of a solution.

"Chemical dependency is not a moral weakness," notes Dr. Unger. It's a disease. While emotional pain can contribute to addiction, according to Dr. Burke, it's far more likely to happen if you have a "vulnerable physiology," too. "And some people seem more susceptible to a physiological addiction than others, although no one is sure why."

HITTING BOTTOM

"It got to the point that I was afraid to go out when I was going to drink, because I'd get into so much trouble," says Patricia. "So instead, I'd stay in my room with my remote control television and my phone nearby. I had practically no contact with the outside world. I also was sleeping a lot—another means of escape from my real world. Then I started losing touch with reality and had trouble telling the difference between my dreams and my wakefulness. I found out later that I was in a state of toxic psychosis."

Women who are chemically dependent live on the brink of catastrophe, according to Carlene Hunt, Ed.D., who has studied women with addiction problems. Like Patricia, the stories they tell have underlying themes of desperation and despair, instability and excruciating loneliness. For the women she studied, chaos went on for "long periods of time without any evident search on their part for treatment," notes Dr. Hunt, who has a private counseling practice in Nashville. "It took some major critical incident or critical kind of experience for the person to make a decision to seek treatment."

FACING REALITY

What Patricia calls her moment of clarity came one night while staying at the home of a close friend.

"After she went to bed I sat in front of the television and drank until I ran out of wine," she recalls. "I was making lots of noise slamming cupboards looking for more. My friend came into the kitchen, and I told her I had to go home. She pleaded with me not to drive my car, and finally I agreed to take a cab. I just had to get out of there and get some more to drink. After I left she called my father, knowing full well that I would probably never speak to her again.

"I took it as a huge betrayal on her part, but in reality, she saved my life. My father called and asked to see me the very next day. He told me he knew of someone that was a heroin addict, and that she had gone to a treatment center for help. He said he knew I was in deep trouble, and he was afraid that I was going to kill somebody else or myself. And then he asked me if I wanted to go to one of those treatment places. I said yes, and, to this day, I don't know where that yes came from."

Patricia says that that simple yes opened the floodgates. "I started crying and thought I'd never stop. I told my father that I just couldn't take it anymore, that I was terrified, out of control and thought I was going crazy. I went in for treatment a few weeks later."

THE HELPING HANDS

It's one thing to rid your body of the addicting chemical. It's quite another to rid your mind of the desire for it, admits Dr. Burke. Indeed, the physical withdrawal from an addictive substance may be the easiest part.

"We know from Vietnam veterans that a physiological addiction is relatively easy to overcome," says the psychologist. "Many vets became addicted to heroin while they were over there, but not that many remained addicts once back in the States. That's because they were out of the stressful situation that created the psychological need. So once their physiological addiction was treated, they no longer craved the substance," explains Dr. Burke.

Granted, withdrawal from a chemical addiction is no picnic, adds addiction counselor Gaunt. "Depending on the substance, detoxification can take a few days to more than a month. Patients can suffer from fatigue, depression and agitation. Sometimes there are quite odd withdrawal symptoms, too, like feeling that your arm is detached from your body. And with some drugs, you can have a seizure if you withdraw too quickly. So we monitor everyone carefully and medicate only in order to keep the patient stable and safe."

Because most people have a physiological as well as a psychological addiction, programs such as the one at the Betty Ford Center concentrate on a holistic approach to recovery. Generally, that means that a multidisciplinary team of physicians and nurses cares for your physiological needs while a team of counselors and psychologists helps you uncover and deal with the stresses and life experiences that are working against you. Simultaneously, says Gaunt, other members of the team start you on health-promoting nutritional and physical fitness programs.

COULD YOU BECOME AN ADDICT?

Take this quiz developed by the American Holistic Medical Association and find out where you stand.

- Do you feel you never quite measure up?
- Has your pleasure in life become centered around one substance (food, alcohol, drug) or activity (sex, exercise, work)?
- Are you highly self-critical?
- Do other people see you as strong, self-sufficient and controlled (but you know it's not true)?
- Do you avoid conflict?
- Do you feel powerless in many areas of your life?
- Do you have a high need for approval?
- Do you have difficulty in making decisions?
- Do you have difficulty in expressing or identifying feelings?
- Do you find yourself frequently feeling responsible for others' behavior?
- Do you have difficulty in forming close, intimate relationships?

According to the association, you're at high risk of developing a dependency on a substance or activity if you answered yes to five or more of these questions. Contact a local chapter of one of the anonymous groups (alcohol or narcotics) for information, or consider seeing a therapist for some advice and counseling.

"Recovery centers around every part of your being," says Gaunt. "The whole recovery process is based on group therapy. Everything we do is structured around our patient community, and that's because there's something extremely therapeutic about recovering people working with each other," she points out. "It's why Alcoholics Anonymous has been so successful."

FEELING GOOD AGAIN

Patricia says that withdrawing from alcohol was not that difficult. "It was not nearly as uncomfortable for me as what I had just left behind," she admits. "I simply knew I was done drinking, that I just couldn't do it anymore. I had reached the bottom emotionally and spiritually. Almost immediately I started to feel better because I wasn't hung over anymore."

Eventually, says Gaunt, the lifestyle changes that each person is required to make during the recovery process have an extremely positive impact on their lives. In fact, for many, the recovery process leaves them healthier than they've ever been.

Patricia spent five weeks at the treatment center. "I remember when I reached 30 days clean and sober—a milestone when you're in recovery—I started crying because it had been so many years since I had drawn a sober breath," she says. "There was hope, and there had not been hope in my life before. It was exhilarating, but it was scary, too. What did I know about hope?"

In Dr. Hunt's study of alcoholic women, there also was the sense that leaving alcohol behind was the easy part. It was the long process of change and growth that presented the greatest challenge. These women pointed out that recovery was "an ongoing experience that included a growing realization of previously undiscovered parts of themselves. They often became conscious of painful parts of the past that their drinking and denial systems had long covered. Recovery meant a new awareness of reality."

"When I quit drinking, I made a conscious decision to accept whatever life dealt me," says Patricia. "Over the summer, for example, I had a brief relationship with a man, which then fell apart. I was in tremendous agony over it. My therapist explained to me that I had merely had the kind of summer romance that any junior high school student might experience. But because I was an alcoholic by age 12, I had never had a chance to learn what these situations felt like or how to cope with and recover from them. It was like starting over—emotionally—from adolescence."

CHAPTER 25

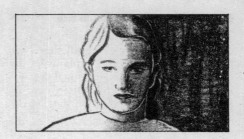

DEPRESSION

WOMEN OUTNUMBER MEN 2 TO 1

*D*epressed? You're not alone. In fact, even if you're *seriously* depressed, you're not alone.

One-fourth of all women have a major bout with depression at some time in their lives, but sometimes the symptoms are so masked in illness that they don't realize that depression is causing their problems, according to Margaret Jensvold, M.D., director of the Institute for Research on Women's Health in Washington, D.C. "Instead, a woman might go to her family physician with complaints of headaches or backaches or the blahs."

Major depression is far more than unrelenting sadness or an inability to enjoy life's pleasures. The classic symptoms include severe disturbances in appetite and sleep patterns, namely insomnia and drastic weight loss. Some women, however, overeat—especially sweets and other carbohydrates—and sleep excessively.

Everyone feels down on occasion, and usually there's a good reason for it. You lose at romance, you lose your job or you don't get the one you want. And it's normal to feel depressed after the death of someone close. But in cases such as these you eventually climb out of the doldrums and get on with living. That's because these are things that go with the ebb and flow of life. It's fleeting depression—more a case of what's commonly called the blues.

BEYOND THE BLUES

Then there's chronic depression, when your symptoms become increasingly severe until they begin to impair your normal everyday routine, explains Dr. Jensvold. It's a feeling that puts you in an emotional vise. And the worst thing is, you don't know why. Often you may not be able to pinpoint a cause or situation that precipitated the depression. And you find that all the things you would normally do to lift yourself from a sad mood just aren't working anymore.

Besides persistent sadness or an "empty" mood, you may also have feelings of guilt, worthlessness or hopelessness, says Dr. Jensvold. Or you may feel restless or irritable and have difficulty concentrating, remembering or making decisions. Not everyone who is depressed experiences all the symptoms, though. According to the National Institute of Mental Health, some experience only a few, and some experience many. What's more, the severity of symptoms varies from woman to woman. What's consistent with depression, however, is that the symptoms occur all or most of the time for at least two weeks.

WHY WOMEN?

"There are currently at least seven million women in the United States with a diagnosable depression," according to Ellen McGrath, Ph.D., chairwoman of the American Psychological Association National Task Force on Women and Depression and executive director of the Psychology Center in Laguna Beach, California. Studies show that women have double the risk for depression. Dr. McGrath and her associates found a number of possible explanations for this gender difference.

One factor may be that women tend to dwell too much on their feelings. "Women will think and think about their feelings and the causes of their moods to the point that it actually amplifies and prolongs their depressive episodes," says Dr. Jensvold. "Men who get depressed, on the other hand, are more likely to shut out their feelings, often by turning to activity. Women should be encouraged to use more 'action mastery,' go out and do something, *anything*, rather than just thinking about their feelings. Men and women need to learn how to adopt a bit of each other's styles. Men should be encouraged to get more in touch with their feelings."

Physical and sexual abuse are also major factors in women's depression, notes Dr. McGrath in her book *Women and Depression: Risk Factors and Treatment Issues*. "One study estimated that 37 percent of women have had a significant experience of physical or sexual abuse before the age of 21. Several task force members felt these figures were an underestimate and the real numbers may be as high as 50 percent," she writes. For many women depressive symptoms may, in fact, be long-standing effects of post-traumatic stress syndrome, she maintains.

Marriage, believe it or not, may also be a risk factor for women, but not for men. According to the American Psychological Association, women in unhappy marriages are much more likely to be depressed than either married men or single women. Mothers of young children are highly vulnerable as well. Poverty is also a "pathway to depression," according to Dr. McGrath. And more women than men are poor.

Biology plays a role, too. Besides the possibility of a hereditary factor, infertility, menopause, menstruation and childbirth may also play a role. In fact, researchers are still investigating the link between the hormonal swing of the menstrual cycle and mood swings.

LEARNING TO COPE

The most effective way to deal with chronic depression, agree the experts, is through counseling and/or medication. These treatments have been found to significantly help reduce depressive symptoms for 80 to 90 percent of people in 12 to 14 weeks, according to Dr. McGrath.

Through counseling, women can learn how to reverse negative thinking, feelings of helplessness and low self-esteem. "They learn to gain control and competence in their

SELF-HELP ADVICE FOR THE MOODY BLUES

Whether it's a mean bout of the blues or deep depression, experts say there are a number of things you can do for yourself to dig your way out. The secret is to stop the excuses and *do something*. And that includes seeking professional help. In the meantime, here's what you can do for yourself right now.

- Do not set difficult goals for yourself or take on a great deal of responsibility. Expecting too much from yourself only increases chances of failure, which will only make you feel worse.
- Break large overwhelming jobs into small manageable ones, set some priorities and deal with things as you are able to do so.
- Don't make major decisions, such as moving, changing careers, getting divorced, without talking things over with close friends or trusted relatives. Try to put off making important decisions until your depression is over.
- Avoid being alone. Spend time with other people. Try talking to them about something other than depression.
- Participate in activities that make you feel better. Try going to a movie, a ball game or other social activities.
- Exercise. Studies suggest that people who are depressed feel better when they exercise on a regular basis. Aerobic exercises, in particular (jogging, walking, swimming, biking), generate a significant antidepressant effect.
- Eliminate caffeine and refined sugar from your diet. One study showed that those who did experienced a significant decline in their depression, and they maintained that status at a three-month checkup.
- Don't binge on junk food and don't skip meals. Instead, maintain a healthy, well-balanced diet.
- Indulge yourself. Give yourself a treat once in a while, something just for you, just because it makes you feel good—a hot bubble bath, a night at the opera, square dancing, whatever.
- Don't get upset if your mood is not greatly improved right away. Feeling better takes time.

lives," says Robin Post, Ph.D., a clinical psychologist in Denver. "They learn how to be assertive and communicate their needs. They learn the coping skills they need, ways to solve problems and how to grieve for the losses in their lives. They learn how to recognize and accept the feelings they have, whether they are ones of anger, sadness or fear."

For some women, antidepressant medications, most notably fluoxetine (Prozac) and tricyclic antidepressants, such as nortriptyline (Pamelor), are sometimes prescribed to get them through the worst times. But taking drugs is not without its drawbacks. They can have unpleasant side effects, such as dry mouth, constipation, bladder problems, sexual problems, blurred vision, dizziness, drowsiness and disturbed sleep.

"Of course, the medication prescribed and the length of time it needs to be taken depends on the individual and on what type of depression she has," says Dr. Jensvold. "If you can't sleep and can't eat, for example, your doctor may prescribe nortriptyline, a drug known for its sedating quality, which helps you sleep. For those who eat and sleep too much, the antidepressant fluoxetine is most commonly prescribed. Sometimes a combination of drugs is needed for best results," says Dr. Jensvold.

Although occasionally drugs may be taken for the long term, usually they are part of a short-term treatment plan. The primary goal is to learn the necessary coping techniques to pull life together again. And what works for one person may not work for another.

The thing to remember, says Dr. Jensvold, is that fighting depression can take time. But it *can* be licked.

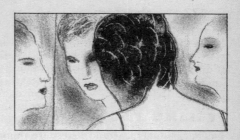

DIETING

FOR MANY, IT'S A SECOND CARRER

*L*osing weight is such a way of life among American women, dieting is considered "normal" eating. In fact, some researchers have found so much in common between dieters and women with eating disorders, they have come to see anorexia and bulimia as simply "the extreme end of the continuum" of female eating behavior, according to Kathleen Pike, Ph.D., a psychologist who studies and treats eating disorders at the New York Psychiatric Institute at Columbia Presbyterian Medical Center.

Many dieters have the same skewed body image as people with eating disorders, seeing fat where others see slimness. If you are not one yourself, you know a chronic dieter. She may have 5 or 10 or 20 pounds to lose—or none at all. But for all the blood, sweat and tears (and occasionally, pounds) she sheds dieting, it might as well be 100. Many dieters suffer from what therapist Kim Chernin, author of *The Obsession: Reflections on the Tyranny of Slenderness*, calls pseudo-obesity. At or near their ideal weight, they are nevertheless driven "toward a condition of ruddy-cheeked emaciation" idealized by models and actresses who are unusually tall and thin.

Like anorexics and bulimics, chronic dieters are *always* dieting, yet thinking, dreaming, obsessing about food. "If I really wanted to let myself go, I would weigh 400 pounds," claims Delia Bogart, 46, who at 5 feet, 8 inches tall weighs about 145 pounds, a desirable—though not to her—weight for her height. "I have a big appetite and I love food. I start looking at my watch at breakfast to see how long it is until lunch. My best friend tells me that ever since she's known me, I've been trying to lose the same 10 pounds."

FEELING FAT

Not surprisingly, chronic dieters are almost always women. "For an overwhelming number of women in our society, being a woman means feeling too fat," write Yale University researchers Judith Rodin, Ph.D., Lisa Silberstein and Ruth Striegel-Moore, who have explored some of the pressures on women to "pursue thinness like a career."

For females, the heat is on by the time they're 9. A study done by a University of California researcher of 494 girls between 9 and 18 found that an astonishing number—31 percent—were already binge eating by age 9, with another third admitting they were afraid of getting fat. By the time those girls reach college, according to another study, more than half are engaging in unhealthful dietary practices, such as bingeing and vomiting. And it apparently never ends. In a study on elderly women conducted by Dr. Rodin and her colleagues at Yale, their greatest personal concern, next to memory loss, was their weight.

WHERE IT BEGINS

There was a time, not so long ago, when abundant flesh was considered sexy. And we're not harking back to the round and rosy nudes of the painter Rubens. In the 1950s, the ultraslim, ultrasleek Audrey Hepburn was considered beautiful and glamorous, but it was Marilyn Monroe who had sex appeal. Except during her illnesses, Marilyn's figure was padded, soft and voluptuous, packed into tight, revealing dresses like sausage in a casing. Today, Marilyn might serve as a before picture for Weight Watchers.

Today, there are millions of women who were raised on the images of virtual 98-pound weaklings, like 1960s supermodel Twiggy, whose figures were decidedly boyish—or prepubescent girlish—and strikingly like the cadaverous silhouettes of anorexics whose disorder some researchers see as a backlash against maturation and womanhood. In fact, several researchers have suggested that the quest for thinness is an expression of sexual liberation, since a thin body represents athleticism and androgyny—if not down-right masculinity—rather than motherliness.

There are other reasons, too. Fat is considered unhealthy and has been associated with a variety of ailments, includ-ing heart disease. Studies have also shown that even as children, we think of fat as "bad," a virtual moral transgres-sion. Fat people are so stigmatized that we regard over-weight with almost as much dread as mortal illness. In one telling study, when children with juvenile diabetes were asked if they would trade their life-threatening disease for obesity, most said no.

Unfortunately for most women, attractiveness is cur-rency. It's what buys acceptance, the best man, the best job, the best life. With few exceptions, most people don't consider a fat woman beautiful.

OUR BODIES, OUR SELVES

Why do ordinary women aspire to the angularity of say, model Paulina or actress Julia Roberts, whose bodies are tools of their trade and who have body sizes natural to only about 5 percent of the population?

For most women, genetics makes the attainment of that particular body type nearly impossible. And therein lies the rub. Our culture, says social historian Roberta Pollack Seid in her book *Never Too Thin*, "has set up a female body standard that is antithetical to female biology." Although we may resist the idea that biology is destiny, when it comes to our bodies, it is. A woman needs a fat-to-lean ratio of about 22 percent to start and maintain menstruation. Under that figure, we risk bone-thinning amenorrhea (an absence of the menstrual cycle) and infertility.

We are also circumscribed by what some diet experts call our setpoints, the weight we can maintain without conscious effort. When we go below our setpoint weight, our bodies ruthlessly seek the former status quo, conserving energy and boosting our appetites, one of the major reasons dieting is nearly always a losing battle.

One dieter finally realized the futility of her constant efforts to slim down to model size when, she says, she read a magazine article about movie stars and their clothes. "Before I read it, I didn't know there were grown people who wore a size 4!" she marvels. "I couldn't get a forearm into a 4. I decided that unless I went on the concentration camp diet, I'd better be happy being a 12."

CAUTION: DIETING IS BAD FOR YOUR HEALTH

There are other reasons to jump off the dieting treadmill. For one, chronic dieting is a form of malnutrition. It's not healthy. "Losing weight can certainly be as harmful as overweight, with an impressive array of health hazards accompanying it," according to eating disorders researchers Janet Polivy, Ph.D., and Linda Thomsen. Although overweight can be a serious health problem for certain people, notably those with high blood pressure and diabetes, there is accumulating evidence that for most people the dangers of fat have been overestimated. In fact, some researchers believe that being moderately obese—up to 25 percent above standard body weight—doesn't affect long-term health.

There's also evidence that dieting—particularly very-low-calorie or bizarre diet plans—can *cause* a variety of ailments including gallstones, headaches, nausea, muscle aches, fatigue, anemia, cardiac disorders and even death in rare cases. You can feel tired and unable to concentrate even on a balanced diet. Studies, including the famous Framingham Heart Study, have found that so-called yo-yo dieting may shift body fat to the abdominal area, where fat is associated with more diabetes, high blood pressure and heart disease.

DIETING MAKES YOU FAT

There are psychological hazards as well. Many dieters may recognize what experts call the dieting depression syndrome

HOW TO BE A HAPPY LOSER

What if you really need to lose weight? How do you shed the lose/gain, lose/gain syndrome and end up a winner at losing?

"Any diet that works is going to have to teach you new eating habits you can carry out for the rest of your life," says New York psychologist and eating disorder expert Kathleen Pike, Ph.D. "As soon as you begin thinking you're going to be on a diet for six weeks and then the diet is over, you are set up to gain weight again. People say they go to diet programs because 'I don't have to think about it. I just open the box and eat it.' The problem is that in order for it to work long term, you have to think about it."

One relatively painless way to lose weight is to stop counting calories and begin counting fat. In a 22-week study at Cornell University, 13 women who ate a low-fat diet (getting 25 percent of their calories from fat), without restricting how many calories or how much food they ate, lost weight slowly for months without having to give up any goodies. They could eat pizza, ice cream and cookies, as long as they were low in fat. Researchers estimate you can lose 10 percent of your body weight in a year just by cutting back on fat.

And you have to exercise. Exercise, along with firming and building muscles and burning calories, is what allows you to eat more. You can burn roughly 200 calories or more, depending on your weight, just by taking a brisk (3½ miles per hour) half-hour walk every day. It can mean the difference between listening to your stomach growl on 1,000 calories a day and feeding it a couple of snacks to tide it over at 1,200 calories a day.

In fact, researchers have found that the difference between long-time weight losers and those who gain it back is exercise, as little as 3.3 hours of it a week, according to one expert.

Just be wary of taking exercise to the same extremes that many take dieting. Just as eating too little can make you ill and doom you to a fat future, exercising too much can lead to injuries, depression and fertility problems. In fact, when it comes to weight, the best diet advice comes from the ancient Greeks: Nothing in excess.

as those feelings of irritability, anxiety, depression, apathy, mood swings and fatigue that accompany all those carrot sticks and 8-ounce glasses of water.

Dieters may also be oversensitive to stress and turn to eating to relieve it. Not only do they find comfort in eating, but many choose sugar-laden, high-carbohydrate foods, which research has found increase mood-elevating chemicals in the brain—the Twinkie as a natural high. In fact, a number of studies have found that dieting can lead to binge eating, which may account for why so many dieters who "took it all off" put it all back on again. In other words, dieting can *make* you fat.

"When you go on high-restraint diets that essentially are unsustainable, you set yourself up to binge or eat compulsively," says Dr. Pike. "Once you get into that cycle—restraint then bingeing—ultimately the restraint loses and the eating wins out."

You become the victim of "weight cycling." Once you stop your diet, your body goes into famine-survival mode. Your metabolism is slowed down and your body has become more efficient at storing fat. If you go back to your old eating habits—hunger is such a primal urge, most people do—you often find yourself weighing more than you did when you first started. You can diet again, says Dr. Pike, "but your body has become so efficient you don't lose as much weight."

REALITY CHECK

How do you know if you need to diet or are simply a victim of the current quest for ultrathinness? You need to do a reality check, says Dr. Pike. Ask people you know and trust—a friend, your doctor or nurse—if *they* think you need to lose weight. Some studies have found that many women—95 percent in one research project—overestimate the size of their bodies more as a result of how they feel about themselves than of how they see themselves.

You may also be doing some "magical" thinking, says Dr. Pike. Many women believe that thinness equals happiness. "Sometimes a certain weight is associated with a happy time when you were that weight. You think, 'If I go back to that weight, I will achieve that level of happiness.' Often women believe there is some kind of cause and effect, that reaching a certain weight will guarantee them all kinds of happiness and pleasure."

Comforting—or distressing—as it might be to think, "If I lost 20 pounds, I'd be happy," the truth is you will still be you. The thin person inside every fat person is the same person without cellulite.

See also Body Image, Eating Disorders, Overweight

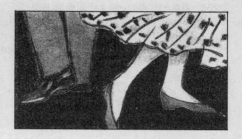

DIVORCE

THE END IS OVERWHELMING

*W*hen my best friend told me she was getting a divorce, I felt a sudden rush of envy. Yes, *envy!*" admits Alice Jordan, a 47-year-old medical technologist. "I think that's when I knew for sure that my marriage was over, too. And in fact, three months later, I got the courage to do something I had been contemplating for 14 of the 16 years my husband and I had been together—I told him that I wanted a divorce."

That emancipation proclamation is being heard by more spouses than ever before in the United States. Forget "until death do us part." According to the most recent estimates, one out of every two marriages now ends in divorce. "The soaring divorce rate has sometimes been blamed on the women's movement," says Constance Ahrons, Ph.D., professor of sociology at the University of Southern California in Los Angeles and associate director of its Marriage and Family Therapy Program. "And in part that may be true. The fact is, as women have become more economically independent, they've been financially able to leave bad marriages."

Perhaps that's why you'll find that today, women walk away from their marriages far more often than men do. Indeed, 65 to 68 percent of those calling it quits are women, says Dr. Ahrons.

THE ERA OF NO FAULT

Clearly, the stigma surrounding divorce has lessened, says Diane Medved, Ph.D., a clinical psychologist from Santa Monica, California, and the author of *The Case against Divorce*. "In some circles it's almost considered fashionable. True, most people don't eagerly embrace it," she admits, "but they don't see it as something that's necessarily tragic, either."

Dr. Ahrons agrees. "The fact that the concept of no-fault divorce has been widely accepted is a way of stating that two people do indeed have the right to dissolve a marriage if they so choose. And no one has to be 'blamed' for the breakup with accusations of adultery or mental cruelty," says Dr. Ahrons, who is also the coauthor of *Divorced Families: Meeting the Challenge of Divorce and Remarriage*. "Today the most common reason given is lack of communication." Meaning, whatever the couple fought about—whether it was money, cheating, child rearing, household responsibilities—is really irrelevant. It all boils down to the same thing—communication breakdown, a growing apart of basic values.

Divorce may be more acceptable these days and easier to obtain, but that doesn't mean that dissolving a marriage is a breeze. On the contrary, it's one of the most wrenching experiences you can go through, with aftereffects lasting for years, no matter who does the leaving.

WHEN YOU DO THE LEAVING

It's not always easy to garner sympathy from friends and family when you're the one who wants out, especially if your husband was a "nice guy," says Dr. Ahrons. And if ever there's a time you need a little sympathy, this is it.

"Women feel very responsible for the pain that their husbands and children go through during a divorce," says Dr. Ahrons. "They feel they're being selfish by addressing their own needs, and so they suffer a great deal of guilt.

"On the positive side, the one who does the leaving usually makes a quicker adjustment than the one who was left," explains Dr. Ahrons. "That's because leavers experience most of their pain prior to the separation. They've suffered through the painful decision-making process previously and are more in control when it actually happens."

Sometimes the decision to leave can take years, says Dr. Ahrons. "The leaver may see that her marriage isn't going well, so she'll go back to school or get a job or try numerous other activities—even an extramarital affair—in an effort to get her needs met someplace else," she says. "Eventually she may start to fantasize about the realities of a separation, what it might feel like, where she might live, even how she'd decorate a place of her own. It's an attempt to normalize the divorce process."

WHEN YOUR HUSBAND WALKS OUT

When the shoe is on the other foot and your husband walks out of the marriage, however, your experience may be more painful.

There's no greater rejection felt than when your husband tells you he wants a divorce, says Dr. Ahrons. "No matter how much he tries to soften the blow, there's no getting around the fact that he doesn't want you any longer," she says. "There's usually a loss of self-esteem, especially for those whose identities have been wrapped up in their marriages.

"Women typically go through a period of not knowing who they are and having to rediscover themselves. Out of this trauma can come some profound growth. I'll hear a woman proudly announce that, 'this week I balanced the checkbook,' or 'last week I fixed the toilet.' They're meeting and mastering each new challenge. A man, on the other hand, might say, 'this week I learned to make a meat loaf.' Each one has to pick up the roles that the other person carried during the marriage."

Eventually you do come out of the pain of divorce, says Dr. Ahrons, although it can take anywhere from two to five years. You find yourself moving on in your life.

Painful emotions are not the only factor to deal with while you're getting accustomed to the single life, either. This is one place where economics really rears its ugly head.

THE DOLLARS AND NONSENSE OF DIVORCE

To put it bluntly, a woman's standard of living generally takes a nosedive after divorce, says Dr. Medved. Not so for men.

According to certain estimates, women's standard of living goes down 73 percent after divorce, while a man's *goes up* 42 percent. Indeed, the prospect of a grim financial future often keeps women bound to marriages that are unfulfilling or worse.

"If she's been a stay-at-home wife, and he's been out working, he's the one with a retirement fund and years of employment experience," says Dr. Ahrons. "When she enters the job market, she enters at a lower pay scale, and it's unlikely that she'll ever catch up. And while it's true that women suffer these inequities in marriage, too, we don't see them because there's a shared income."

The inequities are sure to surface during the divorce, though. "Even though the couple's property is usually split fairly equally now, it doesn't take long for the economic discrepancy to show," says Dr. Ahrons. "She may get some support for a few years while she's getting on her feet, but she is still going to be way beneath him in earning power. Five years down the line, he's going to be looking a lot better financially than she is."

And the money problems are compounded if you have children. In fact, if you have children, the whole divorce experience can become painfully complicated.

TELLING THE KIDS

You're going through your own agony, but at the same time, you have to be strong and supportive for your children—not an easy task. But the kids need to be told what's happening, and depending on their ages, you can tell them a little bit about why, too.

Your children will also have immediate questions that should be answered explicitly and as often as they are asked—which could be dozens of times over the course of the divorce and after. Questions such as: Why are you doing this? Where will I live? Will I have to go to a new school? Where will my dad live? When will I see him? Experts say that kids need to be reassured that their needs will continue to be met.

With older kids, you can give them more information about the reason for the divorce—skip the intimate details, though, and be careful not to disparage the other parent, warns Dr. Ahrons. "No matter how angry you get, don't tell your children that you hate their father," she advises. "After all, your kids are part of him. If you hate him, then you're saying you hate a part of them, too."

Don't expect your children to blithely sail through a major upheaval like divorce. Even infants and toddlers can react negatively with sleep, toilet training and feeding problems. Preschoolers may start hitting or biting their playmates or throwing temper tantrums. Younger school-age kids may react with sadness, school phobia, bed-wetting or hyperactivity. Meanwhile, older children and teens may feel depressed, lonely, devalued, rejected, hurt, anxious or ashamed. It's almost enough to make you stay married. And some people do.

You can be your child's biggest source of help when it comes to recovering from the divorce. A lot has to do with how you and your husband handle the process, which means, of course, that both of you have to act like grown-ups—not always possible in the heat of the battle. And all too often, there *is* a battle.

Dr. Ahrons has identified four types of ex-spouse relationships—Fiery Foes, Angry Associates, Cooperative Colleagues and Perfect Pals. "What's best for the children is for their parents to find a way to cooperate with each other, especially around parenting issues," she states. "Otherwise the children are constantly involved in loyalty conflicts, and that can be disastrous."

One 15-year-old girl told Dr. Ahrons that she doesn't believe in religion. The reason? Her dad is Jewish and her mom is Catholic. If she had to choose a religion, it would mean choosing one parent's or the other's, and she couldn't do that, she said.

MAKING IT EASIER

To help you—and your children—achieve the smoothest divorce possible, the experts have a few other suggestions.

Listen to your children's anger. They will feel it and display it. After all, they didn't ask for this to happen in their lives.

Realize that your kids will have sad feelings. A divorce is not something they'll get over quickly. It takes 2½ to 3 years for them to get over the worst of it.

Try to remain patient. Your kids will no doubt ask you questions every day. Pointed ones, accusatory ones, repetitive ones. Answer them all as best you can.

Understand your children's reunion fantasies. Most kids dream about their parents reuniting, even if the marriage was a disaster. Don't feed into those fantasies, but realize they are normal.

Set up a regular visitation schedule. Research has shown that frequency of visits has no effect on child adjustment, but regularity of visits does, according to Marla Beth Isaacs, Ph.D., a psychologist in private practice in Philadelphia and author of *Difficult Divorce: Therapy for Children and Parents.* Children whose parents had a visitation schedule in the first year of separation are apparently more socially competent by the third year than are those kids whose parents do not have a visitation schedule. The researchers believe that a schedule provides evidence for the child that the family will still be there despite the many changes brought about by the divorce.

Talk to your ex-spouse about the children. Parents who talk about the kids (school problems, music lessons, birthdays and so forth), especially during the first year of separation, have children who adjust better to the divorce.

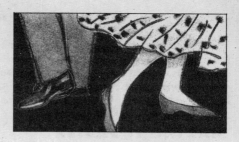

DUAL CAREERS

WORKING UP TO THE CHALLENGE

*I*n a book on dual-career marriages published a decade ago, the authors—two psychologists—called the then-budding phenomenon "probably the most important social change of the twentieth century," comparable in magnitude to the domestication of animals and the Industrial Revolution.

Only the hindsight of history will bear out whether that is fact or hyperbole. But for today's couples who are juggling careers and marriages and sometimes kids—an estimated 38.7 percent of 26.3 million families, according to latest statistics—the more immediate question is, "How do we do it?" For many, it's like being stranded in the wilderness without a map.

"Before I got married, I had trouble with the concept of the joint checking account," jokes Helen Bergey, a 39-year-old school librarian who is married to a high school history teacher and is the mother of three children.

"Imagine my confusion," says Helen, "when I was suddenly faced with the modern problems of finding two good jobs in one place and divvying up laundry, cooking and chauffeuring kids, between two people who put in long hours away from home. My mother never had to do this. I think things were far easier for her than they are for me. She lived at a time when the division of labor was something etched in stone. Today, we're making up the rules as we go along."

In fact, some dual-career couples admit to a sense of longing for a simpler time in simpler places—the mythical Mayberrys or Lake Wobegons—where men were men and women were housewives and everyone knew what to do. For some the stress of balancing two careers, a household and a family is so great that one or the other—usually the woman—bails out of the work force.

But far more stay. The dual-career family has become both an economic and social fact of life. While the media image of the two-career couple is that of a pair of yuppies struggling to make the payments on the Volvo and the Saab and the house in the Hamptons, many couples need two salaries just to get by in an era of $100,000 handyman's specials and economy cars that cost more than the houses they grew up in. But many women need careers—not just jobs—for the fulfillment, sense of self-worth and economic independence they offer. Necessary or not, the dual-career lifestyle is not an easy one.

CONFLICT IS COMMON

The opportunity for conflict to arise in a two-earner family is enormous. Studies show that no matter how prestigious and lucrative their careers, women still do the bulk of the housework and parenting, a situation that may spawn the most bickering in dual-earner homes. There are other, even more serious considerations than who dusts and who takes out the trash. What happens when one or the other of you is offered a fabulous job in another state? What if you begin making more money than your spouse or climb far ahead of him on the career ladder? What if you stop being the woman he married? Like housework, these can be power issues that can explode a marriage like a land mine.

There are no easy answers to the conflicts that plague two-career marriages. A lot more negotiating and compromise goes on in dual-earner marriages—over everything from who has diaper duty to whose career takes precedence this week. Too often, busy couples give their marriage only what time is left over, leading to anger, resentment and loneliness. If the marriage ceases to be fulfilling, couples sometimes turn to their careers for greater satisfaction. Then you risk making decisions based on feeding your career, and your marriage can die of starvation.

"Many two-earner couples feel they are always tired," says Matti Gershenfeld, Ph.D., director of the Couples Learning Center in Jenkintown, Pennsylvania. "It's not an accident that for many of them sex is bad."

As in any good marriage, couples work out their differences over time, tinkering with the glitches the way they learn to tolerate each other's idiosyncracies. But for a two-career relationship to work, it has to be healthy. "Your only insurance is to have a really good, caring, loving relationship in which you can talk about these things honestly," says Gisela Booth, Ph.D., a clinical psychologist and assistant clinical professor of psychology at Chicago's Northwestern University. "It is essential that two people accept and respect each other's career commitment and needs."

Unlike the give-and-take relationships of yesteryear— she gives, he takes—the giving and taking are reciprocal in the modern two-career marriage. It's a marriage built of teamwork, on mutual support.

Gay Hirshey got her first taste of how a mutually supportive marriage works when she married her second husband, Tom, nine years ago. "In my first marriage, my husband wanted me to do things for him. I want to do things for Tom, too, but the difference is, he wants to do things for me just as much. When I lost my full-time job a few years ago, I thought it might be a good opportunity for me to start my own business. I was worried about all the financial pressure that would put on Tom. But he said, 'Go for it.' He reminded me that when he lost his job a few years earlier, I supported us for six months. He said, 'If you can do that for me, I can do the same for you.' Well, this was not in the rule books when I grew up. What a concept!"

Feeding the marriage is essential. Along with keeping up a running dialogue, Dr. Gershenfeld often recommends that couples go on "mini-vacations," taking advantage of the special weekend rates many hotels and motels offer to attract business during slow seasons. "Basically, you need to get out of the rat race, away from the schedule that runs you," she says. "It's good for the marriage and will ultimately be good for your kids. Otherwise, you take your frustrations out on them."

CAREER VERSUS MARRIAGE

There will be times when your career will take precedence over your relationship, but not in a way to mortally wound it. There may come a time, for instance, when you have to choose between staying home with a sick husband who is longing to be nurtured and going to work because a project is due. "You may have to decide to go with your career demands, knowing it won't jeopardize the relationship, although it might hurt your spouse at the moment," says Dr. Booth.

You don't want to consistently sacrifice your job to your relationships because you or your spouse expects it. In doing so, you might lose out on advancement opportunities that could make your career less satisfying and you unhappy.

"I think the relationship has to come first in the final analysis," says Dr. Booth, "but it need not always come first in each instance."

POWER AND STATUS

Making this marriage work is not always going to be easy. You're asking a man to enter into a whole new kind of relationship for which he has probably had no role models and no experience. And both of you will likely find that the culture has deeply embedded in you subliminal messages about the way men and women are supposed to think and act. You may discover, as if for the very first time, that men and women are truly different. And it's not only plumbing. It's also wiring.

Like it or not, men are socialized to assume power, says Lucia A. Gilbert, Ph.D., professor in the Department of Educational Psychology at the University of Texas in Austin

CAREER CONFLICTS: SOLUTIONS THAT WORK

Thirteen years ago, Jacqueline Fawcett, R.N., Ph.D., got an offer she couldn't resist. The University of Pennsylvania offered her a plum job that would allow her to teach and pursue research in the field of maternity nursing. The problem was, Dr. Fawcett's artist husband was firmly and happily ensconced in his job at the University of Connecticut.

The problem of job relocation is one of the stickiest that face dual-career couples. But as it turned out, it was no problem at all for the Fawcetts. Dr. Fawcett took the job and her husband remained in Connecticut. Their commuter marriage was born.

Dr. Fawcett spends two nights a week in Philadelphia in a house she shares with a colleague. The rest of the time she lives in Connecticut with her husband. "It's the best of all possible worlds for a married woman who works," claims Dr. Fawcett. "I have what is my own life three days a week—I have time for myself and my career—and the rest of the time I have my married life. It's great. We have our own time and space, and then we have our time together."

Rather than damaging her marriage, Dr. Fawcett says, commuting has enhanced it. "I sometimes think we'd be divorced if I hadn't done this," she admits. "The time and space apart makes us able to appreciate each other more. On the nights I'm home, I'm happy. I don't mind cooking and doing a little housekeeping. I probably would have more responsibilities, more expectations if I lived in Connecticut full-time. Now, I can have a social life with my female colleagues that doesn't interfere with my marriage."

The commuter marriage certainly isn't the best solution for every relocation problem. The Fawcetts have jobs in cities only slightly more than a 1-hour airplane flight apart. Couples who are bi-coastal, for instance, might only be able to get together once every few weeks and, unfortunately, that kind of absence doesn't always make the heart grow fonder. The Fawcetts are also, as she says, "voluntarily child-free." Couples with children might find this solution quite stressful—or impossible, if the children are in school.

Career conflicts need to be talked about, but other than that, there's no rule of thumb—nor a limit to the creative solutions couples come up with, says University of Texas Health Science Center psychiatrist Diane Martinez, M.D.

Here, as in other aspects of their lives, two-career couples need to put their relationship first, weighing career opportunities against the sacrifice their partners may have to make.

Dr. Martinez says one couple she knows—both doctors—have solved their conflict by taking turns "choosing from a set of options that were viable to both." He chose the medical school they both attended (tricky, since she had to get in) and she got the next choice, where they went for their residency. But, Dr. Martinez points out, neither partner ever felt he or she was making a big sacrifice.

and author of *Sharing It All: The Rewards and Struggles of Two-Career Families*. They grow up with what she calls a sense of "entitlement," a belief that what they do or want should take precedence over the needs of women. Some feel it more, some less.

For some men, studies suggest, power is central to their self-image. Even the most sensitive man may be surprised to realize that, when push comes to shove, he considers his wife's career as secondary to his own.

He may resent a wife who makes a lot of money or is traveling faster up the career ladder than he is. He may see you as usurping the power he's been led to believe, by cultural inculcation, is rightly his, says Diane Martinez, M.D., a psychiatrist at the University of Texas Health Science Center in San Antonio. A man with this strong a sense of entitlement isn't a good candidate for a two-career marriage.

Most men in two-career marriages struggle with these feelings of "male specialness," says Dr. Gilbert. Raised to be the breadwinner, a man may unconsciously believe he can put his work first to fulfill this important role, which, in reality, he's now sharing with you. Especially if he's ambitious himself, he may be surprised to find he resents your bigger paycheck or longer title, because men traditionally have made more and achieved more in the work arena. Or he may expect you to just drop everything and come along if he gets a good job offer in another city, because he's made the assumption that your career plays second fiddle to his.

"We live in a society in which relatively few married women hold positions of power and leadership, although many may have interesting careers," says Dr. Gilbert. "Men are well aware of their spouses' abilities and ambition; they just don't take their careers as seriously as their own."

Men committed to making their two-career marriages work make the effort to recognize these subliminal time bombs and defuse them—something that takes a lot of soul-searching, discussion and occasionally, professional help. Remember, it's going to be hard, warns Dr. Gilbert. He's going to be challenging traditional notions of what a man is supposed to be—notions you might hold, too.

SUBTLE SABOTAGE

Even if you go into a marriage with the best intention of making it equal, your upbringing may sabotage you. Like your spouse, you may unconsciously accept certain assumptions about sex roles.

"Men and women internalize the same messages," says Dr. Gilbert. Even in today's culture, women still "marry up." They look for men who are older and wiser and probably more powerful. Stereotypes die hard. When Dr. Gilbert and her colleagues questioned soon-to-be university grads about their future mates, the results were surprising. "Women not only want men to be warm and sensitive, they also want them to be successful," says Dr. Gilbert. And the men? They want their wives to be warm and supportive, too, but success is not an issue.

Many women subconsciously accept the idea that the man is the breadwinner, even when they have well-paying careers themselves. Without knowing it, you may think it's your birthright to stay home and you may be subtly transmitting the message to your husband that it is the woman's right to have someone take care of her, says Dr. Gilbert. "Think of it. If a man felt like that, you'd call him a failure."

You may also unconsciously believe your career is secondary to your husband's. Traditionally, women have been expected to be altruistic, reading cues and filling needs even before they're expressed, says Dr. Martinez. Because of your upbringing, you may also be more likely to fear placing your job over your relationships and may sacrifice your career aspirations to keep your family happy, something that may be central to *your* self-image.

How *do* you fight this enemy in your mind? Knowing these outdated messages may suddenly leap from your unconscious to your actions will help. It will also help if you and your spouse talk about them. Examining your motives will help keep you from switching to autopilot.

LOOKING FOR MR. GOOD GUY

You ease your chances of having a successful dual-career relationship if you first marry the right man. It may sound funny, but the phenomenon of the dual-career family has added a new dimension to the idea of marriage compatibility. Before you tie the knot, you need to know if you're marrying a man who is honest, kind *and* willing to vacuum and change diapers.

If you're going to make a dual-earner relationship work, you also need a man who supports your career and won't ask you to subordinate your goals to his.

And you need to find out if he's Mr. Right during courtship, says professor Lucia A. Gilbert, Ph.D., of the University of Texas.

"The first thing a woman should do during courtship is discuss with her future spouse what his plans are," says Dr. Gilbert. "People are different in terms of how much they want to be involved in parenting and in their career ambitions. But regardless of these differences, most women are not going to want to be in a two-career family where there isn't going to be a certain degree of role-sharing and involvement in parenting and household work. If it looks like there isn't compatibility there and he's not the least bit interested in doing any of that, then it is not going to work. If you're so desperate for this man that you're going to marry him anyway, that's your choice, but it's going to be a struggle."

FAIR'S FAIR

There are no tidy little prescriptions for working out the details of a solid two-career marriage, but there is a goal to shoot for. It's not equality, says Dr. Gilbert, but equity, a sense that everyone is doing and getting their fair share. "When you think about it, when in a relationship do two people make exactly the same amount of money or have exactly the same amount of demands on their time?" she points out. "In the past, what we researchers have done is looked for equality in a marriage, so all the research shows that marriages aren't equal."

But equal isn't everything. Good marriages are not necessarily based on equality or on evenly divvying things up but on a sense of fairness. It's an overall faith in the relationship that your needs will be met. If not now, then later.

Carolyn Roberts has one of those marriages. Both she and her husband, David, hold executive jobs in Fortune 500 companies and share in the raising of their two boys. Their division of labor is strictly along sex-stereotyped lines. "I don't think he's ever cleaned a toilet bowl in his life," says Carolyn. "On the other hand, I've never changed the oil in the car. In our marriage, I take care of most of the 'women' things, he takes care of most of the 'men' things, and we both share parenting. I'd say it all works out. I'm very happy."

Carolyn and her husband—along with the more than 38 million other two-career couples in America—are blazing new trails in our mutable social system, an act that takes courage and vision. They are challenging a restrictive set of rules that once doomed women to the kitchen and the nursery and men to early, stress-related deaths. They are the vanguard of a new revolution, people who are liberating each other from those rules and, as Helen Bergey put it, making up new rules as they go along.

See also Housework, Superwoman Syndrome

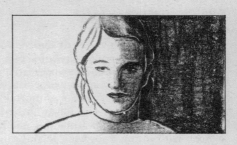

EATING DISORDERS

PUZZLING PROFILES IN ANOREXIA AND BULIMIA

*A*t 77 pounds, Anna thought she was fat. Then, one day, as she emerged from the shower, her young daughter stared at her and screamed. "I said, 'Honey, what's wrong?'" recalls Anna, 36. "She was sobbing and she said, 'Do you have any idea what you look like? Mom, you're a skeleton.' That's when I knew I was out of control."

At 20, Janine was an insulin-dependent diabetic who would eat large quantities of food and vomit it up. She began manipulating her insulin so she would urinate more and lose weight. As a consequence, she lost control of her diabetes and damaged her kidneys. But she didn't accept that she had a problem until "one day I realized I had to go to sleep to have enough energy to take a shower."

Anna and Janine both suffer from eating disorders. Anna is an anorexic. Anorexia nervosa typically strikes young women, often in their teens, who, like Anna, use starvation diets, often in conjunction with strenuous exercise, to whittle themselves down to skeletal thinness yet continue to see themselves as fat. Janine is bulimic. Bulimics, most often young women, typically binge and purge, either through forced vomiting, the use of laxatives or emetics, such as Ipecac syrup, or rigorous dieting and exercising. They, too, have distorted body images and a morbid fear of being fat.

Both anorexia and bulimia are considered psychiatric

disorders that are just as poorly understood as other mental illnesses and can respond poorly to treatment. Both disorders may be on the rise. Anywhere from 2 to 5 percent of adolescents and young adult women suffer from anorexia, which, if untreated can have a mortality rate of nearly 20 percent. Another 5 percent are believed to suffer from bulimia, although death from this condition is rare. But women with eating disorders can suffer from a wide range of ailments from heart irregularities to amenorrhea, a potentially serious condition in which the menstrual periods cease, to long-term complications such as osteoporosis, a bone-thinning disease that usually strikes women after menopause.

WHO IS AT RISK?

Most experts agree that a number of factors put a young woman at risk for an eating disorder. What alarms many researchers and clinicians is the fact that the current thin ideal for women—unattainable for all but a very small percentage of the population—may be making an increasing number of women vulnerable. "Many women already use food as something more than just a means to satisfy their hunger, and they are deeply concerned and distressed about their weight," says Lisa Silberstein, Ph.D., former clinical director of the Yale University Eating Disorders Clinic who is now in private practice in New Haven, Connecticut. "The issues of weight and food are a weak link for so many women."

In fact, some eating disorders programs are reporting an increase in the number of older career women seeking treatment. According to Dr. Silberstein, they are Superwoman "wannabes"—women who have absorbed society's message that success requires women to be smart and beautiful. And they must also be a size 6. "There are some studies that suggest that women who embrace the ideal of being and doing it all are also going to be at risk for eating disorders," she says. "The superwoman image creates an impossible goal."

As does trying to be model-thin when your genes dictate

otherwise. "There are also biological variables that come into play," says Dr. Silberstein. "At least in terms of weight, the body shape that people come to occupy is determined by genetic disposition. If someone is genetically programmed to occupy a larger body type, she may be at more risk than somebody else of developing an eating disorder because she may always feel slightly heavy."

A LITTLE GIRL FOREVER

One of the reasons researchers believe so many eating disorders start at puberty is because that tender time, when girls begin to notice boys, is when their bodies begin the process of maturation by laying down more fat. Unfortunately, nature's ideal of womanliness isn't society's. "Girls are programmed at puberty to put on the bulk of their increase in fat and boys put it on in terms of muscle and lean tissue," says Dr. Silberstein. "At puberty, boys start to have bodies that more approximates the male ideal. For them, a growth spurt is desirable. We did studies of body dissatisfaction among college males and we found they are likely to want to be heavier instead of thinner. With women this is virtually unheard of."

In fact, some researchers theorize that anorexia is a young woman's way of canceling puberty. Probably because they lack an adequate amount of body fat, anorexics don't get their periods and often lose some of their sexual characteristics such as pubic hair. They remain, in effect, little girls. Their fear of fat is, in essence, fear of life. Other researchers point out that by becoming anorexic or bulimic, a woman may feel she is finally in control of her life—or at least has found a part of it she can control, usually better than anyone else. It may be her best stab at perfection.

THE MOST VULNERABLE

Although we're all subject to society's whims of fashion and body size, very few women actually do develop eating disorders. For those who do, other factors may be at work. "There are some people who are more vulnerable to incorporating cultural messages about body ideal, such as dancers and models," says Dr. Silberstein. "Also at greater risk are women who are unusually dependent on external sources of praise and external standards. Also the generic risk factors for mental problems, in general, such as low self-esteem and depression, increase risk for eating disorders."

Studies have also found that in some, though not all, cases, there may be a higher incidence of family instability.

BE ALERT TO THE WARNING SIGNS

The signs and symptoms of eating disorders can be subtle and insidious. They can include:

- Refusal to accept and maintain body weight, particularly if you are of normal or below normal weight
- Distorted body image (you think you are fat, although those around you assure you that you are not)
- Excessive exercising
- Preoccupation with weight and diet
- Loss of three consecutive menstrual periods
- Loss of pubic hair
- Binge eating, especially of "junk" foods
- Changes in mood, particularly preceding or following binge eating
- Significant weight loss (at least 15 percent below normal)
- Significant weight fluctuations (10 pounds or more in a month)
- Inability to recognize basic feelings, such as hunger or sadness
- Aversion to certain foods or unusual food preferences
- Food hoarding
- Sensitivity to cold
- Abuse of laxatives, diuretics and emetics
- Erosion of dental enamel (caused by gastric acid during vomiting)
- Withdrawal from family and friends
- Inability to concentrate
- Depression and loss of sleep

"There is a higher incidence of other types of psychiatric illness in the family, including alcohol and substance abuse," says Dr. Silberstein.

In one study of 78 women with eating disorders, researchers found that 30 percent reported they had been sexually abused. However, when the researchers probed deeper, expanding the criteria for abuse, the figure rose to 64 percent. Several other studies found that one-third to two-thirds of all women who suffer from eating disorders were sexually abused as children or teens.

Other researchers, including Judith Rodin, Ph.D., and Kathleen Pike, Ph.D., of Yale, have looked at the relationship between women with eating disorders and their mothers. "These young women developing eating disorders today are the daughters of the first generation of weight watchers," Dr. Silberstein points out. And, in fact, the Rodin-Pike study found that young women with eating disorders were more likely to have mothers who were excessively weight-conscious and who, because they believed their daughters weren't attractive enough, encouraged their quest for thinness.

DISTORTING THE FACTS

Common to women with both anorexia and bulimia is a distorted body image. No matter how thin they become, they still think of themselves as fat, although they're aware that by objective criteria they are underweight. Along with this perceptual distortion comes denial. Many women with eating disorders refuse to admit that they have a problem, and so treatment may be difficult. "Their denial is very powerful," says Dr. Silberstein. "Bulimics often continue to tell themselves for years that their bingeing and purging is not a serious problem but a good way to lose weight."

In fact, for both anorexics and bulimics, the control of their body weight serves an important purpose in their lives. Although inappropriate and, in some cases, life threatening, it is a way to cope with their problems. Bulimics, for instance, often use food as a way to "modulate their emotions," says Dr. Silberstein. "For them, eating may be a way to numb their feelings and to relieve stress. For many, food keeps them company when they're lonely."

Another reason treatment is so difficult is that it usually involves refeeding, which can be a painful experience both physically and emotionally. Some centers use drugs to ease the gastric upset and abdominal distension that sometimes accompany refeeding and psychotherapy to help reduce the fear of gaining weight most women experience. Group therapy is used to help women regain some accurate sense of their own body size and to reduce their feeling of isolation and "freakishness," which may cause them to deny that they have a problem. In one study of a self-help group, one woman told the researcher, "The group helped me feel I was not bad as a person."

OUT OF TOUCH WITH REALITY

Though women with eating disorders are usually preoccupied with food and diet, many have little knowledge of basic nutritional facts and need nutritional counseling. They are also out of touch with their feelings, using food or severe deprivation to control—in fact, stave off—their underlying feelings of anxiety and depression. "Often they need insight-oriented psychotherapy," says Dr. Silberstein, to help them learn to identify and cope with their feelings.

Some clinicians have found that antidepressants can be helpful in the treatment of eating disorders, particularly bulimia, and increasingly the drug of choice for women who binge and purge is fluoxetine, marketed under the name Prozac. No one is certain why it works, but fluoxetine—used in the treatment of everything from depression to obsessive-compulsive disorders—does regulate a mood-altering brain chemical called serotonin, which can suppress appetite. In those with amenorrhea, in which the menstrual cycle comes to a halt, doctors may recommend estrogen replacement therapy to guard against premature bone loss.

In some cases, family therapy is called for "because the families continue to act in ways that may have contributed to the development of the eating disorder in the first place," says Dr. Silberstein.

Depending on her medical condition, a woman with an eating disorder may be seen on an inpatient or outpatient basis. Even after successful treatment, there may be some residual effects, "although a woman who has had an eating disorder may continue to experience some struggle with food," says Dr. Silberstein. "The goal of therapy is for her to control food rather than food controlling her. Treatment helps move her out of medical danger and can improve functioning in other aspects of her life."

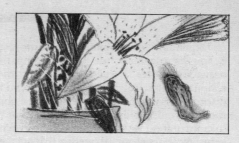

ENDOMETRIOSIS

PRIME SUSPECT IN PELVIC PAIN

*M*ary Lou Ballweg spent 15 years baffling doctors before she found out what was causing her agonizing menstrual pain. "The pain got so bad that many times I couldn't get up and down the stairs in my house," says Ballweg, who was finally diagnosed with endometriosis at age 31.

Long before any doctor said so, Ballweg was convinced she had endometriosis. She had already rejected the notions that her symptoms were psychosomatic, that she was a hypochondriac or, as one doctor put it, "just the nervous type." She decided to do some research on her own.

"Almost everything I read or heard about endometriosis turned out to be contradictory, confusing and often wrong," she says. "Nobody seemed to know anything about this disease," which was one of the main reasons she went on to co-found the Endometriosis Association. "Even today, an estimated 70 percent of the women who come to us complain that their doctors try to blame the symptoms on something psychological."

THE UNWELCOME GUEST

Doctors don't know what causes endometriosis. They are also at a loss to explain why some women get it and others don't, although there is some evidence that it may be inherited. It's also the first suspect when a woman has trouble conceiving. Basically, endometriosis is your menstrual cycle gone amok. Each month, in preparation for a possible pregnancy, the tissues lining your uterus thicken with blood to form a nourishing nest. When conception fails to occur, the lining (called the endometrium) is sloughed off and sheds through your vagina—in other words, you menstruate.

Sometimes, though, normal endometrial tissue backs up through the fallopian tubes, escapes through the fringes into the abdominal cavity, implants and grows *outside* the uterus, explains Dorothy Barbo, M.D., professor of obstetrics and gynecology at the University of New Mexico School of Medicine and medical director of the university's Center for Women's Health in Albuquerque. It can attach to the ovaries, fallopian tubes, bladder or even the rectum. Like endometrial tissue that remains inside the uterus, these fragments respond to signals from ovarian hormones. When the ovaries signal for the endometrial tissue to begin its cyclic growth, this stray tissue also becomes engorged with blood. As a result, you may experience severe pain during your period, while having sex or even when trying to go to the bathroom. Or you may experience no pain at all. In fact, you can have endometriosis and not even know it.

Unlike menstrual fluid, which flows from the uterus and out the vagina each month, blood from the abnormal endometrial tissue has no place to go. Inflammation sets in. As the inflammation subsides, it is replaced with scar tissue. As this process continues month after month, the patches of endometriosis may get bigger. Sometimes it can even cause organs to malfunction or cause adhesions that bind organs together.

THE ALL-IN-YOUR-HEAD DIAGNOSIS

The worst thing about endometriosis is that it is insidious. It can play sneak for years, doing its damage without your ever knowing it. An estimated 1 to 2 percent of all women who have not yet gone through menopause have some degree of endometriosis. That's more than five million women in the United States. It can start at any age, although it's most common in women in their thirties and forties. And symptoms subside once a woman reaches menopause—if she can wait that long without surgical intervention.

Although severity of symptoms can vary from woman to woman, "the typical complaint of those suffering from endometriosis is a deep, constant ache that often precedes, accompanies and outlasts your period," notes Ellen L. Yankauskas, M.D., director of the Women's Center for Family Health in Atascadero, California. Indeed, a survey by the Endometriosis Association reports that 83 percent of the women who have this condition suffer pain throughout their cycle.

As if the pain isn't bad enough, most women have to contend with a long delay between seeking help and being appropriately diagnosed and/or treated. "Most people seem to find it difficult to believe that women with endometriosis are subjected to the widespread disbelief and disrespect that occurs," says Ballweg, who is also the author of *Overcoming Endometriosis*. But a preliminary study conducted at the Institute for the Study and Treatment of Endometriosis at Grant Hospital of Chicago points out the problems.

The researchers found that women with endometriosis who complained of painful periods or painful intercourse were usually not treated—or treated with over-the-counter medications—without further investigation. One woman stated that her doctor patted her hand and said, "It's part of being a woman." Another said her doctor prescribed a mild tranquilizer because he thought maybe college was getting to her.

When these women were finally diagnosed, most expressed feelings of relief, say the researchers. "The women were glad to have proof that their pain was physiologic in origin," the researchers noted. "They felt vindicated."

TREATMENT OPTIONS

"As with any illness, education and support are the foundation of the treatment," maintains Dr. Yankauskas. For starters, your doctor likely will suggest using antiprostaglandin and anti-inflammatory medications—over-the-counter Advil or its extra-strength prescription sister Motrin—for pain relief. But long-term treatment most likely will include hormone therapy or surgery.

Hormone therapy in the form of birth control pills keeps endometriosis under control for many, says Dr. Yankauskas. Most birth control pills consist of progestin and estrogen, the amounts of which have been decreased over the years. Since it's the progestin that is helpful in shrinking endometriosis, the amount of estrogen should be kept at the minimum. Stronger hormone treatments are sometimes prescribed to temporarily quell the condition until surgery or, if you're close in age, menopause. Pregnancy can put symptoms on hold, too, but it does not cure endometriosis as doctors once thought. On the contrary, says Ballweg, symptoms often reappear with a vengeance a few months after delivery.

Danazol, a synthetic male hormone, suppresses the ovaries' production of estrogen and creates a false menopause. But according to Dr. Barbo, it often produces undesirable side effects—weight gain, depression and hot flashes. Another medication—Gn-RH agonists (gonadotropin releasing hormone)—is used in a similar way, and most women find the side effects more acceptable than those of danazol. None of these drugs like danazol can be given for more than six months because of the consequences of a false menopause, including the risk of bone-thinning osteoporosis.

Conventional surgery in the past involved opening the abdominal cavity and cutting tissue out with a scalpel or cauterizing it. A newer, high-technology technique is called laparoscopy. Performed with an instrument known as a laparoscope, the procedure, either with a laser or electrical cauterization, is done through tiny incisions in the abdomen, explains Dr. Barbo. Because the abdomen is not opened there is less risk of infection, scarring, bleeding and pain, and the patient can go home the same day. The procedure appears to be more successful than conventional surgery for severe endometriosis.

And, of course, there is hysterectomy—removal of the uterus, and in the case of endometriosis, the ovaries. Almost 20 percent of hysterectomies are performed to treat endometriosis. It is also a procedure clouded in controversy because of the numbers performed each year. But, say some doctors, even this major operation is not a certain solution to the condition, because a small piece of the ovary can remain in the body, generating estrogen. What's more, post-hysterectomy estrogen replacement therapy can bring back endometriosis, especially in severe cases.

See also Fibroids, Hysterectomy

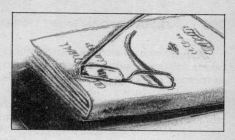

ESTROGEN REPLACEMENT THERAPY

THE GOOD, THE BAD, THE UNKNOWN

*S*hould you or shouldn't you? Is it safe or isn't it? Will it help or won't it? Your menopause has come—or maybe it's even gone—so you need to know, and you need to know soon. Does it make sense to take estrogen when your body's own natural supply runs out? It could be one of the most important decisions you make during your middle years—a decision that could have lasting effects not only on your future health but also on the quality and quantity of your life.

Marie Califano speaks for many. "When I reached menopause about four years ago, my doctor suggested I take estrogen," says the 55-year-old librarian. "But I didn't want to. I had almost no hot flashes or any other symptoms for that matter. And it just seemed unnatural to me to replace the estrogen that my body doesn't want to make anymore. I consider menopause just a normal part of aging, something my body is going through. Perhaps I'd feel differently about it," Marie speculates, "if I were burdened with unbearable symptoms."

Roseanne Dwyer had a different reason for her decision not to take estrogen. "I did take it for two years right after I had a surgical menopause at the age of 28," says the now 38-year-old hairstylist, "but then I decided to stop." (Surgical menopause results from the removal of the ovaries and uterus in a hysterectomy.)

"I was more concerned about the long-range effects of taking estrogen than I was about the hot flashes I started to have again. All the research studies that I saw had been done on women who had started estrogen in their fifties and sixties. Nobody seemed to know what would happen to someone who started taking estrogen in her twenties and then continued it for 30 or 40 years," she says. "On top of that, I read that estrogen increased the risk of breast cancer and endometrial cancer. If my doctor could have shown me one study—something in black and white—that said even for long-term usage the benefits outweighed the risks, then I might have felt differently."

Clarice Harrell, on the other hand, feels that estrogen replacement therapy gave her back her life. She suffered wild menopausal mood swings and hot flashes that left her literally exhausted, irritable and "bouncing off walls." "This is now the easiest time of my life instead of the most difficult," says Clarice, a 46-year-old flight attendant. "I feel feminine, my sex drive is as good as ever, I don't have to deal with the aggravation of the monthlies and, most important of all, I don't have those awful mood swings. Even if I found out today that estrogen was bad for me, I'd still take it."

SOMETHING TO CROW ABOUT

Estrogen replacement therapy—ERT—usually involves a regular program of estrogen to replace the natural estrogen that wanes at menopause. Sometimes another hormone, progestin (a synthetic form of progesterone), is added to the estrogen regimen. When a combination is taken, it's then referred to as hormone replacement therapy—HRT. The hormones are available in pills, although sometimes they are administered through creams, skin patches, injection or vaginal suppositories. Millions of menopausal and postmenopausal American women are now on ERT or HRT, and many physicians believe that most women could benefit from the treatment. In this country patches come in two strengths. Your doctor will help you decide which patch to use.

In fact, today it's hard to find a doctor who isn't crowing over the health benefits of ERT. "There's not a physician in the world who knows the literature on ERT who wouldn't encourage every single woman who qualifies to take it," claims Deborah T. Gold, Ph.D., senior fellow in the Center for the Study of Aging and Human Development at Duke University Medical Center in Durham, North Carolina. "And that's by and large the vast majority of women."

It's no secret, for example, that estrogen replacement therapy can improve menopausal symptoms. With the decline of estrogen, about 25 percent of women experience hot flashes, insomnia, mood swings and vaginal atrophy. For some, like Clarice, the symptoms are severe. ERT can relieve those symptoms by as much as 95 percent. It's especially helpful if your menopause is the result of a hysterectomy. Symptoms of estrogen withdrawal following surgical menopause can be particularly severe.

Doctors have also known for years that ERT begun at menopause is considered the best preventive treatment available for osteoporosis, the bone-thinning disease common in older women. Bone density dwindles rapidly after menopause. The result can be debilitating fractures. But if estrogen treatment is begun at or immediately after menopause, it minimizes that bone loss for as long as a woman stays on the hormone.

"I can see the difference between taking estrogen and not taking estrogen when I look at my own mother and then at her sister," says Dr. Gold, who is also an assistant professor of psychiatry and sociology at the medical center. "My aunt had a surgical menopause and didn't take estrogen because she was concerned about cancer. My mother went through a natural menopause and decided to take estrogen," says Dr. Gold. "Today, my aunt has a terribly humped back and has had fractures in her spine, wrist and hips. My mother, on the other hand, has perfect posture and has had no fractures. Now here are two women with essentially the same genetic material, and it's estrogen that's made the difference in their health.

"Even if you were to put aside the tremendous effect

that estrogen has on menopausal symptoms and bone health," adds Dr. Gold, "there is enough research to show that ERT would still be worthwhile for women to take."

YOU GOTTA HAVE HEART

Dr. Gold is referring to the impressive body of research that has demonstrated estrogen's life-enhancing and heart-saving properties. In one seven-year study, researchers from the University of Southern California found that women who take estrogen can add up to three years to their lives— mostly because it dramatically reduces their risk of dying from heart disease and stroke.

After studying the mortality rates of almost 9,000 estrogen users and nonusers, the researchers found that the women who took estrogen—no matter how long they took it—were less likely to die of heart disease and stroke. In fact, even short-term use—3 years or less—that was discontinued more than 15 years before participation in the study was associated with some reduction in mortality. But women who had taken the drug for 15 years or more benefited the most. Researchers believe the beneficial effect of estrogens on heart disease risk may be due in part to a favorable alteration in blood cholesterol levels.

THE (NOT SO) DOWNSIDE

What about those nagging concerns that women still have about the potential side effects of estrogen replacement therapy? They haven't gone away. Especially the fear of breast cancer. "I'm absolutely terrified of getting breast cancer." says Lucinda Mikulsky. "My mother's sister died from it, and I saw how she suffered," says the 49-year-old junior high school teacher. "Since the doctors don't all agree about the breast cancer risk of taking estrogen, I'd just as soon sit it out. At least I know there are other things I can do to exert some control over my risk of getting heart disease and osteoporosis. But I feel totally powerless when it comes to avoiding breast cancer."

It's true that some previous studies have suggested a link

between ERT and breast cancer. But these early studies were done when estrogen dosages were much greater than they are today. Doctors now know that ERT can have the same benefits at half the dosage. A recent analysis of the research on the connection between ERT and breast cancer has found that women who take 0.625 milligrams per day—the most common dose administered today—had no increased risk of developing breast cancer over those who did not take estrogen. What's more, say the researchers, at this lower dose there is no convincing evidence that duration of treatment increases breast cancer risk, either.

The research done so far, however, still leaves open the possibility of an increased risk of breast cancer in those who had taken the higher doses (1.25 milligrams per day) in the past. Still, the experts insist that the risk is very small.

Unfortunately, the same cannot be said for the part estrogen—no matter what the dose—may play in developing another type of cancer.

THE QUESTION OF RISK

Studies have established that taking estrogen alone for more than two years significantly increases your risk of endometrial cancer (cancer of the uterine lining). But doctors have found that prescribing the lower doses of estrogen combined with progestin eliminates that risk. Indeed, studies have shown that the incidence of endometrial cancer in women on the combination of hormones is even below that of women who get no hormone treatment at all.

There is a catch-22 here. Researchers are still unsure what effect progestin may have on breast cancer risk and whether it may interfere with estrogen's bone-building and heart-strengthening benefits. "We do know that taking progestin along with estrogen can adversely affect blood cholesterol by lowering HDL cholesterol—that's the good kind—and raising LDL cholesterol—the bad kind," says Donna Shoupe, M.D., associate professor of obstetrics and gynecology at the University of Southern California in Los Angeles. Estrogen, by itself, has a beneficial effect on cholesterol.

These questions may be answered by a long-term clinical trial now under way that's known as the Postmenopausal Estrogen/Progestin Interventions. Researchers supported by the National Heart, Lung, and Blood Institute are measuring HRT's effect on the four main indicators of heart health—HDL cholesterol, insulin, blood pressure and fibrinogen (a clotting factor)—along with bone mass and changes in the breasts and uterus. They hope to find out which estrogen regimen is most effective and least risky.

In the meantime, there are some promising results from a study that evaluated a continuous combined low-dose regimen of estrogen and progestin on menopausal women. Researchers from the University of Arizona Health Sciences Center in Tucson found that a combination of 0.625 milligrams per day of estrogen and 2.5 or 5 milligrams per day of progestin improved menopausal symptoms and protected the endometrial lining, while maintaining the beneficial effects on blood cholesterol levels that estrogen alone is known to elicit. What's more, say the researchers, there was a marked decrease in annoying episodes of period-like bleeding with this low-dose combination, a frequent occurrence when higher doses of progestin are used.

Dr. Shoupe is also experimenting with a new way of delivering progestin to menopausal women that appears to eliminate its unsafe and unpleasant side effects. She studied a group of women who used a progestin-releasing intrauterine device (IUD). "With the IUD, progestin is delivered locally, in the uterus—the only place it's needed—and the side effects of oral progestin are avoided," she says. Dr. Shoupe hopes that eventually a device will be developed—it could be called a progestin uterine implant—that would be made of biodegradable materials that could last for five to ten years.

WEIGHING THE ODDS

The decision to have estrogen replacement therapy or hormone replacement therapy is an easy one for many women. Clarice Harrell is far from alone in her whole-hearted recommendation. In fact, even skeptical Roseanne Dwyer started to take estrogen again, after a seven-year absence, when her new doctor found that she had lost a great deal of bone density. "He scared the living daylights out of me," she says. "Now I wear my estrogen patch faithfully. As a side benefit, I must admit my sex drive has taken a leap forward, too."

And there's no denying the heart-saving benefits of ERT. Trudy L. Bush, Ph.D., an epidemiologist at Johns Hopkins University School of Hygiene and Public health, notes that heart disease—not cancer—is the leading killer of post-menopausal women. Each year, heart disease accounts for 12 deaths per 2,000 in women over age 50. Breast cancer, on the other hand, accounts for only 2 deaths per 2,000.

Still, estrogen replacement therapy isn't for everyone. Marie Califano, for example, says she's satisfied that she can live just fine without estrogen. In spite of her increased risk of heart disease—she admits she's 30 pounds over-weight and heart disease runs in her family—she'd still rather use nonhormonal alternatives. "I just don't like the idea of taking drugs," she insists.

Even if you want to take estrogen, most doctors will tell you that if you have had breast cancer, it's best to find an alternative to hormone therapy. (Many give that same advice to women who are at high risk of developing breast cancer, too.) If you have a history of blood clotting or strokes—and especially if you are a heavy smoker—you may also be told to avoid ERT.

In addition, if you suffer from fibroids or endometriosis (estrogen fuels both conditions), liver disease, migraines, gallbladder disease or a seizure disorder, you may be well-advised to avoid hormone therapy.

If you are not a candidate for ERT, there are many nonhormonal options that can help you reduce your risk of heart disease and osteoporosis as well as decrease most unpleasant menopausal symptoms.

THE DECISION IS YOURS

ERT is not without its annoying, albeit minor, side effects. Fluid retention, breast tenderness and weight gain are some

HORMONES AND PREVENTIVE CARE

If you decide to take estrogen or a combination of estrogen and progestin, there are a few health precautions that the experts recommend.

- Get a mammogram *before* you begin.
- Closely monitor your breasts during hormone treatment. That means having a mammogram once a year, a breast examination by a physician twice a year and doing a breast self-exam every month (for instructions see "How to Perform a Breast Self-Exam" on page 45).
- Schedule an endometrial biopsy if you're taking estrogen without progestin and you still have your uterus.
- Report any unusual bleeding to your physician immediately. It can be a warning of endometrial cancer.
- Monitor your blood pressure closely if you have a history of high blood pressure.
- Take the lowest effective dose of hormones that you can.

of the most common complaints. And, if you're taking progestin along with your estrogen, you might also be faced with menstrual-like bleeding. Roseanne says that weight gain and water retention are her biggest complaints, although she's willing to put up with it because of her fear of osteoporosis. As for the weight gain, she says her doctor told her, "If you don't put it in your mouth, you won't put on extra pounds."

Look at it this way. Today women are living a large part of their lives—about 30 years—after they go through menopause, says Dr. Gold. "Given the changes in our life expectancy, we need to modify our health behaviors in order for our bodies to accommodate that extended time."

Estrogen replacement therapy is just one health behavior to consider. As Clarice points out, "it's a personal decision that you make with your doctor. You must balance all the scientific evidence with your own health needs."

See also Heart Disease, Menopause, Osteoporosis

CHAPTER 32

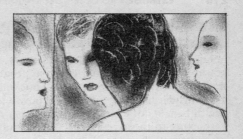

EXERCISE

ADVICE FOR THOSE WHO "HATE TO SWEAT"

What would you say if your doctor told you that by adopting one single good health habit, you could lose weight, reduce your risk of heart disease, cancer and osteoporosis, eliminate premenstrual syndrome symptoms, manage stress, alleviate depression, banish feelings of hostility and improve your sex life?

When her doctor told her that, Josie Alberts responded, "I hate to sweat. But then," laughs Josie, 42, who finally did follow her doctor's recommendation to exercise, "I didn't realize a little sweat could do so much!"

According to a plethora of studies, it's clear it can do all that and more. But some women seem to resist exercise the way cats do water. Are they suffering from what some are calling fear of fitness?

"We run into a number of women in their forties and fifties and some even younger who say, 'I hate to sweat,'" says Ronette Kolotkin, Ph.D., clinical psychologist at the Duke University Diet and Fitness Center in Durham, North Carolina. "They perceive exercise as something jocks do. They see it as unfeminine. It messes up their hair or nails. Also a lot of women are concerned about being criticized for doing it wrong. Or they're self-conscious about going to the health club where everyone is wearing a size 6 leotard."

VIEW FROM THE COUCH

At least 40 percent of the population falls into the "couch potato" category—completely sedentary. Of those who do get involved in structured exercise programs, about half drop out within a few months. Shocking statistics when you consider how convincing and how widely reported the health benefits of exercise have become. And it's certainly perplexing to those researchers who study the psychology of exercise adherence. Why aren't people taking to the roads and gyms in hordes?

A piece of the answer—at least where women are concerned—can be found by looking at exercise in a historical context. In the early part of this century, it was considered unhealthy and inappropriate for women to exercise because of the misguided belief that it would damage their reproductive systems or make them appear masculine. Women were permitted to participate in the Olympics in 1920, and then only in certain "ladylike" sports. Old notions die hard: It was only in 1984 that a women's marathon was finally added to the Olympic games!

Even in the 1960s, when physical fitness became the rage, most girls seemed to regard exercise as something you didn't really have to do once gym class was over. "Most women weren't brought up to think that exercise is a regular part of one's lifestyle," says psychologist Joyce Nash, Ph.D., author of *Maximize Your Body Potential*. "Now things have changed somewhat. My stepdaughter is learning to play basketball and doing things that I never would have dreamed of because when I was a teenager, girls didn't play basketball. Girls were cheerleaders, and even that was being more vigorous than most people."

THE KLUTZ SYNDROME

If you grew up in the 1960s and weren't blessed with natural athletic talent, you probably have a traumatic exercise story to tell. And it's probably the reason you may shy away from exercising today. Beatrice Robinson, Ph.D., now an avid tennis player, admits she has suffered from "the klutz syndrome."

"I can remember in seventh grade being in a volleyball competition and not being able to serve," says Dr. Robinson, an assistant professor of psychology at the University of Minnesota Medical School in Minneapolis. "The humiliation! The worse I felt, the more unable I was to serve. Having the whole team look at me and really get annoyed traumatized me to the extent that I didn't try to do anything physical for ten years. I was convinced I was an athletic moron. I think a lot of women have at least one incident that convinced them they were athletic morons, too."

Overweight women, who could benefit greatly by exercise, may have had a lifetime of exercise traumas that cause them to make a wide arc around the health club. "When I was young, I was fat, clumsy and didn't use my body," says Dr. Kolotkin. "I was the classic last one picked for teams. How do you tell someone to exercise when her body is a source of embarrassment and they can't do the things they need to do in gym class?"

TALKING HEADS

In fact, many women, fat and otherwise, are so frustrated by their bodies they virtually become disembodied. "I see a lot of people who live in their heads, who avoid looking at their bodies and doing anything physical," says Dr. Robinson, who conducts therapy groups for obese women. "They seem to feel that if they ignore their bodies, which they hate, it will be less painful. Fortunately, that doesn't work very well. But that kind of thinking makes you more inactive."

Yet the thing we fear may very well be our salvation. In her therapy groups, Dr. Robinson and her colleague psychologist Jane Bacon found that once their obese clients did begin to exercise, their self-esteem began to soar. "In the beginning we didn't focus on it, but eventually we began to see how important exercise was in terms of liking your body. If you exercise, it's something about your body you *can* like. When you see your endurance and strength building up, it almost forces you to look at something else other than how your body looks. It makes you realize that your body was designed not to be looked at, but to function and move."

Dr. Robinson's experience with her clients jibes with research that has found that exercise is an antidote to depression and can even raise the mood of nondepressed people. One of the most hopeful findings of the latest research is that it's the act of exercising, not fitness, that gives the mood-raising benefit, meaning you don't have to have the cardiovascular fitness of a marathon runner to experience "runner's high." A study done at the Institute for Aerobics Research in Dallas, Texas, reported a similar finding related to longevity. The study, involving more than 10,000 men and 3,000 women, revealed that even a slight increase in exercise—a half-hour brisk walk every day—can significantly reduce your risk of dying from heart disease, cancer and the other killer diseases.

BECOMING PART OF THE CLUB

Now that you know it doesn't take much to feel better and live longer, what else can you do to motivate yourself? Here's what the experts say.

Do something fun. If you regard exercise as roughly equivalent to having root canal done, you're doing the wrong exercise. "I think finding something you like is very important, and varying it is, too," says Dr. Robinson. If running makes you sore and the stationary bike bores you to tears, try walking or a lifetime sport such as biking, tennis or racquetball. Exercise shouldn't be a chore. It should be a good time.

"Running always seemed like a chore to me, which is why I play tennis," says Dr. Robinson. "Running is work and tennis is fun. You may not love it when you first start, but once you get better at it, it becomes more enjoyable. You should also try to find a couple of different things you like to do so you don't get bored."

Be realistic. If the last time you laced on sneakers was in your senior year of high school, you certainly don't want to set up an exercise program of Olympic magnitude. You're setting yourself up for failure. "If you set yourself up on this really ambitious exercise plan, you'll do it for a couple of weeks and then drop it," says Dr. Robinson. "Do something moderate that you can easily fit into your life." Most studies that examine the physical and psychological health benefits of exercise have found that a little goes a long way. A brisk walk a few times a week is all you need.

If you're not particularly athletic, shy away from competitive situations. You risk injury *and* a blow to your self-esteem. "Take it one step at a time," says Dr. Kolotkin. "You don't have to be the best one in aerobics class. In our society, competition and competitive sports are overemphasized. If you're not particularly athletic, you may not feel good about your body or yourself."

Also, if you set your goals a little lower than "triathelete," you're more likely to experience the kind of self-perpetuating success you need to stick to your exercise program. You want to achieve *your* personal best, not surpass someone else's. Go easy on yourself.

"You've read all the exercise books and you know to get these great cardiovascular effects you need to exercise at least three or four times a week for half an hour," says Dr. Robinson. "So if you do it two times a week for 15 minutes, that's still better than nothing. Take a look at what you can really do and what you can sustain."

Incorporate fitness into your daily life. This one should be easy, because it's probably something you already unwittingly do. "Walk the stairs, park the car a little farther away and walk to the store," advises Dr. Robinson. "When you're in the house, instead of storing up all your loads and running up and down the stairs once, run up and down the stairs every time you think of something."

And if you're charting your exercise progress, give yourself credit for every extra thing you do.

Reinforce yourself. To get a horse to move, you suspend a carrot at the end of a stick and dangle it in front of its face. Find your own self-reward. One exercise expert suggests picking a spot where you'd like to go, calculating its distance from your home and setting out to exercise your way there. Record the number of miles you put on walking, biking or swimming and plan a celebration for when you finally "get there." You can reward yourself with a real trip, a party, a new outfit—whatever seems appropriate.

Create a supportive environment. Exercise with a friend or family members. Keep your exercise clothes always at the ready. Drive to the health club on days you really don't want to exercise (once you're there, it will be easy enough to walk in). Keep an exercise diary so you can see physical proof of your commitment and progress. Your daily life should remind you that exercise is a part of it.

Talk yourself into it. Exercise is a habit that takes, according to one expert, 60 to 90 days to work into your life. During those early months, you'll find it very easy to find excuses not to exercise. That's why you have to be vigilant, replacing self-defeating thoughts ("I'm too tired," "I'm too busy," "I'll never get off this plateau") with positive thoughts ("I always feel great after I exercise," "I enjoy walking with my friend").

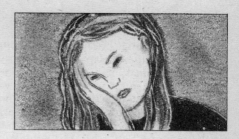

FATIGUE

FIGHTING THE I'M-TOO-TIRED BLUES

*T*ell the kids to answer their own phone calls."

"Hire a cleaning lady."

"Get somebody else to change the toilet paper roll. And pick up those dirty socks!!"

"Let the dog walk himself."

Sound familiar? If you're barking at the dog and the bags under your eyes are so big they qualify as carry-on luggage, maybe you're just running on empty. We all know the feeling, that worn-down-to-your-bones sensation of fatigue. When you're feeling that low, it's hard to be high on life, let alone pick up socks. But it doesn't have to be that way. You can banish fatigue and reinvigorate the old you.

Fatigue may be associated with mood swings or increased stress. It can also be a signal of a physical illness. But it's definitely a clue that something's wrong somewhere, says Dedra Buchwald, M.D., assistant professor of medicine at the University of Washington and director of the Chronic Fatigue Clinic at Harborview Medical Center in Seattle. Chronic fatigue is a symptom that should never be ignored.

ALL TOO COMMON

Sure, it's normal to get tired. Everybody does. Normal fatigue occurs after a 50-mile bike race. Normal fatigue occurs after you've been awakened five times by a feverish child. Normal fatigue occurs after a stressful day at work. And normal fatigue disappears after a good night's sleep.

It's not normal, on the other hand, to feel tired when you first get up in the morning or after walking to the end of the driveway to pick up the mail. It's not normal to have to rest up before performing a simple task like vacuuming the rugs. And it's not normal to live with fatigue week after week no matter how much rest you get.

Yet fatigue is a way of life for many Americans. And doctors get plenty of complaints about it. In one study, 28 percent of women and 19 percent of men who visited their doctors complained that fatigue had been a "major problem" for a month or more.

What are some of the most common problems that give women the I'm-too-tired-to-do-anything kind of feeling? Here's what the experts had to say.

TRASH THAT DIET

They don't call them "crash" diets for nothing. Diet or not, you have to eat if you don't want to wind up nose-down on the pavement. Simply put, crash or fad diets can leave you feeling fatigued.

Because they offer so little in the way of balanced nutrition, crash diets can turn your muscle mass into mush. The destruction becomes so pronounced after a short time that the muscle tissue can no longer efficiently process calcium, according to studies done at the University of Toronto. If you're on that kind of a diet, your body will not be able to function properly. It will slow down and conserve energy by making you slow down.

To get a good start on a diet that will leave you feeling fresh and exhilarated, bear in mind these basic rules established by doctors and nutritionists.

Eat a variety of foods. Avoid diet plans that force you to live on one specific kind of food, like grapefruit. We need a wide variety of nutrients from all kinds of food. No one food supplies you with all the nutrients your body needs to maintain health.

Women, in general, shouldn't eat fewer than 1,200 calories a day. According to diet and nutrition experts at Stanford University, you can't get all the nutrients you need if you eat less than that. Diets in the super-low 800-calorie range may pose a particular threat to health, which can result in a breakdown in heart muscle.

Also, you shouldn't eat big meals late at night. You probably won't be able to burn off the calories as quickly by bedtime as you would earlier in the day.

Don't skip meals. If you do, you'll only be hungrier later. When you do sit down to eat, you probably will eat more than you should.

GET SOME QUALITY SLEEP

It seems so obvious, but if you haven't slept well the night before, you're very likely going to feel tired the day after.

Half of all Americans have trouble dozing off at some time in their lives, and an astonishing 35 million have chronic insomnia. Scientists believe sleep disturbance is a common response to changes in our lives, from trouble at the office to serious illness. For most of us, normal sleep patterns return after the daytime problem that is the source of worry goes away or gets better.

If occasional sleeplessness troubles you, follow these simple suggestions from Patricia Prinz, Ph.D., professor of psychiatry and behavioral sciences at the University of Washington School of Medicine.

- Try not to drink coffee, cola or other caffeine drinks after 6:00 or 7:00 P.M.
- Go to bed at the same time every night.
- Get regular, moderate exercise.
- Skip alcohol after dinner. Booze interferes with sound sleep.

THAT'S NO EXCUSE!

If your body isn't exercised regularly, it probably doesn't use oxygen very efficiently. Your muscles need that oxygen or they don't work as long or as hard as they can. The result of all this sitting around: When you need muscle power, you don't get it, and you tire quickly.

What's more, as your muscles sag, so does your self-image. Your emotional state can become a mirror image of your physical condition, adding to your fatigue.

That's why exercise benefits you in two ways, say the experts. First, it improves your physical condition, enabling your body to deliver more efficiently oxygen to your muscles, increasing your endurance. Second, exercise stimulates an overall feeling of well-being. Studies show that as you exercise, your body becomes better able to handle the every-day emotional and physical stresses of life.

DE-STRESS YOUR LIFE

It takes a lot of energy to deal with the pressures of everyday life. Especially if you're a wife and mother and hold down a job. After expending all that energy, you may be left with a gnawing, overwhelming sense of fatigue.

Not all of the stresses of life leave us feeling emotionally drained, say doctors. It's a certain kind of stress, the kind in which you have no choices, no options, no alternatives. The classic example is the woman who finds herself in a dead-end job. She has a tough boss she can't talk back to. She has to do the same things day after day. She has no sense of control. She may have a family who needs her, so she has even more work to do when she gets home. She feels trapped.

There are some actions you can take that may alleviate the symptoms of fatigue associated with stress.

Ask your doctor, or consult a stress therapist, about relaxation techniques. They may take only 10 to 15 minutes to learn. Once you have the techniques, use them to take a couple of 10- or 15-minute "vacations" from your work around the home or office every day. Doing these exercises and paying attention to your feelings can break that all-day feeling of tension.

THINK INTERNALLY

Fatigue is also a symptom of a host of physical ailments. After assessing nonmedical sources of your fatigue, your doctor will most likely want to run some tests to see if you have an underlying condition.

Fatigue is the number one symptom in a number of conditions affecting women. Iron-deficiency anemia, for example, is common in menstruating women. Thyroid disease also can cause significant fatigue.

In fact, many diseases can cause fatigue, says Dr. Buchwald. So if it's not your lifestyle that's getting you down, you owe it to yourself to get to your doctor—whether you feel like it or not!

See also Chronic Fatigue Syndrome

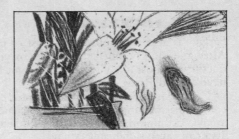

FIBROCYSTIC BREASTS

THE WRONG KIND OF TENDERNESS

What's in a name? If the name is fibrocystic breast disease—or its alternatives, benign breast disease, mammary dysplasia, fibrocystic mastopathy or chronic cystic mastitis—not much at all. Fibrocystic breast disease (FBD) is a meaningless umbrella term, a wastebasket into which doctors throw every breast problem that isn't cancerous, says Susan Love, M.D., director of the Faulkner Breast Center in Boston and clinical assistant professor of surgery at Harvard Medical School. FBD and its aliases are nothing more than intimidating names for "noncondition."

Until you know better, a diagnosis of fibrocystic breast disease sounds ominous. But it's not.

What we're dealing with here are breasts that are painful and feel lumpy or tender. Breasts that can swell or discharge a bit of fluid from the nipples. But *not* breasts that kill—even though we know of at least one woman who admits that there have been times during her menstrual cycle when she "wanted to rip them off."

NORMAL OR ABNORMAL?

"The breast changes that doctors call fibrocystic disease often have little or nothing to do with either fibrous tissue or cysts," explains Kerry McGinn, R.N., author of *Keeping Abreast: Breast Changes That Are Not Cancer*. "The breast is simply carrying out its normal processes, sometimes over-enthusiastically."

Breasts are mainly fat tissue, honeycombed with milk-producing glands and ducts that respond to changes in body chemistry. The milk-producing cells lining the glands are controlled cyclically by hormones. During your child-bearing years, these cells are stimulated to grow and to accumulate fluids during your menstrual cycle, often giving the breasts a lumpy feel. "If there's enough fluid to stretch the tissues and nerves, a woman may feel tenderness or pain, too," says McGinn, who wrote her book with the participation of the Breast Health Center at Children's Hospital of San Francisco.

So, yes, your symptoms are very real, says Dr. Love. It's the diagnosis that's unreal. Actually, what you're feeling are *normal, benign* changes that occur in the breasts of almost all women at some time during their lives, and with varying degrees of discomfort. Experts say at least 50 percent of women at some time will report breast lumpiness or pain to their doctors. And it's estimated that another 40 percent don't report it at all. So what's all the fuss about?

LUMP VERSUS LUMPINESS

"It scares me to death when I feel lumps in my breasts," says Mamie Kessler, a 42-year-old housewife and mother of four. "They're there, then they're not there. Then I think I'm imagining them. Or that I'm just paranoid because the specter of breast cancer is so overwhelming. My doctor says they're just fibrocystic changes and nothing to worry about. But with all that lumpiness, I'm concerned that one of them won't be 'nothing.' "

Of course, there are lumps and then there are *lumps*. But, as Dr. Love points out, "lumpiness is not the same thing as having one dominant lump. The confusion of the two can cause a woman days and weeks of needless mental anguish. Lumpiness is not a disease—'fibrocystic' or otherwise. It's simply normal breast tissue." A general pattern of many little lumps in both breasts *is* perfectly normal.

Cysts and fibroadenomas are fibrocystic changes, too, and even though they feel like the scary kinds of lumps, they're not. A fibroadenoma is a lump of fibrous and glandular tissue, explains Dr. Love. It's usually painless, firm or rubbery and often moves freely in the breast. It's more common in young adult women.

"A cyst typically occurs in women in their thirties, forties and early fifties," says Dr. Love. It's a fluid-filled sac, like a large blister, that grows in the midst of breast tissue. "It's smooth on the outside and squishy on the inside, so that if you push on it, you can feel that it has fluid inside." If there's enough fluid in a cyst, however, it can feel quite firm.

They're sometimes very painful, too, says McGinn, but when they are aspirated with a needle, the cyst collapses as the fluid is withdrawn, and the pain goes with it.

McGinn says she's had lots of cysts that caused a great deal of pain and discomfort. "I would go to the doctor, he would aspirate the fluid, the pain would disappear instantly and that would be the end of it."

Nevertheless, any discrete lump or unusual thickening needs to be checked out by a doctor, stress McGinn and Dr. Love. Even though fibroadenomas and cysts are totally benign, only a doctor can determine that that's indeed what they are—either by aspirating fluid if it's a cyst or by doing a biopsy if the lump is suspicious in any way.

THOSE PAINFUL BREASTS

One woman describes her breast pain as feeling like a "migraine in my chest." Another says she can't sleep on her stomach for two weeks before her period. But with FBD, the pain can be there one month and gone the next, only to come back again and again.

"Just when I think I can't take another bout of painful and swollen breasts, I'll have a cycle that's virtually pain-free," says Shannon Scott, a 29-year-old computer programmer. "I'm rather large-breasted to begin with, but during some months, my breasts swell a whole bra size. And that's when they're usually the most painful, too."

But this too is normal. "Breast symptoms vary from month to month because hormones vary from month to month," explains Dr. Love. "Your ovaries do not produce the same amount every single cycle. They're not little machines, after all. So it's not uncommon to have very painful breasts one month and no pain the next." You can have pain for six months straight, then it will be gone and you may never have another problem.

CONTROLLING FBD SYMPTOMS

Since FBD is not even classified as a disease, you won't be surprised to hear there is no cure. Your doctor might tell

---

A CANCER CONNECTION?

"When a woman is told that she has fibrocystic breast disease she can't help thinking about the possibility of cancer, too. She wants to know if it can become cancer or if it increases her risk of developing cancer," says Kerry McGinn, R.N., an expert on fibrocystic breast disease.

A few years ago, pathologists—the doctors who examine breast tissue microscopically to determine if it's cancerous—had a conference to answer just those questions once and for all. After studying all the research they could find—and there was plenty of it—the pathologists came to this conclusion: In almost all cases, FBD does *not* lead to cancer or increase your risk of developing it.

"Breast cells ordinarily multiply, or proliferate, to replace old cells or to prepare for pregnancy or lactation, but do so within clear limits," explains McGinn. "So when a pathologist refers to 'nonproliferative' changes, it means there is no cell multiplication beyond the limits of normal."

In fact, Susan Love, M.D., of the Faulkner Breast Clinic in Boston points out that in a study of 10,000 benign breast biopsies, only 3 percent fell into a category considered to moderately increase a woman's chances of breast cancer.

you that the pain, swelling, lumpiness and tenderness are something you'll have to get used to. Or that the symptoms may just go away. But there are some lifestyle—mostly dietary—changes that may make a difference.

Try cutting out coffee and other caffeine-containing foods. That includes tea, colas, chocolate and over-the-counter medications such as Dexatrim, Excedrin Extra-Strength, Midol, Anacin, Sinarest and others (check the labels).

Although the connection between caffeine and fibrocystic breast pain is controversial, some studies have found breast pain relief in women who gave up coffee. Linda Russell, a family nurse practitioner with the Department of Surgery at Duke University Medical Center in Durham, North Carolina, says that 61 percent of the patients in her study had a "dramatic reduction" in their breast pain when they gave up caffeine. If your breast pain is severe, you may want to try avoiding caffeine products for awhile and see if you find relief.

Limit sodium intake. This helps reduce swelling. Keep salt to under a teaspoon a day.

Stop smoking. But don't rely on nicotine gum to help you, because nicotine is the suspected irritant.

Eat a low-fat diet. Some preliminary studies show that lower-fat diets may reduce breast pain—and, more significantly, reduce your risk of breast cancer, says Dr. Love.

Consider stress-reduction techniques. Hormones have been known to respond to the stresses in our lives, says McGinn. Anything you can do to reduce those stresses may also help your breast discomfort. That includes meditation, physical exercise and biofeedback training, which uses electronic sensors to detect changes in body temperature and muscle tension.

Take a multivitamin and mineral supplement. It should contain vitamin A, the B-complex vitamins, vitamin E, iodine and selenium. In research trials, all have been shown to have some beneficial effect on breast pain and lumps, even though some of the evidence is inconclusive.

Beware of diuretics. These so-called water pills get rid of the fluid you're retaining everywhere but in the breasts, says Wende Logan-Young, M.D., director of the Breast Clinic in Rochester, New York, and a consultant at the Roswell Park Cancer Institute in Buffalo. What's more, diuretics can actually make breast cysts worse because they have a hormonelike effect that combines with your own hormones. Nevertheless, some gynecologists continue to prescribe them for breast swelling and pain, she says.

Take analgesics. Aspirin, acetaminophen and ibuprofen work for pain no matter where it is.

Wear a firm-fitting support bra. Bouncing breasts can only add to your discomfort.

Use prescription drugs as a last resort. Danazol, a drug that works by interfering with hormone production by the ovaries, should be reserved for those few who are truly disabled by their breast symptoms, says Dr. Love. Danazol can cause serious side effects such as skipped menstrual periods (which can lead to bone loss), acne, oily skin, growth of facial hair, fluid retention and weight gain.

That's *some* help. But will there ever be a "cure"? "Eventually," says Dr. Love, "we will be able to invent something as specific for breast pain as some of the anti-inflammatory drugs are for menstrual cramps, and women will no longer have to suffer from it."

See also Breast Care

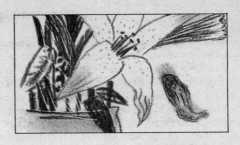

FIBROIDS

TREATMENT OPTIONS FOR
UTERINE GROWTHS

*E*lsa Davidson, a 39-year-old nutritionist, found out she had uterine fibroids during a routine gynecological examination. Although her doctor said she was "filled with them," they had caused her no discomfort. In fact, she had no clue she even *had* them. So she did as her doctor suggested—kept tabs on their growth with yearly checkups. During the next five years, the fibroids grew steadily, and gradually, so did the symptoms.

"My periods became so heavy that I would be in the bathroom every half-hour changing the super-plus tampon and the two extra heavy-duty pads that I needed to wear," says Elsa. "The monthly blood loss left me anemic and literally weak in the knees. Every time I got my period, I was in a constant panic that I wouldn't be able to find a bathroom in time and I'd bleed through my clothes."

Elsa knew decision time was drawing near when the fibroids became so large that they began pushing on her bladder, causing occasional incontinence along with, her monthly hemorrhage. After considering all her options, she decided that a hysterectomy was the right choice for her.

According to the National Center for Health Statistics, fibroids account for 30 percent of all hysterectomies in the United States—almost 200,000 per year. But by no means is hysterectomy the *only* solution to a fibroid problem, even if that's the way it sometimes appears.

THE DO-NOTHING-NOW OPTION

Fibroids are usually benign tumors composed mostly of muscle tissue; they range in size from a pea to a cantaloupe or even larger. They can be outside or inside the uterus, embedded in the uterine walls or attached by stalks (called pedunculated fibroids). Nobody really knows why they appear in the first place, but about 20 percent of women over 35 get them. Black women are three times more likely than whites to get them.

Fibroids are rarely cancerous (only about 1 in 1,000 is). So if you have no symptoms—and many women don't—there's no reason to take action, says Ruth Schwartz, M.D., clinical professor of obstetrics and gynecology at the University of Rochester School of Medicine and Dentistry in New York.

Since fibroids depend on estrogen for their growth, a woman nearing menopause (a time when estrogen production naturally begins to decline) may be able to wait it out. Fibroids are likely to shrink or disappear altogether after menopause. For younger women, it's best to monitor the fibroids to see if they grow, how fast they grow and whether or not they start to cause major discomfort, says Dr. Schwartz.

And for many women, they do. The American College of Obstetricians and Gynecologists says that about a third of women with fibroids complain of heavy bleeding with their periods. Another third experience pressure to varying degrees and pelvic pain.

SEX AND PREGNANCY COMPLICATIONS

Diane Shapiro, a 42-year-old secretary, says that the bleeding and pain from her fibroids increased to the point that she stopped dating. "I'm a single woman, and I was afraid that if I met someone I was interested in, I wouldn't feel right telling him that for me intercourse was painful," she says. "You know, a wife can say to a husband, 'Don't do this, it hurts.' I figured I'd scare any potential boyfriend away with this problem. That's when I knew I had to do something about it. What was I going to do, spend the rest of my life alone?"

Fibroids can also interfere with pregnancy or delivery, although admittedly the vast majority cause no trouble at all, says Carol Ann Burton, M.D., clinical instructor of obstetrics and gynecology at the University of Southern California School of Medicine in Los Angeles.

"If the fibroid is located on the inside of the uterus, the placenta may not implant properly, leading to a first-trimester miscarriage," she says. "Sometimes fibroids grow rapidly during pregnancy due to the hormonal environment. As the uterus stretches, premature labor may occur. Or the fibroid may outgrow its blood supply and die, causing excruciating pain as it degenerates."

AVOIDING HYSTERECTOMY

To get rid of fibroids, a doctor could just take out the whole uterus, fibroids and all. But that may not be necessary. Believe it or not, doctors have been performing myomectomies—the surgical removal of *just* the fibroids—since the 1800s. And what could be called the traditional myomectomy is getting to be the more preferred technique. Each year about 18,000 are performed—perhaps because more women are demanding alternatives to hysterectomy.

During a traditional myomectomy, a physician makes cuts through the abdomen and the uterus. The fibroids are cut out, then the incisions are stitched closed. It is major surgery, however, and like any major surgery, there's the possibility of infection, an adverse reaction to anesthesia or blood loss requiring blood transfusion, says Dr. Burton. In fact, blood loss may be even greater for myomectomy than hysterectomy, although recuperation time is about the same—four to six weeks.

What's more, in about 25 percent of cases the fibroids regrow within five years, either from little "seedlings" that were missed during the initial surgery or from new fibroids that develop after the operation. Then either the operation may have to be repeated or a hysterectomy done after all, adds Dr. Schwartz, who is also a member of the American College of Obstetricians and Gynecologists's task force on hysterectomy. The more fibroids there are to begin with, the greater the chance of recurrence.

And because a myomectomy involves cutting into the uterus, it's possible that adhesions or scarring may cause pregnancy or fertility problems later. Granted, say doctors, these complications are not common. And for women whose fibroids are causing pregnancy problems, the operation is usually beneficial.

THE MICROSURGERY OPTION

If you happen to have very small fibroids, you may be eligible for some of the newer procedures that vastly shorten recuperation time and reduce the potential for complications. The location of your fibroids often dictates the type of technique your doctor can perform to remove them. Consequently, there isn't just one procedure that's right for everyone.

Fibroids that extend into the cavity of the uterus, for example, can usually be handled with a hysteroscope, a telescope-type instrument that is inserted through the vagina and cervix, allowing visual inspection of the inside of the uterus, explains Dr. Schwartz. The hysteroscope can be equipped with a laser that burns away the tumors, or with a resectoscope, an instrument that uses an electric current to shave down the tumors.

Small fibroids that are located on the outside of the uterus, on the other hand, can often be removed with a laparoscope, an instrument that's inserted through a tiny incision near the navel. The laparoscope can also be equipped with a laser or other cauterizing attachment to remove fibroids, says Dr. Schwartz.

Both the hysteroscopic and laparoscopic procedures are done on an outpatient basis—a major advantage. The procedures themselves cost about the same as a traditional myomectomy, but generally, there are no hospital costs. There may be mild cramping for a few days afterward, Dr. Schwartz says, but recovery is quick. A woman can usually return to work in less than a week. The down side is that even with these less-invasive procedures, the tumors can grow back, necessitating a possible repeat performance or a hysterectomy.

SHRINK FIRST, OPERATE LATER

Even if your fibroids are large, you may still be able to take advantage of microsurgical techniques. This is an option to discuss with your doctor. A new class of drugs—called Gn-RH agonists (gonadotropin releasing hormone)—taken for a few months can actually shrink fibroids enough that major abdominal surgery can be avoided.

These drugs block the ovaries' production of the female hormone estrogen. And since fibroids are estrogen-sensitive tumors, they shrink—not all the way, but by 40 to 50 percent on the average. And because the medications also cut down the blood supply in the uterus, says Dr. Schwartz, myomectomies can be performed with less blood loss.

Actually, if you should happen to be near menopause, taking one of these drugs may help you avoid surgery altogether, says Dr. Burton. By the time you finish a course of treatment, your body's natural decline in estrogen production may finish the job for you. Since the drugs put you in an artificial state of menopause, they can only be used for about six months.

Once you stop taking these drugs and estrogen production recurs, so do the fibroids, usually within six months. That may not matter if the idea is to shrink the fibroids enough for microsurgery.

SLOW THE FLOW

If your fibroids are not large, and the only grief they're giving you is heavy bleeding, there are other options you might discuss with your doctor. Drugs such as danazol (a synthetic steroid derived from male hormones) will curb abnormally heavy bleeding, although they'll do nothing to shrink the fibroids. You may, however, find that the side effects of these drugs are more than you care to live with. About 80 percent of women experience some side effects, which include excess weight gain, bloating, hair growth, elevated cholesterol and vaginal spotting. These are mild in most cases.

Another possible alternative is a procedure called laser ablation therapy. Using a laser-equipped hysteroscope, the uterine lining is literally destroyed. No lining, no bleeding. But the fibroids are still there and could conceivably grow and cause trouble in the future. A woman is also considered sterile after this procedure. So clearly, this isn't for everyone. If you've completed your family, however, and the heavy bleeding cannot be controlled by other means, then laser ablation is a possible solution. It's done on an outpatient basis and recovery is very quick. Patients go home the same day and are back to work in just one or two days. Side effects are usually mild.

THE BEST DECISION FOR YOU

There's no one treatment that's just right for everyone. Indeed, there are pros and cons to just about every choice. Question your doctor about what she's planning to do and why. Seek a second opinion if you feel uncertain about her judgment or simply want more information. You may feel, after all is said and done, that a hysterectomy is the right choice for you. It is, after all, the only sure "cure" for fibroids. In any case, though, look for a doctor skilled in the technique that you've decided upon.

See also Endometriosis, Hysterectomy

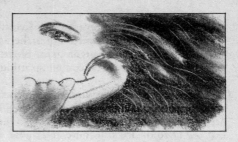

FRIENDSHIP

THE DIFFERENCE BETWEEN THE SEXES

*I*t's ironic that Hollywood is so enamored of the male buddy movie. Some of the most memorable platonic love stories of the screen have paired Newman and Redford, Gibson and Glover, Hoffman and Cruise, not to mention various permutations of the Brat Pack. What's ironic is that this brand of "bond" picture enshrines a relationship that research has consistently shown is about as rare as a hockey game without a fistfight.

Lillian B. Rubin, Ph.D., a senior research associate at the Institute for the Study of Social Change at the University of California in Berkeley, has studied the role of friendship, which she calls the neglected relationship. It's women's friendships, she says, not men's, that ought to be the stuff of film and story.

HERE'S TO GOOD FRIENDS

"Women at all stages of life have more intimate, close, nurturing relationships than men do," says Dr. Rubin, who interviewed 300 men and women about their relationships. "I believe that may be one of the reasons men who are left widowed tend to have higher mortality and morbidity rates than women. It's not because men can't cook an egg but because they usually do not have intimate, close relationships, even with their children. Women who are widowed tend to live out their lives with close relationships and friendships that enrich them and make life worth living."

Women's ability to nurture friendships may even be one of the reasons why they live longer than men. Since the 1970s, study after study has found that friendships and social relationships are good for your health. In fact, many of those studies have implied that without social attachments, you're doomed. In 1979, two researchers who studied the health and social affiliations of nearly 5,000 residents of Alameda County, California, found that they could predict who would die within the nine years under survey simply by counting how many social ties they had. On the strength of this and similar studies, the California Department of Health launched a program exhorting Californians to "make a friend" because "friends can be good medicine."

In fact, researchers now conclude that social relationships may have the ability to alter body chemistry, protecting us from a host of potentially fatal diseases from tuberculosis to cancer to heart disease.

THAT'S WHAT FRIENDS ARE FOR

Friends are the people who are there to throw you a rope when you're drowning. They're also a buffer against stress and loneliness. The phrase "among friends" can bring with it the same sense of comfort and relief as "home," because friends make us feel we're home.

How do we choose the friends we do? Often we choose friends who are like a "second self," says Dr. Rubin. Although the "why" of friendship is as mysterious as the "why" of love, we may gravitate toward those people whom we instinctively know will reflect back to us the person we are, or want to be.

"We're like two streams that flow together," says Stephanie Gordon of her friend, Laurel, who is also her business partner.

Like many friends, Stephanie and Laurel bring out the best in each other. "I never would have dreamed of starting my own business if Laurel hadn't been right there beside me. I never could have done it alone. It's nice to know I have someone to share the ups and downs with, and we complement one another. She's really organized and has good business sense, and I'm very creative. Then we have qualities we share, like a sense of humor and a way of looking at the world—kind of cockeyed. We laugh a lot."

BETTER THAN FAMILY

Friends often do for us what our family can't. We can talk to them about the things that are taboo among family members. "Friends are not judgmental," says Sarah Garrison, 47, a mother of two who recently married for the second time. "I could tell my best friend that I had an affair when I was married, but could I have told my mother? I don't think so. 'Hey Mom, guess what, I'm cheating on my husband.' I hate to think what my mother would have said."

As Dr. Rubin points out, our friends often serve as a more accurate mirror than our family, who are more likely to see us as we were, not as we are.

Sometimes, Dr. Rubin says, friends make up for deficits in our lives, are the surrogate parents or siblings we need to help us fill in the blank spots and learn to grow. "One of the major benefits I have seen in friends outside a marriage is that it takes the heat off inside," says Dr. Rubin. Friends can provide everything from intimacy to another point of view, even affection missing from a marriage, putting less pressure on both spouses to meet all the other's needs.

Friends also fill a special need for those who may be isolated—the elderly, for example. In a study of the health effects of forced relocation on 401 older people in New Haven and Hartford, Connecticut, researchers at Yale University found three factors that helped keep elderly people alive when they became ill: having a child living within 50 miles, belief and participation in religion and at least two good friends. Another study found that having close female friends, even more than marriage, children and grandchildren, was vital to a woman's sense of well-being in her later years.

STAYING FRIENDS

Few people need to be taught how to make friends, but in these busy days of "have your answering machine call my answering machine," keeping friends can be tough. Like other relationships, friendship takes time and work.

Lilly Keane, 44, puts a lot of effort into keeping her friendships going. She has a few good friends scattered around the country, and she keeps in touch with all of them. "I send a lot of cards," she says. "I'll see cards that remind me of my friends and I'll buy them and send them with a little note to let them know I'm thinking of them. And I am thinking of them. Part of me is always aware of the people I want to keep in my life."

Though she's "not a phone person," she also makes it a point to call regularly, even if it's just to check in. "Even if I haven't been in touch with someone for a while, I've never been too embarrassed to call."

In her book *Among Friends*, journalist Letty Cottin Pogrebin writes of a group of friends who actually do keep in touch through their answering machines, leaving messages "that are warm but brief." One woman writes letters over the lunch hour at work, and two friends meet on Saturday for a morning cup of coffee before they begin housecleaning—both their houses, together.

One segment of society that desperately needs friends but has trouble keeping them is new mothers, who are often too tired and too busy to keep up a social life. Studies have shown that new mothers are happier and more confident when they meet regularly with other women, particularly other mothers.

"You often lose old friends when you have a baby because you're less available to them," says psychologist Ellen McGrath, Ph.D., executive director of the Psychology Center in Laguna Beach, California. "People can feel rejected."

To help your friendships stay intact, she says, you need

CAN HARRY BE FRIENDS WITH SALLY?

Can men and women be friends? That is, *just* friends, pals, buddies, chums—with no sex?

That question was the premise of the movie *When Harry Met Sally* and the answer in Nora Ephron's witty script was an equivocal, "Well, yes and no." Harry and Sally were friends, and then became lovers, which almost ruined a beautiful friendship *and* a beautiful love affair.

But can men and women really be friends? The research proves they can. But friendship with a man tends to be a different kind of relationship than women have with one another, in large part because men and women regard friendship in very different ways. For women, friends are those people to whom you bare your innermost thoughts.

The hallmark of women's friendships is intimacy. Very few men have intimate relationships with one another. They *do* things, rather than *share* things with one another. Instead, men save their intimacy for the women in their lives. In her study of over 300 people and their friendships, social researcher Lillian B. Rubin, Ph.D., found very few men who could name a best friend, but those who did most frequently named a woman.

Male friends, says Dr. Rubin, allow a woman to express her "harder edge," the part of herself that she may hide from her women friends. "Sex is almost always an undercurrent in all cross-sex friendships. It's part of what makes such friendships attractive and even titillating.

"But most women and men agree that acting on the attraction by becoming sexually involved with each other would risk the friendship, since sex tends to stir longings that are inappropriate for friendship," she adds.

Some men and women are able to successfully mix friendship with sexual pleasure, but most male/female friends carefully skirt the whole issue. Sex can confuse and change a friendship forever. Not every good friend can make the transition to lover, Harry and Sally notwithstanding.

to do some preparation beforehand. Coach your friends and let them know you're not going to be available as much. When the baby actually comes, get together as often as you can, but don't spend the entire time talking about the baby.

It's important, she says, no matter how busy you are, to make time for your friends. "You need to be especially sensitive to your friends and yourself." This is particularly true when your life paths begin to separate—perhaps you work and she doesn't or you're married and she isn't. Stay sensitive to each other and don't disconnect from her experience because it's so different from yours. You're just at different times and different stages in your lives. Soon you may be back sharing the same experiences again.

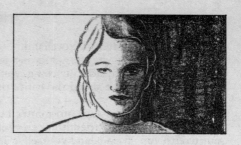

GRIEF

IT'S OH, SO PERSONAL

*B*uddhist legend tells of a young woman who grieved for her infant son so intensely that she would not give up the body for burial. Clutching her precious burden, she approached the wise and compassionate Buddha and asked for his help. He agreed to help, on one condition. She must go down into the nearby village and return with a mustard seed (a common spice for that time and place) from a household that had never been touched by death.

She returned to the Buddha that night without the seed. And, after arranging for her son's burial, she became one of the Buddha's disciples. Her door-to-door quest had taught her an all-important lesson—that grief is universal.

At some point in our lives, each one of us will experience grief. But for all its universality, it's one of the least understood emotions.

Although most of us think of grief as the vortex of painful feelings that follows the death of someone close to us, psychologists have long recognized that grief accompanies other significant losses—divorce, the loss of a job, a home, friends, a pet, our health, our dreams, even our sense of who we are.

GRIEF HAS MANY FACES

According to University of Michigan researcher Camille Wortman, Ph.D., grief often involves "a permanent change that cannot be altered or undone." And the "changes" that can create this devastating sense of loss can be surprisingly varied. For example, fertility experts have identified the profound emotions that accompany a diagnosis of infertility as a grief reaction, generated as a couple struggles to come to terms with the loss of their dreams of parenthood. Even something positive, such as getting a new job or marrying, can trigger grief. Although a new job or a marriage are certainly not the end of a life, they can be the end of life as you know it. At a time when you expect to be so happy, feelings of grief and sadness can be confusing, as Rita Harper learned.

A few years ago, Rita left the newspaper where she had worked for eight years for a job as an editor at a national magazine in New York. "I should have been thrilled out of my mind. It was what I wanted more than anything in the world. But all I could think about was leaving the people I had come to know and love over those eight years," says Rita. "I cried all the time. I couldn't sleep. I alternately stopped eating or overate. I knew enough to know that those were the signs of depression, but I couldn't figure out why I was depressed. I finally went to a counselor who helped me realize that I was grieving for the life and the people I was leaving behind."

What makes a loss painful and hard to bear, says therapist Alla Renee Bozarth, Ph.D., is the meaning we have given—sometimes unconsciously—to what we have lost. The more of ourselves we have invested in a person, place or thing, the more deeply we feel the loss. "In being cut off from that someone or something," writes Dr. Bozarth in her book *Life Is Goodbye, Life Is Hello*, "I am in fact cut off from that part of me that the other represented. I have lost a part of my own self. Finding my way back to the missing part of myself, reclaiming it from the person or thing now gone, is the process I have called grieving. It is, literally, a lifesaving process."

AS YOU LIVE AND GRIEVE

It is also a painful and frightening process. Although it's generally accepted that the grieving process is a series of phases that range from shock and confusion to the regaining of equilibrium, it's clear that each person makes her own individual and solitary journey.

"We grieve as we live," says Elizabeth Harper Neeld, Ph.D. Her book, *Seven Choices: Taking the Steps to a New Life after Losing Someone You Love*, was written after dozens of interviews with people who survived the loss of someone close and also chronicles her own struggle to deal with her husband's death.

"There is no *proper* way to grieve," says Dr. Neeld. "If you display a lot of emotion normally, you may respond with a lot of emotion. A quiet person may respond with increased quietness. An efficient person may become more efficient. Some people become ill, some become very angry, some people act as if nothing has happened. Some people will clean the house from top to bottom, and some won't be able to move off the couch. They act that way because something profound has happened and that's their way of responding. It's ridiculous to think there is a proper way to react. The only thing that's proper is to take into account that something has happened that has snapped the thread of continuity in our lives."

GIVE IT TIME

Just as there is no prescription for grieving, there is no timetable for grief.

Studies that have looked at the course of the grieving process have found that a significant number of people do not "get over it" or resolve their feelings for years, if at all. Researchers at the University of California at San Francisco School of Nursing interviewed families that had experienced what may be the most grievous loss of all—the loss of a child. They found that a surprising number of families that had lost a child to cancer continued to feel a sense of pain and loss—often described as an empty space in their lives—seven to nine years afterward. Although the families had gone on with their lives and no longer felt intense pain on a daily basis, they viewed the loss as part of themselves and their grief as a connection to the child who had died.

"Scars are always, always there," one mother explained. "Part of that I don't ever want to lose, because I feel connected."

Although these families represented the largest segment of the study group, the researchers found that other families had dealt with the loss of their children in much different ways. Some felt they had truly "gotten over it," accepting the death as God's will, or as one parent explained, as "a thing that happens." Others tried to fill the void by becoming involved in projects such as doing charitable work, building a house or by having or adopting a child.

A CHAOTIC PROCESS

In her work, Dr. Neeld has found that those who successfully deal with the losses in their lives go through a process of healing that is, at best, chaotic. "It's not a straight line. You go back and forth through phases. At times it seems you have no direction, but it's all headed toward integrating the experience, of making some sense of it. It's not a matter of 'getting over it.' We don't ever put the loss behind us or get over it. It becomes part of who we are for the rest of our lives, but not in a dominating way. The people I interviewed had integrated their losses into their lives and weren't undone by them."

For many people, the initial reaction to a loss is one of shock and denial. But it's not true denial. The initial "numbness" we feel is a self-protective device, an "anesthetic of the heart," as Dr. Bozarth describes it. This merciful numbness allows us to absorb the reality gradually. One woman recalls repeating the word "no" over and over again after learning that her best friend had died in a freak accident. "Somewhere inside I understood what I was hearing," she says, "but I didn't want it to be true."

After the shock wears off, you may pass through phases of profound sadness, anger, guilt, depression, helplessness, confusion and erratic or impulsive behavior. You may find yourself thinking obsessively about the person you lost.

You may also experience physical symptoms. Appetite loss, insomnia and even more serious illnesses are common.

Even though we know that life is ephemeral, we are still shocked, both mentally and physically, by death.

REBUILDING A LIFE

In her research, Dr. Neeld found that most people go through what she calls a second crisis once the initial distress seems to be over and they come to grips with the long-term implications of their loss. This second crisis may be even more painful than the first. It's like childbirth, but the new life you are giving birth to is your own. "Those longer-term tasks of building a new identity, new patterns, new behaviors, taking new action, will resurrect your grief because, if nothing else, they will remind you of what you have lost," says Dr. Neeld.

"What's hard is you're not leaving the loss behind," she says. "You're building a new identity that's you—you *plus* the loss. You've lost your assumed future and now you need a new one. That's called hope. That's called life. You don't get that overnight."

You may even resist building a new life for yourself, out of loyalty to the loved one you lost. "It's hard, because we don't know how to love a dead person," says Dr. Neeld. "We think holding on is the only way. You don't have them, and so you're in this never-never land. It's very seductive because it's easier to stay there than to do the next half of the grieving process, which is forging a new identity."

In fact, working through grief can be as tough as a second job, says Dr. Neeld. It's hard work, during which you often make imperceptible progress, and the relapses can be many. Although your grief is uniquely your own, those who specialize in helping others work through grief have some suggestions for reaching the stage of acceptance.

FEEL THE PAIN

"You have to tell the truth about your feelings and you have to feel them," says Dr. Neeld. No matter how painful it may be, the first and best way to grieve is to allow yourself to feel it fully.

"Pain has a stubborn habit of not going away just because we deny it exists," explains Dr. Bozarth. "Pain is an essential part of any growth process—the processes of growing up, growing old, growing beyond grief. . . . Ultimately, the only way to get through something is to get *through* it—not over, under or around it, but all the way through it. And it has to take as long as it takes."

Allow yourself to cry, to yell, to throw things, to feel numb or angry or scared. Realize that it's normal to feel angry at your loved one, at God or at the world for hurting or abandoning you. It's normal to be afraid of life alone or to be afraid about your future.

"It all comes with the territory," says Dr. Neeld. Trying to put up a brave front or hiding your feelings from yourself and others may simply force them to emerge elsewhere in other, more destructive ways, she says.

Don't be afraid if you think or do "crazy," impulsive and seemingly self-destructive things after you lose a loved one, explains Dr. Neeld. Some people have hallucinations or other "supernatural" experiences after they lose a loved one, she says.

"After I broke up with my fiancé, I went out with and slept with anyone who asked me," confesses one woman. "I don't know why I didn't come down with a disease, I was that indiscriminate. After a few months of that, I realized how dangerous that was, and I stopped. But for a while, the whole world seemed out of control, and I didn't see why I shouldn't be, too."

Another woman whose best friend was killed says for months afterward she would dial her friend's phone number, hoping she would pick up the phone. "I knew she was dead and I know it sounds nuts," she remembers, "but part of me still hoped that if I called, she would answer."

When you have a hard time coming to grips with your feelings, talk about it. A counselor or an understanding friend can help you enormously.

"You need someone who is comfortable with your doing your grieving in any way you want to do it, as often as you want to, as long as you need to," says Dr. Neeld. "You need someone who doesn't say, 'you cried about that picture *last* week,' but instead who says, 'you may cry about that picture any time and as many times as you want to.' "

DO WHAT FEELS RIGHT

In her interviews, Dr. Neeld asked people what they did to deal with the healing process. The answers were varied—from gardening to going to an aquarium. "For each of them it was different, but for each of them it was a way of moving back into life," she says. Some found rituals—either religious or their own—meaningful and comforting. Some people exercise, others write in journals. Some turn to their faith for comfort, while others find that their faith is shattered, and they need to rebuild that faith.

"For months after I lost my dad and my oldest friend, who died within hours of each other, I felt like driving to the ocean and tossing flowers in," says one woman. "I didn't know why—I still don't—but I felt I wouldn't be 'finished' until I did. I finally did it on vacation. It was a handful of wildflowers at a Nantucket Sound beach. I felt something was truly laid to rest that day."

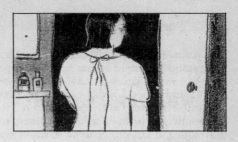

GYNECOLOGISTS

FINDING A PHYSICIAN WHO CARES

*A*my Glass says she can't remember her first date, the day she graduated from college or half the men she dated before she got married. "But I can remember my first trip to the gynecologist as if it were yesterday," says the 41-year-old schoolteacher.

She was 19, had recently become sexually active with the man she would eventually marry and wanted to get birth control pills.

"I was the kind of person who didn't even get undressed in front of my sister or best friend," she recalls. "As I lay there with my legs up in stirrups, I could feel my face grow hot and my heart pound. I wanted to cry from embarrassment when the doctor told me to spread my knees. I opened them an inch or two, and then he had to pry them open the rest of the way. It was all so matter-of-fact for him. He had no idea what a nightmare it was for me."

Twenty years and three kids later, Amy still dreads her annual trip to the gynecologist. And she's far from alone. Even women gynecologists hate it.

AN ANNUAL ORDEAL

Naked and flat on your back, with legs high and spread-eagled, and *not* being face-to-face with your doctor—who is practically a stranger and most likely a man—can be a mortifying experience, even in the best doctor/patient relationships.

"Women will tell me, 'I love you, Dr. Thornton, but I can't stand having to get into that position, so hurry up,' " says Yvonne S. Thornton, M.D., associate professor of obstetrics and gynecology at Cornell University Medical College in New York City. "And I can relate to that, because I have to go through it once a year, too. It's probably the biggest reason why women don't come in for yearly gynecological examinations, even though they should."

And while no one will ever admit to enjoying the medical care necessity known as the annual, the right doctor can actually help make it as easy as possible, says Dr. Thornton. A caring doctor, for example, will talk to you at length before the actual physical exam. "I want to know the psychological makeup of my patient," says Dr. Thornton. "Does she seem very nervous? Does she cry easily? Has something made her unhappy during a previous gynecological examination? Is she a virgin? Does she have three children? There's no rushing the patient. I feel it's important to take as much time as is needed."

And the right doctor will also make it as comfortable as possible. Dr. Thornton has mink-covered stirrups (actually fake fur and washable), mobiles of balloons and seashells suspended from the ceiling just above each examining table and comfortable cloth dressing gowns. Not paper.

Cheryl Hogan says she has such a gynecologist and wishes she had met her 20 years ago. "I don't ever get nervous anymore," says the 39-year-old housewife. "My doctor asks me lots of questions about *me* and what's going on in my life, not just about my symptoms and body parts. She knows what I do for a living, and she knows all about my husband and daughter. Then during the exam, she tells me exactly what she's doing and why. There's always time for her to answer all my questions. And I come in with a written list!"

Cheryl admits to an initial encounter similar to Amy Glass's. "I purposely chose a woman because I figured I'd get some empathy. Instead I got a Nazi general! She was rough with me and barked orders like, 'You *will* relax!' I was 21, a virgin, and petrified. I *hated* when I had to go back."

PERSONALITY MINUS

Dr. Thornton can smile at Cheryl's description of her first doctor because it so typically fits one of the categories of obstetricians/gynecologists she has formulated. She calls it the female-insensitive. And it's the worst type there is.

"This female drill sergeant-type is such a disappointment because you've gone to her with the expectation that she'll be *more* compassionate, not less," says Dr. Thornton. "Yet here she is as rough and gruff as any man. You feel betrayed by your own sex."

The second worst in Dr. Thornton's book is the male-insensitive type. "To him you're just a pathological specimen upon which to practice his craft," she explains. "He does the exam, declares you healthy or sick, tells you to get dressed, says good-bye, boom, and he's out of there."

One woman, who'd been seeing the same gynecologist for ten years, said he stared at her blankly one night at a fund-raising event but gave her husband, whom he knew from a health club, a big hello. "He had no idea who I was," she says.

Another woman says that her gynecologist whistled while he worked, and then declared, based on his exam, that she would probably never be able to conceive a child. "I was 24 years old at the time and devastated by what he said," she says. "I hated him even more when I found out later from another doctor that he was wrong."

LOOKING FOR DR. RIGHT

The best kind of doctor to have is one who is compassionate—and it doesn't matter if it's a man or woman, says Dr. Thornton. But, she admits, the female-compassionate type is probably the best of them all.

"The truly nice male obstetrician/gynecologist has raised his level of consciousness and will listen and try to understand and solve your problems. He will not say your symptoms are all in your head," says Dr. Thornton. "The female-compassionate is the best, however, because she has all those qualities, plus she herself has been through vaginal labor, menstruation, infections, pelvic exams and mammograms. She has a keen insight to the feelings that are never written in books—the sort of unspoken thread that binds all women into a sorority. She *knows* for example, how you feel when you find out you have herpes, or when your heavy, painful periods ruin half of every month."

In fact, it's more important to investigate the type of person a doctor is than to inspect the degree on his or her wall. All gynecologists, no matter where they went to school, are trained to a certain standard, states Dr. Thornton. So, medically speaking, you can feel fairly secure as to the kind of care you'll receive. "But how that care is dispensed is another thing," she says. "The level of sensitivity to your feelings can vary from doctor to doctor. Does your gynecologist use a smaller speculum for smaller vaginas? Does he or she try to do a manual exam with one finger (instead of two) in a young woman whose vagina is so narrow that it can't even accommodate a pencil?"

If you're a healthy woman, an annual examination should *not* be painful. "You and your physician need to work out a plan so that you're relaxed. The more tense you are, the tighter your muscles become, and you wind up fighting against each other. When a patient tenses up, I tell her to hold the nurse's hand, take deep breaths, try to make her tummy as soft as possible. When she's relaxed, then I continue the exam."

A LOOK, A FEEL AND A PAP

Obviously, the purpose of a gynecological exam is not just to measure your embarrassment quotient. It's the best preventive medicine money can buy, and sometimes the only routine medical care women get. Often a woman's gynecologist also acts as her primary care physician.

"When I do a physical, I do it from top to bottom, because I know I'm probably the only doctor my patients see," says Dr. Thornton.

In addition to a pelvic and breast exam, both of which are important, a caring physician will also check your heart

SYMPTOMS THAT SAY SEE YOUR DOCTOR

Ideally, a woman should have her first pelvic examination by about age 18 or when she becomes sexually active—whichever comes first.

After that, many doctors, including Cornell University Medical College's Yvonne S. Thornton, M.D., recommend one every year.

But preventive care isn't the only reason you should see your gynecologist. A trip to the doctor is also warranted for the following female reproductive system symptoms.

- If you haven't begun menstruating by age 16.
- If your mother took the now-banned drug diethylstilbestrol (DES), once used to help problem pregnancies come to full term. Daughters of DES mothers have been found to be at an increased risk for uterine and cervical cancers.
- If you've been suffering from severe menstrual cramps.
- If your menstrual flow is very heavy or lasts longer than ten days or you experience any other vaginal bleeding.
- If you experience any burning, itching or unusual discharge.
- If you've been experiencing painful intercourse, especially if you also have chills or fever.
- If you are sexually active and have missed one period.
- If you miss three or more periods and are abstaining from sex.
- Any time you have burning when you urinate.

and thyroid. And the pelvic exam should also include a Pap smear. This is a painless procedure in which cells are scraped from the cervical wall and tested for cancer. Cervical cancer is one of the deadliest cancers in women.

A Pap smear, however, carries a 15 to 30 percent rate of false negatives. That is, the results may indicate that your cervix is normal when, in fact, it isn't. For these reasons, Dr. Thornton and most other specialists recommend a pelvic exam and Pap test every year as a safeguard.

If you prefer to be under the care of only one physician, it doesn't necessarily have to be a gynecologist, notes Lila A. Wallis, M.D., clinical professor of medicine at Cornell

University Medical College in New York City and past president of the American Medical Women's Association. "There are many internists who can do a comprehensive job and are skilled in office gynecological skills and have more psychosocial skills than gynecologists," she says. "There are also many women physicians who care and are well-versed in the reproductive tract as well as other systems. If a women prefers, she does *not* have to go back and forth between doctors."

See also Medical Care

CHAPTER 39

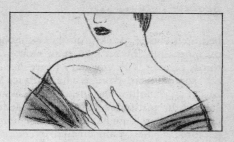

HEART DISEASE

WOMEN ARE A PRIME TARGET

*I*n a revealing Gallup survey, 501 women were asked, "What, in your opinion, is the number one killer of women 50 years of age and older?" Sixty-five percent of them said cancer. They were wrong.

The answer is heart disease. And only 15 percent got it right, which really isn't all that surprising. Until recently, heart disease has always been considered "a disease that kills men."

According to the American Heart Association, an estimated 247,000 of the more than 520,000 yearly deaths from heart attack—that's 47 percent—occur in women. And more than 90,000 women die each year of stroke. One in nine women from the ages of 45 to 64 has some form of cardiovascular disease, and the ratio climbs to one in three at age 65 and beyond.

SHAMEFUL NEGLECT

Startling statistics. So why then has heart disease always been thought of as something that happens mostly to men? And why has most of the focus been on men when it comes to winning the war against heart disease?

In part, say researchers who are presently examining the issue, because heart disease only becomes a problem to women later in life. Statistically, women generally lag 10 years behind men in developing heart disease and 20 years behind for heart attacks. Another is that heart disease comes on more suddenly in men than women. For almost two-thirds of men with coronary heart disease, their first sign that something is wrong is a heart attack, says Renee Hartz, M.D., a cardiothoracic surgeon and associate professor of surgery at Northwestern University Medical School in Chicago. But more than half the women first experience angina pectoris, a chest pain created by increasing pressure on arteries slowed down by the buildup of plaque.

The famous and long-standing Framingham Heart Study found that 75 percent of men with angina had a heart attack within five years—twice the rate of heart attack in women with angina. "These data fostered the widespread perception that angina pectoris was a benign problem in women," says Nanette K. Wenger, M.D., professor at Emory University School of Medicine and director of the cardiac clinics at Grady Memorial Hospital in Atlanta. "This flawed myth of better tolerance of angina fostered less attention to women with this symptom, and less concern with their preventive care and coronary risk modification."

THE MAKING OF A MYTH

If the medical profession itself can take a good deal of the blame for perpetuating the myth that women don't get heart disease, then so can the media and the advertising community. Think of the commercials you see on television. The one for a particular heart-healthy oil is typical. A wife tells how she is watching over her husband's heart health by preparing meals low in cholesterol. The message? It's only her husband who's at risk. She's watching his diet for his—but not her own—good.

"Women are not sensitized to think of themselves as being at risk of heart disease," says Nancy Norvell, Ph.D., a clinical psychologist who specializes in behavioral medicine at the University of South Florida in Tampa. "It's something men look out for. With women the buzz word is cancer. Television dramas give a leading character ovarian cancer, not heart disease, because that's what women will respond to," she states. "Women are constantly misled, and they mislead themselves by believing that they are somehow protected from heart disease because they are female."

IT'S ALL IN YOUR HEAD

And when women do experience chest pain, the complaint is often dismissed as nothing serious by their doctors. Dr. Hartz's own mother, who went to the emergency room of her local hospital with chest pain, was sent home with a few pain pills for what later turned out to be a heart attack. The next day she was in the cardiac intensive care unit.

"Women often tend to put off seeing a doctor when they experience chest pains," says Dr. Norvell. "In part that's because they've bought the myth that women don't get heart disease, especially not young women. But it's also because women are more likely to be dismissed by their doctors as being neurotic." One study found that women were twice as likely as men to have their cardiac symptoms attributed to psychiatric or other non-heart-related causes.

"There's also no stigma attached to a man whose chest pain turns out to be unrelated to a heart condition," Dr. Norvell adds. "It's accepted, in fact, expected for a man to be concerned about his heart."

ODD WOMEN OUT

It all adds up to some pretty peculiar thinking, especially when you consider that the odds are in favor of men—not women—when it comes to beating the disease.

"Women rarely show symptoms of heart disease before menopause, though it probably develops earlier," says Dr. Hartz. "Because of that, it has not received the public attention that it has in men, who are often stricken in their prime."

Consequently, the stakes are a lot higher. In one study of 5,839 people hospitalized for heart attack, 23 percent of the women died during their initial stay in the hospital, compared with only 16 percent of the men. And the American Heart Association reports that women who have heart

WOMEN, STRESS AND HEART DISEASE

Stress. It's a twentieth-century word created by twentieth-century pressures. In the house, on the job, from the boss, spouse, peers and the bill collectors. It was once the sole burden of men. But not anymore.

Some experts will argue that for women, especially working women, it's even worse. Women tend to have the need to be all things to all people. On the job or at home, the work never seems to end. Neither do the demands made by others on their time. It all goes into that pressure cooker known as stress, a contributing factor to many diseases, including the number one killer, heart disease.

"Women experience greater role conflict between work and family than their male counterparts," according to Margaret A. Chesney, Ph.D., associate adjunct professor in the Department of Epidemiology at the University of California School of Medicine in San Francisco. "Even in cases where men share tasks in the home, women, more than men, assume responsibility for seeing that these tasks are done.

"Employed men and women both show cardiovascular arousal during the workday," Dr. Chesney notes, "but they show distinctly different patterns in the evening. Men experience a decrease in arousal—'an unwinding'—that begins when they arrive home. Women, on the other hand, show an increase in arousal that extends into the evening." In other words, women don't "unwind" at the end of the day but continue their "workday" in the home environment.

What does all this stress add up to? Chest pain, says Linnea Lindholm, Ph.D., a research manager in the Department of Medicine, Division of Cardiology at the University of Florida in Gainesville. Women who have heart disease or who are at risk of developing it need to understand what being overworked, overburdened and overwhelmed can do to them. "Women can have such a hard time saying no that sometimes the only way they get a rest is when they get physically sick," says Dr. Lindholm, who counsels women with heart disease. "That's quite a price to pay."

Women must learn to pace themselves, delegate work and learn how to say no. "Saying no is the hardest. I ask the people I counsel, 'How likely is it that you will lose your job or make enemies if you say no once in a while?' And then we problem solve ways to change behavior patterns," says Dr. Lindholm. "When someone approaches you with another request or another project, get in the habit of saying, 'Can I get back to you on that?' Then go to a quiet place—your office, the lounge—and think about it for a while. It's so easy to get caught up in the moment and say yes before you know what you've gotten yourself into. Taking a few moments to look over your work load gives you the opportunity to realistically assess the time the project would take. It's easier then to call the person back and politely refuse."

Dorothy Metzger knows how hard that can be. But with Dr. Lindholm's help, she's succeeding. "I guess you could say that I was a compulsive worker, and I always worked under a great deal of stress. This used to go on for months at a time, until my body would rebel with chest pains," admits Dorothy. "I always understood the connection between diet and heart disease, but I had no idea of what stress could do."

Dr. Lindholm helped Dorothy become conscious of what that pressure was doing to her and taught her a few simple stress-reduction techniques. "Now I recognize within a day or two when the work load is piling up again, and I can fix the problem before my heart is affected," she says. "I don't get chest pain anymore."

attacks are twice as likely as men to die within the first few weeks.

What's more, women undergoing coronary artery bypass surgery have a mortality rate that's at least twice that of men who undergo the same operation. Dr. Hartz says that one of the reasons for this higher mortality risk may be due to size: Women are more difficult to operate on because they're smaller and their coronary arteries are smaller. Also, women are generally older and sicker than men when the surgery is eventually performed.

THE ESTROGEN CONNECTION

The operative word here is *older*. Women tend to get heart attacks and develop heart disease later in life. There's a reason for this: estrogen.

Researchers have known for a long time that this female hormone provides women protection against heart disease. (Interestingly, researchers who gave experimental doses of the hormone to men found it gave them no protection.) When hormone levels start to fall off and then stop at menopause, a woman's risk of heart disease starts to go up. But researchers have also discovered that she's at a lot less risk if she's taking estrogen replacement therapy (ERT). Women who use ERT have about half as many heart attacks as women not using estrogen, according to Trudy L. Bush, Ph.D., associate professor of epidemiology at Johns Hopkins University School of Hygiene and Public Health in Baltimore.

Experts believe that estrogen promotes higher levels of HDL cholesterol—the heart-protecting kind. They've found women who take estrogen have higher levels of HDL and lower levels of LDL cholesterol (the bad kind) than nonusers. "It's high levels of LDL that cause the heart and blood vessels to become clogged with fatty deposits," explains Dr. Bush. But high levels of HDL actually protect the heart and blood vessels against this fatty buildup.

But ERT is not risk-free. For one thing, it is suspected of increasing the risk of certain kinds of cancer.

GETTING HEART SMART

So there you have it. Heart disease is an equal opportunity killer. It doesn't favor men; it doesn't discriminate against women. And it doesn't have to get *you*.

Unless you were asleep through the 1980s, you already know that there is more evidence today than ever before that the way you live your life has a great deal to do with whether or not you'll become another statistic. But just in case you need a reminder, here's some advice you should take to heart.

Stop smoking. Women who smoke have a risk of heart attack that's 2 to 6 times that of a nonsmoker. If you smoke and use oral contraceptives, you are up to 39 *times* more likely to have a heart attack. If your husband smokes, get him to stop—for your sake. Statistics indicate there is a higher risk of death from heart disease among nonsmoking married women whose husbands are smokers than among women who live in nonsmoking households.

Keep your cholesterol level low. Preferably at 200 or below. Close to one-third of all American adult women have cholesterol levels that put them at increased risk of developing heart disease. Cholesterol is the substance that creates plaque buildup in the arteries. If your level is over 240 milligrams per deciliter (mg/dl), the risk of heart disease is twice what it would be if the level were below 200. One study suggests that coronary atherosclerosis (narrowing of the arteries in the heart) can actually be reversed by reducing blood cholesterol levels.

Lose weight. People who weigh 30 percent or more over their desirable weight are more likely to develop heart disease and stroke, even if they have no other risk factors. In the Framingham Heart Study, each 10 percent reduction in weight resulted in a 20 percent drop in the incidence of coronary heart disease.

Keep your blood pressure in check. More than half of all women over age 55 have high blood pressure, according to the American Heart Association. But it's by no means limited to the middle and upper years. If yours is high, you may be able to bring it back down to normal by losing weight and reducing salt in your diet. Or you may need to take a special prescription medication to control it. In the Framingham Heart Study, each 10-point decrease in blood pressure was accompanied by a 30 percent reduction in the incidence of heart disease.

Keep on the move. That is, exercise. Research has shown over and over again that you have to work your heart to make it work for you. In particular, aerobic exercise (and that includes walking, jogging, swimming and biking) has been shown to lower blood pressure, lower total cholesterol and raise beneficial HDL cholesterol.

Cut out the fat. Especially the saturated kind. Doctors agree and research has concluded that a high-fat diet is the key factor when it comes to inviting heart disease. You can do this by increasing your intake of fruits, vegetables and grains and decreasing your intake of red meats, luncheon meats and fried foods.

Ask your doctor about taking aspirin. Doctors have known for years that regular use of aspirin cuts the rate of heart attacks in men. But since none of the studies showing that included women, doctors were reluctant to recommend the same thing for women. But now a study, which followed more than 87,000 nurses for six years, shows that women can benefit by taking aspirin, too.

Consider estrogen replacement therapy. It isn't for everyone, but if you have any of the risk factors that contribute to heart disease, you may want to consider estrogen as an option. Talk it over with your doctor.

Build a network of social support. Research indicates that women lacking social ties are more than three times as likely to die from heart disease as women who have strong social ties.

See also Estrogen Replacement Therapy

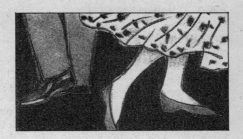

HOUSEWORK

WINNING THE CHORE WARS

*T*raditionally, housework has been woman's work, a domestic task of no inherent value—until you have to pay someone else to do it.

While women, by moving into the work world, have been able to gain "male" power and independence by earning a paycheck, there's no traditionally masculine payoff for cleaning toilets or diapering a baby. A man might cook—since most chefs are men, that might be viewed as an "important" job—but balk at cleaning up, a minimum-wage job in most places. Only money and power equal prestige, as working women have come to understand. This may explain some of the reluctance men show toward taking on domestic duties, possibly one of the lowest-prestige jobs around.

Or it may be even simpler than that, suggests Diane Martinez, M.D., a psychiatrist at the University of Texas Health Science Center at San Antonio and a working wife and mother. Men, she says, are just not tuned-in to domestic tasks. In all likelihood, if they helped out around the house as children, they were given sex-stereotyped roles—trash-hauling as opposed to dusting. They may not ever know without being told that the dirtiest place in the house is the top—or bottom—of the refrigerator. Being born a woman doesn't mean you're genetically tidier than a man, but it's the rare men's college dorm that gets the Good Housekeeping Seal of Approval.

WHO CARES?

"A lot of men really don't care if the floor is vacuumed," says Dr. Martinez. And it's more than just stubbornness, she says. "It just doesn't bother them. They're not organized in the same way as women are in terms of keeping track of when the dog needs a bath or the kids need their immunizations. Even when my husband does the dishes, he doesn't wash the pans, clean the food out of the drain or let the dirty dishwater out of the sink. It drives me crazy, but it doesn't bother him at all," she says. "Men don't often do things to our standards even if they are well-intentioned and trying as hard as they can."

One often-overlooked clue that you are defeating yourself is when you criticize or reject your spouse's efforts to be helpful, sensitive and supportive. You need to give him a break—after all, he's new at it, says Dr. Martinez.

THE EASY WAY OUT

Phyllis George, former beauty queen who has done everything from being a sportscaster to serving as first lady of Kentucky, probably offers the best solution to the housework dilemma that plagues most two-career couples. "The most popular labor-saving device is still money," she says.

The experts all agree. If you can afford it, buy your way out of some unnecessary bickering: Hire help.

Dr. Martinez says her life has been saved by her housekeeper of three years. "She can drive, she can think, she can speak two languages. I can literally ask her to do anything, even the most complicated task. She can't see my patients for me. I haven't asked her to do that. But she can do everything else and with her there the house runs smoothly."

But you can grow too dependent on outside help. When her housekeeper gets sick, Dr. Martinez says, "things just go to hell. Fortunately, she rarely gets sick."

But you don't need a housekeeper to make your life easier. Helen Bergey, a career woman, mother and wife, hired a woman to clean her house once a week. "It costs me $35 and it is money well spent," she says. "My husband and I don't argue about who's going to do what on our only days off, and frankly, our cleaning woman is a better housekeeper than I ever was. The funniest thing is, though, my cleaning woman is in a two-paycheck family, too, and even *she* has to hire a cleaning woman!"

There are other tasks you can foist onto others for a fee unless you live in the hinterlands. Many dry cleaners also do laundry. Some supermarkets will deliver (and you can fax them your shopping list!). And, with the trend toward healthier foods, once or twice a week you can have a nutritious take-out meal that isn't fried and packed in Styrofoam.

NEGOTIATING POWER

What if you can't afford even occasional outside help? Your other option may be less of a sure thing. You need to negotiate with your family, an often delicate transaction that, for many women, achieves only middling success.

What most of the experts recommend is that you and your spouse sit down and draw up a detailed, explicit plan for who does what and when and post it in a public spot in your house. The operative word here is explicit.

"If you've made a deal with your husband that you'll cook dinner if he gives the kids baths, you had better make it clear that he has to clean up the towels in the bathroom afterward," says psychologist Matti Gershenfeld, Ph.D., director of the Couples Learning Center in Jenkintown, Pennsylvania. "Many men will do the fun part of the bath and leave the bathroom a mess."

If who does what is a sore spot in your relationship, you really need to make your discussions heart-to-heart. Tell your spouse what you want and ask him how he feels. Chances are, says Dr. Martinez, you'll be met with a flood of anger and resentment because he thinks you don't appreciate all the things he *does* do.

Best of all, she says, he's likely to suggest a plan of action that, because it's his plan, he's more likely to follow.

It's important to remember that men doing housework is a recent phenomenon. In many cases, men and women have very different ideas about what "cleaning the house" means. "To my husband, cleaning the house means picking up the clutter," says top flight executive and mother Carolyn Roberts. "To me, it has something to do with a bucket of water and soap."

The Roberts' compromise seemed obvious to them. David picks up the clutter. Carolyn follows after him with a bucket of water and soap.

One important caveat: Once your husband and family agree to pitch in, don't criticize. "He doesn't have to do it the way you do it," says Dr. Gershenfeld. "It's not important if you dust first and then vacuum and he vacuums first, then dusts. It doesn't matter if he loads the dishwasher from the front to the back or the back to the front. What matters is he's doing it."

See also Dual Careers

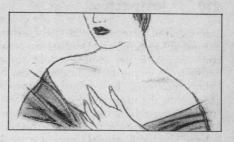

HYSTERECTOMY

CONTROVERSY AND CONSEQUENCES

*E*ach year, 650,000 American women have a hysterectomy, a major surgical procedure that removes the uterus and puts an end to a woman's childbearing years. It's an operation so prevalent in the United States, in fact, that the odds are that one out of every three women will have the operation by the time she reaches age 60, according to the National Center for Health Statistics.

And it is an operation planted in a hotbed of controversy. Concerned doctors and other health care practitioners say that up to 90 percent of all hysterectomies may not be necessary. It's a concern based on the fact that hysterectomy is the second most common major surgery performed in the United States—rating up to five times higher than in other developed countries such as France, Denmark, Sweden, Norway and the United Kingdom. The difference between the United States and other countries is so significant, in fact, that one joke reportedly circulating among doctors is: "What do you call a woman in San Diego who still has her uterus?" Answer: "A tourist."

THE CRADLE OF CONTROVERSY

Is there something about the American uterus that makes it more likely to require removal than a womb bred in France?

No, says Ruth Schwartz, M.D., clinical professor of obstetrics and gynecology at the University of Rochester School of Medicine and Dentistry in New York. A hysterectomy is specifically indicated only for complications that result from giving birth, uncontrolled bleeding for which other treatment has failed, cancer, and precancerous changes in the uterus, she says.

Unfortunately, these are not the main reasons for which hysterectomies are performed in the United States. Figures released by the National Center for Health Statistics reveal that 30 percent of all hysterectomies are to remove fibroids, which are usually benign tumors often causing pain or excessively heavy periods. Twenty percent are performed for a variety of miscellaneous reasons, such as urinary incontinence or "menstrual disorders"—a gynecological catchall that may include uncontrolled bleeding but that also covers almost anything else.

Almost 20 percent are performed to alleviate endometriosis, a condition in which clumps of the uterine lining grow outside the uterus. Prolapsed uterus accounts for another 16 percent, and cancer—the chief indication to *have* a hysterectomy—accounts for a mere 10 percent.

These statistics indicate that 75 percent of hysterectomies are done for non-life-threatening conditions and that somewhere between 80 and 90 percent may not be necessary at all. But these percentages are based on assumptions coming out of only one corner, because not all doctors agree as to what is just reason for removing the uterus, notes the American College of Obstetricians and Gynecologists.

DO YOUR OWN THINKING

Dr. Schwartz acknowledges the difference of opinion from doctor to doctor. One reason, she explains, has to do with the training given at various American medical schools. Doctors at some schools are quite conservative and will teach their students to make medical judgments that help a woman keep her uterus unless it endangers her health. Doctors at other schools are less conservative and will teach their students to judge a uterus that is acting up as though it is excess baggage.

The result is a difference of medical opinion that varies from region to region across the country—a difference that may explain, for example, why women in the South have twice as many hysterectomies as their Yankee cousins.

Your best defense against an unnecessary hysterectomy? Information—and a second opinion, says Nora W. Coffey, president of Hysterectomy Educational Resources and Services, an educational organization in Bala Cynwyd, Pennsylvania. Educational organizations can supply information about the surgery and its options and give you someone to talk to who has gone through the experience of surgery.

"Women often feel as if hysterectomy is some kind of rite of passage, something that will happen in their lifetime," Coffey adds. "Their mothers had one, their sisters, grandmothers or aunts had one, and so what if they have one, too?"

But much of the time, women may not need the surgery. "Of the women whom we referred to specialists for second opinions, 98 *percent* did not need to have hysterectomies," says Coffey.

WHEN OVARIES ARE REMOVED, TOO

Nearly half of all hysterectomies performed also include removal of the ovaries, a procedure Carol Ann Burton, M.D., refers to as castration.

"It's the equivalent to removing a man's testicles," says Dr. Burton, clinical instructor of obstetrics and gynecology at the University of Southern California School of Medicine in Los Angeles. "The ovaries are the chief sex hormone-producing organ in the body. When the ovaries are removed, it produces an instant and intense menopause, with all the typical symptoms." And although estrogen replacement therapy can usually help the body adjust, it's still not as good as producing your own hormones.

"Even 'old' ovaries are vital sex hormone producers," according to Winnifred B. Cutler, Ph.D., author of *Hysterectomy: Before and After*. "At any age, their loss produces a significant bodily deficit. You should try to keep your ovaries, regardless of your age." Keeping them, she notes, does not increase your risk of ovarian cancer as was once thought. Ovarian cancer in and of itself is rare.

POST-OP PROBLEMS

Although most physicians say that the women they operate on rarely experience post-operative problems, studies show that hysterectomy is more frequently associated with depression than other major surgery. And other research suggests that this operation—even without ovary removal—may increase the risk of heart disease, early ovarian failure, bone loss and sexual dysfunction. Conversely, still other research indicates that women who have hysterectomies live longer than women who don't. Unfortunately, the research in these areas remains inconsistent and inconclusive. But it does raise some serious concerns.

Coffey claims that she has counseled thousands of women suffering from post-hysterectomy depression as well as a wide range of other long-term problems, such as loss of sex drive, joint pain, insomnia, weight gain, urinary problems and fatigue. "Doctors will tell you it's all in your head, or that you're the only one they've ever heard with these complaints," she says. And it's simply not true.

"There are some reports that hysterectomy dramatically affects sexual desire and functioning," agrees Dr. Schwartz. "But in my own personal survey of patients during 35 years of practicing medicine, hysterectomy seems to impact the lives of those women who have had sexual problems before their surgery."

To minimize the possibility of such an impact, says Dr. Schwartz, she always discusses with each patient what the woman's uterus means to her, and—since her husband's opinion can play a role in how she feels—how he feels about it, too.

THE POSITIVE SIDE OF SURGERY

Of course, for some women, surgery is not only the only resourse, it also has a very happy ending. For Barbara Paulson, having a hysterectomy resulted in a renewed life.

Barbara, a 34-year-old legal secretary and mother of three girls, had problems with her periods from the time they started at age 13.

"The pain and bleeding were so heavy that I'd throw up and have to miss school," Barbara says. And the periods themselves never seemed to stop. "By the time I reached my midtwenties, I was bleeding three weeks out of every four."

Barbara's doctor attempted to alleviate her bleeding by performing a D and C (a common surgical procedure in which the cervix is dilated and the lining of the uterus removed) on three separate occasions.

"It would help for a month or two," she says, "but then I'd be back to gushing again. I got so tired of waking up in a bed full of blood that I finally started sleeping on towels. Finally my doctor said, 'Barbara, you spend half your life bleeding. When you've had enough, I'll do a hysterectomy.'"

Barbara says she thought about a hysterectomy for some time before agreeing to it. But she admits to being apprehensive about two things: that she'd have a nervous breakdown and that she'd gain a lot of weight. "Those were the two things I had heard could happen," Barbara says.

Not only did neither happen, Barbara says her sex life picked up after the operation—a response echoed by other women. "Since I wasn't bleeding all the time, and there was no threat of pregnancy, we just dove into it with pure pleasure," she says.

"I was a little scared the first time we made love after the surgery, though. I thought I might wreck something inside. But my sexual response was exactly the same. And my husband said it felt the same to him, too."

Joan Cantrell, a 49-year-old real estate saleswoman and mother of two grown sons, says she, too, was afraid there might be a problem with sexual response after hysterectomy. "A few weeks after the surgery, I asked my doctor if I could have an orgasm," she recalls. "Even though he said I could, I wasn't convinced until it happened. I must admit, though, that intercourse isn't quite the same as before. Still, I'm not complaining," says Joan. "Sex is still great for me—just a little different." Doctors warn, however, that this will not be the experience for all women. Some women have complained to their doctors that they can't have an orgasm or that the sensation is not what it used to be.

WHICH WAY OUT?

How you feel after a hysterectomy also depends on which kind of hysterectomy you have: the traditional surgery, in which the uterus is removed through an incision in the abdomen, or the procedure in which it's removed through the vagina.

Removing the uterus through the vagina is the preferable procedure, says Dr. Burton, because the vaginal approach results in a faster recovery and leaves no visible scar.

"It's like recovering from a vaginal birth," she explains. You'll be in the hospital about three days, and be back to full activities in about three or four weeks. With abdominal surgery the hospital stay is about five days and full recovery takes close to six weeks.

Not all women are candidates for a vaginal hysterectomy, though. A woman who has never been through a vaginal birth, for example, or one whose uterus is too large doesn't qualify, says Dr. Burton. Neither does someone with extensive endometriosis or endometrial or ovarian cancer.

You should expect some post-operative pain no matter which procedure you have, says Dr. Burton. Barbara Paulson says that after her abdominal hysterectomy she had "more pain than I ever imagined. I guess I had in my mind that it was going to be like a D and C. But when I awoke, I was screaming, 'Pain, pain, pain,' " she says, incredulous now that she could have been so naive. "The doctor said,

MAKING ALTERNATIVES WORK

If hysterectomy isn't the answer to your problem, than what is the alternative?

It depends on what is wrong with you, explains Ruth Schwartz, M.D., a professor at New York's University of Rochester School of Medicine and Dentistry. There really isn't an alternative to hysterectomy. But there are options to explore for conditions such as fibroids, prolapsed uterus and the other female health problems that often result in hysterectomy but don't have to.

To explore the options to a hysterectomy, you'll need the best doctor you can find. Seek out a physician certified by the American Board of Obstetrics and Gynecology or an internist certified by the American Board of Internal Medicine who specializes in endocrinology—preferably one who is on staff at a teaching hospital or major medical center.

When in doubt about the diagnosis or recommendation, don't hesitate to get a second opinion—or a second diagnostic test. Your best defense against an unnecessary hysterectomy is obtaining information before you meet with the doctor. Read books, find people who've had the surgery (or the alternatives), contact support groups, locate medical literature. And then show them to your doctor, says Nora W. Coffey, president of Hysterectomy Educational Resources and Services in Bala Cynwyd, Pennsylvania. "That's the way to get a doctor's cooperation, and not hostility."

And take control in making the decision, she encourages. Get comprehensive information about the condition you have, your options and the risks and dangers of the options.

'Well, of course you have pain; I just cut into you. What did you think was going to happen?'"

Nevertheless, Barbara was able to return to work in six weeks feeling completely back to normal. Joan Cantrell had her share of discomfort, too, even though her operation was performed vaginally. "I remember taking lots of pain medication, which helped a great deal," she says. "But it left me feeling so out of it, even depressed. Once I quit the drugs, I snapped out of my doldrums and was back to my old self right away."

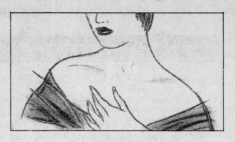

INCONTINENCE

ONE OF WOMEN'S BEST-KEPT SECRETS

*I*t's seldom a major problem, but women commonly find it just too hard to handle.

"Many women won't talk about it, even to their doctors," says Kathryn L. Burgio, Ph.D., research assistant professor of medicine at the University of Pittsburgh School of Medicine. "It's embarrassing. They find it an unacceptable problem, and they choose to hide it rather than deal with it."

Yet the reality is that there are many medical reasons why adults may have a leaky bladder, a condition known as urinary incontinence.

And it's a problem more common than you might think. It afflicts millions of adults. And women—mainly because of childbearing and the design of their plumbing—outnumber men by as much as five to one.

So why the stigma? "Because wetting your pants is something babies do; they can't help it. But sometimes adults can't help it either," says Dr. Burgio, who also runs the incontinence program at the university where she treats people who have the problem.

A SYMPTOM, NOT A DISEASE

There are two main types of incontinence. The most common is stress incontinence, leakage that can occur when coughing, laughing, exercising or lifting. In one survey of

326 gynecology patients at the University of Michigan, 47 percent of women complained of stress incontinence. The other type is urge incontinence, an uncontrollable need to urinate that results in "an accident." Forty to 70 percent of women who have stress incontinence also have urge incontinence, according to statistics.

"There are any number of possible causes of incontinence," explains Kristine E. Whitmore, M.D., clinical associate professor of urology at the University of Pennsylvania and the director of the Incontinence Center and chief of the Department of Urology at Graduate Hospital in Philadelphia. "But it's important to remember that incontinence is not a disease. It's a symptom of an underlying disorder that affects the bladder. It needs evaluation by a physician." Ignoring it can only help make something that may easily be controlled that much worse.

Women who have had children can have incontinence troubles. Childbearing weakens muscles and can cause the bladder to fall out of its normal position. Lack of estrogen after menopause can cause irritation to the urethra, the opening through which you void. Certain urinary and kidney infections and drugs can also create the problem. Even emotional stress can be a factor.

What incontinence is not, emphasizes Dr. Burgio, is a disease of old age. Although it's more common in the elderly, studies have shown that 31 percent of premenopausal women—those in their forties or even younger—have some degree of incontinence on a regular basis. Dr. Burgio says she has a patient who has been incontinent since she was 13 but didn't seek help until she was 83. "That's my most extreme case," she notes.

SILENT MAJORITY

Incontinence often starts out as a loss of a few drops of urine here and there. And for many, that's no big deal. But it's very common for the condition to get progressively worse over time. "Women will tell me that they've had incontinence for 12 or 20 or more years and that's it's only in the past three months that it's gotten to be a 'problem,' " says Dr. Burgio, who is also the coauthor of *Staying Dry: A Practical Guide to Bladder Control.* "Of course, what constitutes a problem varies from woman to woman. For some, any leakage is intolerable. Yet others don't want treatment even when they're having large-volume accidents."

Even when women are troubled by the problem, however, it's rare for them to seek a doctor's advice. Dr. Burgio says that in her research, only 25 percent of the women studied had talked to their doctors about their incontinence. But other studies say it's even less than that. According to another expert, 11 out of 12 don't even mention it to their physicians.

And this only contributes to making it all the tougher to live with.

EMBARRASSING MOMENTS

Horror stories abound, says Dr. Burgio. "I've heard so many at the continence program. It's safe to say that it can be catastrophic at times." Medical journals report that incontinence contributes to depression, social isolation, feelings of low self-esteem and anxiety. "One woman told me, for instance, that she didn't go to her granddaughter's wedding because she was afraid of having an accident and embarrassing everyone. Another told me she had stopped having sexual intercourse because of leakage."

Dr. Burgio recalled a woman who sold real estate and had to be out in her car showing houses all day. "Her job

---

A SELF-HELP GUIDE FOR A LEAKY BLADDER

Sometimes controlling a leaky bladder is a matter of retraining. Here's what physicians recommend you do.

Keep a voiding diary. For a week, write down what you ate, what you drank, when you went to the bathroom and how often you leaked. The diary will help you and your physician track down causes.

Don't overdo the fluids. Some women discover through their diaries that they've been downing gallons of water a day, usually on a weight-loss program. Drinking less can ease the problem. But don't restrict fluid intake. Drinking too little can have serious consequences.

Put your bladder on a schedule. Start by voiding at regular intervals—like hourly—during the day. Over a few weeks, increase the interval, with the goal of reaching 2½ to 3 hours between voidings. In one study, this practice cured 12 percent of the women, while 75 percent improved 50 percent or more.

Avoid alcohol and caffeine-containing beverages and medicines. Both are considered diuretics and can stimulate incontinence.

Eat plenty of fiber. Fiber helps combat constipation, which can contribute to incontinence.

Don't smoke. Nicotine irritates the bladder surface, and coughing associated with smoking triggers stress incontinence.

Shed excess pounds. Being overweight can put additional pressure on your bladder and make incontinence worse.

Try double voiding. This helps you empty your bladder completely. Remain on the toilet until you feel your bladder is empty, then bend over and push forward over your bladder area. Stand up, sit down and try emptying your bladder again.

Go when nature calls. Empty your bladder on a regular basis, and don't let it overfill, which can lead to an over-stretched bladder. Also, if you have a too-full bladder and a weak sphincter (urethral) muscle, you're likely to leak when you cough or sneeze.

Do Kegels. This pelvic exercise, commonly used after childbirth to strengthen the supporting muscles of the bladder and urethra, can also help with incontinence. Even if you're not incontinent, Kegels may prevent problems. Here's how to do them. First you need to identify the correct muscles to exercise. Go to the toilet and start to void. Once the stream of urine has started, try to stop it. If you can slow the stream even slightly, you are using the right muscles. If you have a hard time isolating a muscle, experts recommend trying it with your arm first. Tighten a specific muscle, then relax it. All you need to do is clench the muscle, hold for a count of 3, relax and repeat. You'll need at least 100 to 200 Kegels per day to get the desired results.

and her life revolved around knowing where the toilets were and how long she could wait before she needed one. There were times that she actually had accidents in front of clients. It was devastating," says Dr. Burgio. "She finally gave up the job."

Although embarrassment may be a big part of the silence, Dr. Burgio said another reason many women avoid bringing up the problem is that they think it's untreatable. The fact is that incontinence *is* treatable, now more than ever.

SUCCESS STORIES

Dr. Whitmore says that 50 percent of incontinent people can be cured outright, 30 percent greatly improved and the rest made to feel more comfortable. It's a matter of determining the cause of the incontinence and then supplying the appropriate treatment. Often treating the underlying cause will cure the incontinence.

Self-help measures, including Kegel exercises (see "Self-Help Guide for a Leaky Bladder" on p. 278), can be very successful and are worth a try, says Dr. Burgio. Biofeedback training, which uses electronic sensors to detect changes in body temperature and muscle tension, has been shown to help or cure the problem in most who have tried it. In more severe cases, drugs or even minor surgery are sometimes warranted. Surgery has a 90 percent success rate.

"Doctors generally start with the most conservative methods," says Dr. Whitmore, "and if these fail to help, then they'll turn to the more invasive ones. The most important thing is to get the proper evaluation from your doctor and discuss what options are available to you."

CHAPTER 43

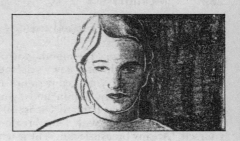

INFERTILITY

TRYING TO MAKE A MIRACLE HAPPEN

For most couples, the real American Dream is summed up tidily in the schoolyard rhyme, "First comes love, then comes marriage, then comes Junior in a baby carriage." But for about 1 in 13 couples, that dream turns into a nightmare when they learn that they are infertile.

The diagnosis of infertility—technically, the failure to conceive after a year of trying or the repeated failure to carry a pregnancy to term—may be one of the most difficult life crises a couple can face. In one study of 200 couples undergoing treatment at a fertility clinic, 40 percent of the women reported that infertility was the most emotionally painful experience of their lives.

For many couples, the pain of not being able to have a child consumes their lives, touching and fouling every aspect of it—their self-esteem, their identities, their sexuality, their marriages, their jobs and their relationships. Pregnancy becomes an obsession, "a full-time job," as one woman put it. Friends, family, career all take a backseat to daily temperature taking, sperm counts, the next medical procedure, the next drug. As one psychologist noted, "There is no balance in their lives. There is, instead, hope one week, grief the next."

Susan Mikesell, Ph.D., who is a Washington, D.C., psychologist specializing in counseling infertile couples, describes the monthly cycle from her own vantage point, both as a psychologist and a woman who struggled with her own fertility problems.

"In the beginning of the month, you are very hopeful," she says. "You feel this is a new cycle and we'll get started and it will work. If your temperature rises the way it's supposed to (a sign of ovulation) and if you have intercourse at the right time, you have this sense of euphoria for the next two weeks, along with some breath-holding. You ask yourself, 'Are my breasts feeling a little tender? Am I feeling nausea?' That rise stays there until the signs of the period. At that point, there is usually a denial kind of response: 'People have spotting when they're pregnant, don't they?'

"Then it sinks in. Your temperature is down for sure and you are definitely not pregnant. The sadness and immediate loss feelings can last from a few minutes to several days or weeks. As the next cycle begins, these feelings fade and hope returns—unless the cycle continues for too long. It repeats itself month after month, a terrible cycle."

THE INFERTILE IDENTITY

In some women, infertility, with its incumbent sense of failure and loss, becomes so central to their identities that even when they do become pregnant they find it hard to shake it off.

"I had a really hard time making the transition from infertile woman to pregnant woman," says Lisa Halloran, 40, who finally conceived her daughter, Colleen, after six years of expensive and high-tech treatments that ate up her life savings and almost destroyed her marriage. "My empathy was with the women who were still trying rather than with my friends who were pregnant. I always felt I could lose the baby and be right back in the pool with those women trying to make a miracle happen."

Infertility carries with it a fundamental sense of failure. The infertile couple can't help but feel "there's something wrong with us." They have not only failed to achieve an important milestone in their lives—parenthood—they are unable to perform a simple biological function that two teenagers can accomplish inadvertently in the backseat of a car. "It's a failure of your will to be unable to produce something you want more dearly than anything else in your life," says Lisa, "something that is so easy for other people."

Your decision to become a mother may have followed months, even years, of thinking and planning, and suddenly you find that it is—perhaps was always—out of your hands. For the first time in your adult life, you may feel a puppet of fate.

THE INFERTILITY SYNDROME

In fact, all of these feelings are part of a grief syndrome experienced by most infertile couples that starts often with surprise and denial. "When they discover that something is not working the way they expected it to, the first thing they think is, 'No, this is not true.' It takes a long time to own the label of infertility," says Dr. Mikesell. "Some people will see fertility experts for years and think all the while, 'It's just a matter of time.' "

Like most couples, Lisa and her husband, Sean, spent years taking measures to avoid pregnancy. They assumed that once they wanted to have children, it would simply be a matter of tossing away the contraceptives. The notion that they could be infertile was so farfetched to them that during the first two years of trying "we had no sense of panic. We lost a lot of time because we had no sense of urgency about it," Lisa says.

Denial is actually a temporary coping mechnism, according to Barbara Eck Menning, who founded the national infertility self-help group, Resolve, and counsels infertile couples. "It allows the mind and body to adjust at their own rate to an overwhelming situation."

Before long, however, denial gives way to anger, a predictable response to loss of control. "For the most part," says Dr. Mikesell, "these are people who have worked hard and organized their lives and have gotten what they wanted by hard work and effort. Now they find that no matter how hard they work, hard work has no correlation to the outcome."

Like many infertile women, Lisa says she grew angry at

herself first. "I thought, 'Why did I spend all those years using birth control?'" Then her anger spread to her husband, who at first dragged his feet about being tested, and to the doctors who she felt were insensitive to her frustration and pain, both physical and emotional. Her anger even took an irrational turn. "I would see teenagers on the street, dragging three kids in tow, and I would want to grab their babies from them and say, 'If you don't want this baby, I'll take it.' I was angry at the world."

THE ADOPTION OPTION

For couples whose desire to parent outweighs their desire for a biological child, adoption can be the solution. "But remember," cautions Susan Mikesell, Ph.D., a psychologist in Washington, D.C., "adoption cures childlessness. It doesn't cure infertility."

And it's not always easy. Fewer babies are available for adoption because of more widespread use of contraception and a diminishing of the stigma attached to single parenthood. Some adoption agencies have age limits and others have waiting lists so long they no longer accept applications. Private adoptions can be quite expensive, and in some cases, heartbreaking.

Marisa Sangiacomo and her husband, Louis, were in their early forties, had undergone 14 artificial inseminations and spent months wrangling over whether they would adopt. "We went through a long and painful process of realizing that this is the only way we're going to have a family," says Marisa, who owns her own graphic arts firm in New York City. "I knew I always would have felt a huge loss in my life if I had not made the decision to adopt."

The Sangiacomos first tried private adoption and spent months negotiating with an unmarried teenager in another state, paying her more than $6,000 for medical and other expenses. When the girl's family called to tell them the baby had arrived, the Sangiacomos got on a plane and flew to the hospital, only to find that the young woman had changed her mind.

"I was furious, devastated and numb at the same time," recalls Marisa. "Driving back to the airport, I was so disoriented I drove right through a stop sign in front of a state policeman. When he stopped us and walked up to the car window, I burst into tears. Then I couldn't believe what I said. I just blurted out, 'I'm sorry, but my baby just died.' And I sobbed even more, because I realized that was exactly how I felt."

Shortly afterward, a friend told them about a new agency that arranged adoptions of children from Central and South America at a cost of $12,500. They applied, and 11 months later they became the parents of 5-week-old Marta from Colombia.

"Since she came into our lives, I've been walking on air," says Marisa. "But although I'm a mother now, I'm still aware that I'm infertile. You do not get past the pain. It doesn't mean it's all over. It's still there, but it's tremendously less."

ALL ALONE

In her anger and pain, Lisa also felt isolated. Many infertile couples keep their problem a secret to avoid unwanted advice and pity. "I didn't want people feeling they had to be careful around me," says Lisa, who waited several years before telling her family and friends. "I would have found that more painful than enduring what I did have to endure."

Another reason some couples keep their infertility a secret is that they feel guilty. The infertility is "their punishment" for some past transgression, says Dr. Mikesell, and their guilt a way to atone and make some sense out of it, to find someone or something to blame. Their past sin may be an affair, premarital sex, use of birth control, anything that makes them feel deserving of this retribution. According to Menning, this reaction appears to have no relationship to a person's educational level. "Some of the most sophisticated people I have counseled have applied a mystical belief in 'God's punishment' to their own infertility, even in the absence of belief in a religion," she notes.

However, as Lisa learned, keeping her infertility a secret also cut her off from the comfort and support her family and friends later offered. She did join Resolve and saw a counselor privately when she found her sense of isolation also included alienation from her husband.

MARITAL TENSION

It's easy for couples to become polarized by their inability to have a child, says Dr. Mikesell, and few marriages are untouched by it. In one study, 71 percent of the couples interviewed said their infertility affected their marriage. Although 56 percent said something positive came out of it, a similar number said the experience had some negative effects. "All said, it either draws people together or pulls them apart," says Dr. Mikesell.

Why the problem pulls a lot of people apart has a lot to do with how couples feel about and cope with their fertility problems. Studies show that women tend to feel the pain more keenly than men, perhaps because motherhood is such an integral part of the female identity. Some experts, however, speculate the results of those studies may be attributed to the fact that women simply express their feelings more readily.

Often problems arise when one partner—usually the woman—needs to talk while the other needs to retreat. In one study of infertile couples, the husbands said they wanted to be helpful to their wives, but the discussions that helped ease their wives' stress only increased their own. There also may be conflict if the husband's and wife's desire for a child is different. A man who has children from a previous marriage, for instance, might be willing to give up the costly fertility treatments long before his childless wife. The two may differ on whether to adopt. "Couples who do pretty well most of the time may have some difficulty when facing infertility decisions, especially if the woman expects her husband is going to have the same kinds of feelings and reactions that she has," says Dr. Mikesell. "He, number one, will not necessarily have the same ones she has and, number two, may not have them at the same time she does."

In fact, what may occur is that the husband, socialized to protect his wife, may feel so overwhelmed by her pain and his inability to stop it that he retreats even further, sometimes withdrawing from the treatment process. His wife then feels abandoned. "We were still in the middle of

INFERTILITY: CAUSES AND CURES

What causes infertility? According to experts, three factors most often contribute to infertility in women: ovulatory problems, blocked or scarred fallopian tubes and endometriosis, a condition in which tissue from the uterine lining separates and attaches itself elsewhere in the lower abdomen. In men, abnormal or too few sperm is the main cause of infertility.

Both men and women can have genetic structural abnormalities that cause infertility. Also, those exposed to the now-banned synthetic hormone diethylstilbestrol (DES) while in the womb may have abnormalities in the reproductive organs that can affect infertility. In 3 to 20 percent of all couples, infertility cannot be explained.

Most couples seeking treatment for infertility are treated with conventional medical and surgical techniques ranging from a simple test to help the couple pinpoint ovulation to surgery to repair structural abnormalities or to treat tubal problems, endometriosis or fibroid tumors. Women with ovulatory problems may be treated with drugs to induce ovulation, such as clomiphene citrate (Clomid) and/or a powerful injectable hormonal drug called Pergonal. Hormone therapy is also used on endometriosis and in some cases of male infertility. Other methods include:

- Artificial insemination with the husband's sperm (if he has some fertile sperm) or donor sperm (if the husband's sperm is inactive or sperm count is low).
- In vitro fertilization, in which eggs are surgically removed from a woman's ovaries and transferred to a Petri dish, where they are fertilized with sperm. The resulting embryos are then placed in the woman's uterus.
- Gamete intrafallopian transfer, in which the woman's eggs are retrieved surgically and mixed with sperm, then placed in the fallopian tubes, where conception occurs.
- Zygote intrafallopian transfer, in which the woman's eggs are collected surgically and fertilized. The resulting embryos are placed in the fallopian tube, through which they travel to the uterus.

in vitro [fertilization in a test tube] when Sean started saying we can't afford this much longer, financially and emotionally," recalls Lisa. "I was panic-stricken. He was ready to pull the plug and I wasn't."

If the infertility is the man's problem, which it is in about 40 percent of the cases, the woman may be angry at him and he may feel emasculated. "There is frequently more turmoil with male infertility because there are fewer treatments," says Dr. Mikesell.

The couple may have to wrangle with the tricky issue of donor insemination, which may be *her* only chance to have a baby. "It's a real dilemma," says Dr. Mikesell, "and frequently it is the woman who is more worried about the man's attitude or feelings about being the father of a donor child. She may also feel that she's being selfish: Here is something I can have that he can't. Is it fair for me to do this?"

THE JOB OF SEX

Even if the marriage grows stronger, there is usually a temporary casualty of an infertility problem—the couple's sex life. In a study in which more than half the couples said their infertility had benefited their marriage, no one said it had a beneficial effect on sex.

According to one study, lovemaking, for many couples, becomes "a coercive 'chore,' " a means of getting pregnant. Sex is divided into two categories: "sex for love" and "sex for doctor," with the latter sometimes taking over. "Foreplay" may include temperature taking and hormone injections, turning what was pleasure into pain. Intercourse is choreographed so that the couple uses the "right" positions—the ones that increase the chances for conception—on the "right" nights.

Not only that, but sex is no longer something private between two people who love one another. It may feel like the whole fertility clinic is invited into the bedroom for a peek. A fertility workup includes a detailed profile of the couple's sex life, from how often they make love to what positions they use. "You lose your sense of privacy. All the experimenting and playfulness that comes with sex is scrutinized," says Dr. Mikesell.

Sex may not even be linked to conception. With procedures such as in vitro fertilization, donor insemination and other technologies, the man and woman don't even need to be in the same room to conceive a child—and often aren't. It can be disconcerting to realize "you don't have to have sex to get pregnant," says Dr. Mikesell. "I have a client who came into my office and said, 'I haven't had sex with my husband in three months and I'm sitting here pregnant with twins.'"

LIFE GOES ON

One study calls infertility a crisis with no resolution, which is not strictly true. "There used to be a natural end point when you did all the available treatments and then there wasn't anything else to do. Now you can have in vitro fertilization until you are postmenopausal," says Dr. Mikesell. "It becomes more a personal choice than it ever was."

How do you know when to stop? Sometimes the decision is made for you when you find you've run out of money. More often, it's a decision you have to make yourselves. "Couples have to weigh how much of an investment—emotional, physical and financial—they're making compared to the percentages for conception," says Dr. Mikesell. "Does it pay to spend all of your life savings, take a second mortgage out on your house and risk your marriage or your career to have a 10 percent chance of conceiving in any given cycle?"

Some take what life deals them and view it in a new way. Instead of accepting being childless, Jean Carter, M.D., a Raleigh, North Carolina, obstetrician and her husband, Michael, an English professor, decided to be "child-free."

"We had to change ourselves from being failed parents to being successful nonparents," says Dr. Carter, whose infertility was diagnosed as "unexplained." "We really changed. We started getting up in the morning not seeing ourselves as people who weren't accomplishing the most important thing in their lives. We had gone for five years believing that life without children was not worth living, a complete failure, and we actually had to turn around and look at it from a different angle and say, yes, life can be good, you can accomplish things, you can make a difference in people's lives, you can be nurturing, you can have a good marriage, you can be a good child to your parents without reproducing. That was sort of a discovery for us. It took some getting used to."

The Carters, who wrote a book, called *Sweet Grapes*, about their experience found that beyond grief and acceptance was a stage they called transformation, in which loss is consciously transformed into a gain. "You need to study what was meaningful to you about yourself as a potential parent to see if you can use that in another way, refocus those nurturing drives in some other sphere of life," explains Dr. Carter. "After grief, you need to make a choice, saying I am now taking responsibility for what happens with the rest of my life."

In the Carters' case, they found they had been refocusing their attention on their careers, "filling in the gap without even knowing it."

"I take all my mothering impulses out on my patients and their babies," something that once gave her more heartache than joy, says Dr. Carter. "Our nieces and nephews get a lot of spoiling from us. Infertility sucks away your energy. After we freed ourselves from being infertile we began to go back to doing volunteer work in our community and church. I do some work with Resolve, helping other infertile couples. And I got back to quilting. It's interesting, the average quilt takes about nine months to make and I just crank them out. So I feel in a way I'm giving birth to them."

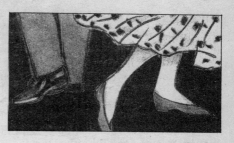

INFIDELITY

WHAT MAKES A SPOUSE UNFAITHFUL

Being married is a lot like going out to dinner. You're satisfied with what you wanted until you see what the other guy has.
ANONYMOUS

*I*t happens in good marriages as well as bad ones. It involves nice guys as well as lecherous ones. It's a leading cause of divorce, but it's been known to mend relationships, too.

Probably at least 50 percent of all married women are living with a husband who has been or will be unfaithful—although some experts and surveys claim the number could be even higher. But what makes the world of infidelity so different today from a generation ago is the number of women who are playing the game.

"When it comes to cheating on your spouse, women are catching up to men," says Judith Slater, Ph.D., a clinical psychologist practicing in Buffalo. "One reason may be that with the majority of women in the work force, they have more contact with men and therefore more opportunity to engage in extramarital affairs."

What doesn't seem to be changing, however, is the toll an affair can take on a relationship. And, as in the past, women are more prone to bear the emotional scars—even when they're the ones doing the cheating.

SEX AND LOVE

When it comes to affairs, men and women feel victimized in different ways. In one study, 202 men and women were asked what would make them feel more betrayed: the idea of their mates having sex with someone else or the idea that their mates were emotionally involved with another. Women overwhelmingly (85 percent) said they'd find the emotional relationship the toughest to handle, while men (60 percent) said they couldn't stand the thought of their women having sex with other men.

The reason, say the researchers, has a lot to do with human nature and the difference between the sexes. Men are inherently more concerned with their partner's chastity, while women are more concerned about their man's emotional commitment.

"Of course, women don't want their husbands to have any kind of affair, sexual or emotional," says Shirley Glass, Ph.D., a clinical psychologist practicing in Owings Mills, Maryland, and a member of the American Association for Marriage and Family Therapy. "But wives are certainly more threatened by their husbands' emotional involvement with another woman than by their sexual involvement. Women are crushed to think that their husbands have shared personal details of their marriage with another woman. It feels like a terrible violation."

Not that the thought of their husbands' having sex with another woman doesn't get to them, too. "Women can be stunned by the thought of sexual competition," adds Dr. Slater. "They can become enraged. I've had women tell me that they felt a level of fury they had never experienced before in their lives, and it astonished them. That may be because a woman's self-esteem often is not very solid, and thoughts of being compared trigger feelings of inadequacy and humiliation."

On top of the overwhelming jealousy, says Dr. Slater, a woman is more likely than a man to blame herself for her mate's affair. She can be hounded by self-doubts: What's wrong with me? Wasn't I good enough?

A husband, on the other hand, often will react somewhat

differently to his wife's liaison. The blow to his sexual ego may be his first thought when he discovers his wife's affair. "Sometimes the husband can't believe that his wife, who hasn't been very sexual with him, is having torrid sex with someone else," says Dr. Slater.

WHY MEN CHEAT

Since men and women feel betrayal in different ways, it's no surprise that they share different agendas when they betray.

Many men are driven by the desire for sexual adventure. "It's not that men don't enjoy the special attention and romance that an affair brings. They do," says Dr. Slater. "But for men there's the undeniable importance of sex."

For many men, an affair can break the monotony of a contented, though ordinary, life of work, home, wife and kids. "An affair offers a kind of escape, an R and R that is tantalizing," says Dr. Slater. "And if there are difficulties in the marriage, lots of arguments, for example, an affair offers a realm in which there is an absence of conflict and a new sense of control."

But not all men are driven into affairs because of sex. "There are men for whom sex and emotional involvement go hand in hand, so an affair can have heavy ramifications," says Dr. Glass. These are the men who usually suffer the most from guilt—and it can be pretty heavy.

"There is also a group of men who believe that having extramarital affairs is acceptable," says Dr. Glass. "It's just part of their set of values, and these men feel no guilt whatsoever."

You can't expect a philanderer to change his stripes, warns Dr. Glass. "If your husband was like that before marriage, the chances are slim that he'll suddenly become the model faithful mate after marriage."

SILENT SUFFERING

And he's probably not fooling a whole lot of people, either, particularly his wife. Women, much more than men, have the ability "to turn the other cheek" when it comes to putting up with a cheating husband. The fact that there are so many cheaters who are still husbands attests to this.

"Sometimes a woman, for whatever reason, just chooses to ignore it, especially if her husband is very good to her in other ways," says Dr. Glass. "This is not uncommon. She may choose to remain in the marriage to ensure an 'intact' household for her children. And let's not forget that divorcing is usually devastating financially for the woman, far more often than it is for the man.

"Often," she continues, "women choose to share their husbands rather than lose them. They don't want to give up the status of being the wife of a wealthy or famous man. Other women have a great fear and dread of being alone."

Unfortunately for the wife, though, sometimes the husband's reason for maintaining the marriage is the same as hers. Therefore, when the kids are finally grown or financial obligations are out of the way, the husband often jumps ship, leaving the wife alone, older and bitter.

"My husband was playing around with every woman he could get his hands on and I knew it," says Stella Jenks, 55 and careerless. "I can remember when I found the bill for the sofa bed he bought for his office. I stayed for the kids, thinking they didn't know what he was like. When the kids graduated from college, he left to marry his most recent girlfriend—a woman my oldest daughter's age. I found out later that the kids knew what he was like all those years. They thought *I* was the one who didn't know."

WHY WOMEN CHEAT

It's a woman's strong emotional makeup that also makes her vulnerable to having an affair.

"Probably most women who have an affair are looking for something that they are unable to get from their husbands," says Dr. Slater. "Special attention, physical affection and communication. When women talk to me about an affair, they almost never emphasize the sexuality. Indeed, that's often the least important part, and in fact it may not even be as good as in their marriages. But the attention,

PRIME TIMES FOR CHEATING

A popular movie from the 1950s called it the seven-year itch. But wanderlust can enter a marriage after 1, 4, 15 or 30 years, says clinical psychologist Judith Slater, Ph.D. But there are times when a marriage is most vulnerable.

When you are newlyweds. Once the honeymoon is over, some couples are shocked by the demands of partnership. They thought the same high level of romance would continue indefinitely and are not prepared to deal with the realities of sharing and compromising, says Dr. Slater.

When you become parents. Sexual interest usually decreases for women for the year after giving birth simply because they are exhausted most of the time, says Maryland psychologist Shirley Glass, Ph.D. The wife often becomes focused on the baby to the extent that the husband can feel left out. It's not uncommon for him to try to balance that by finding someone else who will focus exclusively on him.

When you're in your thirties. Raising families, advancing your careers and the everyday demands of life usually start taking their toll when you're thirtysomething. An affair can be a nice diversion.

When you face middle age. There are all those issues at midlife of aging and achievement, says Dr. Slater. You may feel stuck in your life and you begin to reevaluate what you've accomplished and more important, what you haven't. An affair often seems like it can offer a new beginning.

When you've experienced a tragedy. After the death of a parent or serious illness of a child, for example, people may have an affair to forget—or at least try. It's a fantasy, almost like a vacation from despair, says Dr. Glass.

the romance, the sense of validation they get from their affair is irresistible. Suddenly, their point of view, who they are, what they say, are all important and appreciated by this new man."

One woman, a 42-year-old teacher, says she got emotionally and physically involved with a married colleague quite by accident—or so she thought.

"My husband's idea of affection was to have sex. He didn't much care for spontaneous hugs and kisses and would often peel my arms away from around his neck when I tried to be affectionate," she says. "When I started my affair I didn't realize how wonderful sex could be with another person. I fell head over heels. Only he didn't. It was such a difficult thing to get over. I never told my husband, but I still carry around the guilt."

In fact, guilt is a common side effect in women, says Dr. Glass. "There have been some studies that suggest that women feel more guilt about being unfaithful than men feel."

And it's such an intense emotion, it sometimes prevents women from acting on their desires or needs. "For many women, the guilt often acts as an inhibitor to an affair," she says. "In other words, the guilt of just knowing they have powerful, sexual feelings for another man may be enough to prevent anything from happening. And if they do get sexually involved, they frequently justify their actions by telling themselves they have fallen in love."

IT'S ALL OVER BUT THE ANGER

A marriage damaged by unfaithfulness can survive, insists Dr. Glass. In some cases it can make a marriage stronger. But it's not going to happen overnight, or even in a few months. Infidelity causes a hurt that comes with a slow healing process. Dr. Slater says it can take one to three years to pull the marriage back together again.

But in the aftermath of an affair, a couple has a unique opportunity to grow and strengthen their bond, says Dr. Slater. The wounds *can* and do heal, and if the marriage survives and is a good one, the couple will look back and have a different, less-damaging perspective on it.

If you want your marriage to survive, here's what Dr. Glass and Dr. Slater say can help take the hurt away. And these tips can work for both of you, whether it's the deceived or the deceiver who initiates the reconciliation.

Make sure the affair is over. The deceiver must be able to prove without doubt that the affair is over as a first step to making the marriage work.

Leave ample time for mourning. Remember there's more

than one injured party involved in this triangle. The spouse having the affair is also suffering the loss of a relationship.

Stop the lying. Most people have the toughest time with the lies and deceit that go along with unfaithfulness. One woman recalled that when she was in agony and begged her husband to tell her what was going on, he looked right into her face and lied, insisting that it was all in her mind. That was the bitterest pill, she said.

The betrayed spouse has a right to ask a lot of questions—possibly painful and intimate questions—and the deceiver has an obligation to answer honestly.

Question the motives behind the affair. No matter how angry it makes you, you need to find out what might have been unsatisfying in your marriage that drove your spouse to the arms of another.

Be prepared for setbacks. You both may be doing well and then your spouse gets mysteriously moody. Remember that there may be things in your spouse's life that trigger fond memories of the affair. Such things have the ability to put the injured spouse in an immediate tailspin. The injured spouse will have flashbacks and pain that need to be shared and understood.

Apologize sincerely and often. In other words, be contrite. The injured spouse needs to be reassured about how special she or he is and will want lots of special attention. That's often something they haven't had before or haven't had for years, and it can add some new juice to the relationship.

See also Divorce, Married Men

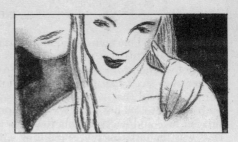

INHIBITED SEXUAL DESIRE

WHEN LIFE INTERFERES WITH YOUR FUN

*Y*ou're frisky. He isn't. You have a headache. He doesn't. Or maybe you both have headaches—all the time. Or you both have jobs and kids to boot, so who has the energy to think about good sex?

Inhibited sexual desire (ISD) is what the experts call it. And New York City sex and marital therapist Shirley Zussman, Ed.D., says it's a concern for about 50 percent of the women who consult her.

How many times have *you* played the numbers game and come up short? You know which numbers. Those statistics that say American couples married five to ten years have sex an average of 2.8 times per week. So you think real hard and maybe you can remember the last time you had sex, but—and this is the part that worries you—it was more like 2.8 *months* ago. And when you think about it even more, you realize you could probably go another few months without so much as a minor blip in your libido. It makes you wonder: "Is there something wrong with me?"

Forget those statistics, says Judith H. Seifer, R.N., Ph.D., associate clinical professor of psychiatry and obstetrics and gynecology at Wright State University School of Medicine in Dayton, Ohio. You may be below average, but this in no way means you're *abnormal*. Look at it this way. By definition, 50 percent of all couples are going to be below average. "The point is," says Dr. Seifer, "it doesn't matter whether you have sex two times a day or two times a year, as long as both partners are satisfied and comfortable with that frequency. You need to learn what's normal for *you*."

"Interest and desire for sex at any given time is as unique for each person as their desire to wear miniskirts or silk shirts," adds Lonnie Barbach, Ph.D., assistant clinical professor of medical psychology at the University of California, San Francisco, School of Medicine. "But how often do you see statistics on what percentage of women wear those articles of clothing? Do you feel bad because you don't own 'enough' silk blouses?"

TOO POOPED TO PLAY

On the other hand, if your formerly lusty libido just kind of lies there—and you miss it—you could well be experiencing ISD. A thoroughly modern condition that strikes women and men equally, this stalled sex drive is often caused by nothing more than your life interfering with your fun.

As one exhausted woman stated, "After juggling 60-hour workweeks and the needs of my children, plus cooking for my family and caring for our home, it's sleep I want when I get into bed." Indeed, today's pressures can sap so much energy from you that sex seems like just one more chore to do before you're allowed to rest, says Dr. Seifer.

Although ISD can spring from many causes, it probably stems primarily from excessive fatigue and stress, says Dr. Zussman.

Is there any way, short of rearranging your entire life, to put a little sizzle back into your sex life? You bet there is.

"If there's one bit of advice I give to couples, especially those over 45, it's to look back and remember when they were dating," says Dr. Seifer. "Intercourse was delayed, often until after marriage, and couples spent huge amounts of time touching—parking, necking, petting.

"I ask couples, 'How often do you pleasure one another in the way you used to, just touching, trailing your fingernails down his back, caressing the inside of her forearm?' Couples look at each other and giggle."

You also aren't going to get in the mood for love if you don't enjoy some time alone together, says Dr. Zussman. She suggests going out on a date. Sit across from each other in a romantic restaurant and have a candlelit dinner for two or go to a movie. Stroll along the beach at sunrise.

GETTING YOUR PASSION BACK

"Built-up anger over the years is the biggest cause of lack of sexual desire," asserts Los Angeles therapist Barbara De Angelis, Ph.D. "When people think they have a sex problem, 90 percent of the time it has to do with little resentments, feelings of frustration about not being loved or acknowledged enough. Work on cleaning out whatever emotional clutter has built up between you. Those things kill passion."

Another wedge is differences in desire. Sometimes one partner wants sex much more often than the other. It's the interpretations that you put on this discrepancy that can cause a problem, says Dr. Barbach. Don't make accusations such as, "you don't love me," "you don't care about me" or "there's something wrong with you" to the spouse whose sexual appetite is limited. Instead, look for alternative ways to satisfy the "hungrier" partner and ways to help the other one keep from feeling under pressure to have more sex than she (or he) feels comfortable with.

"The most common issue I find with midlife couples is sexual boredom," says Dr. Seifer. "Couples get tired of doing the same thing in the same way in the same place."

How do you know if boredom is the problem? Ask yourself this question, says Dr. Seifer: "When you go on vacation and find yourself in a new place like a hotel, do you find that your sexual relationship gets more exciting—then seems to fall back into a rut when you get back home?"

You need to give your sex life as high a priority as you give your workouts or buying a car, says Dr. Zussman. "Don't let anything interfere with the time you've set aside for sex. This may mean restricting time spent on work and worries about family problems, household crises and world concerns."

And when it come to lovemaking, don't let yourself feel the pressure to perform. That means don't be preoccupied with techniques or achieving mutual orgasms, says Dr. Zussman. "Try love play without intercourse. Focus on dancing, touching, massage, bathing. Remember, your only goals should be relaxation, closeness and pleasure."

See also Sexual Dysfunction

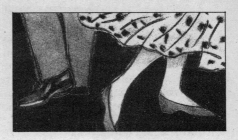

JEALOUSY

A FEELING YOU JUST CAN'T STAND

*I*t's been called a contradictory and chaotic passion. It's an emotion that can strike with sudden intensity, leaving you wracked with a sense of loss and hysteria. It can turn feelings of profound sadness and fear into restless distress, unbearable humiliation and shocking hostility. It's the root of the so-called fatal attraction.

At its worst it's been blamed for suicide attempts, wife-battering, even murder. At its best, it's the twinge you may feel when your best friend tells you she has just bought a second home, while you can't afford to buy your first one.

Jealously is perhaps the strongest and least understood of human emotions.

"It's perfectly normal to feel a bit jealous at times," admits Renae Norton, Ph.D., a clinical psychologist at the Montgomery Center in Cincinnati, Ohio. "You may envy a coworker for her success on the job or because of a particularly satisfying relationship she has. Anytime there's a perceived imbalance or inequality, it's not surprising that the emotion felt is jealousy."

FROM GOOD TO EVIL

Although its connotations are notoriously negative, jealousy can, in fact, be a source of motivation. The envy you feel for your boss's competence can help drive your own ambitions. A twinge of jealousy can help revitalize a romantic relationship when you suddenly notice he's desirable to someone else.

But jealousy can become a treacherous emotion when it overpowers your everyday life. "There's a continuum of jealous behavior," says Dr. Norton. "You may feel reasonable discomfort if your husband shows excessive attention to an attractive young woman. After all, you perceive it as a real threat to your relationship. That's rational."

But there's also the irrational. "I have patients who are unable to tolerate their husbands' viewing a movie with a beautiful woman in it. They are completely obsessed with the idea that their men are having sexual thoughts about another woman. And so they actually screen any movies or television shows before they allow their husbands to watch them. That's quite abnormal behavior, even pathological," she points out.

At this extreme, jealousy might involve imagined threats, paranoid suspicions and much checking up on the suspected partner—following him around, going through his pockets, looking through his mail or his briefcase and extensive questioning. In one study, a jealous patient complained that what she resented most "was the sheer waste of time and effort her jealousy involved her in by the checking on every aspect of her husband's life."

WHY SO PALE AND WAN?

Jealousy, say the experts, is an obvious sign of an insecure woman. "The woman probably grew up deprived in some way—maybe in a way that's not even apparent. And having been deprived she feels entitled to all her wants," explains Dr. Norton. "She constantly scans the environment, checking out who's got what, or if anybody has more than she does. Of course, she will always find that person while ignoring those who have less than she. At this point, she'll experience intense jealousy."

"Jealous women are constantly spending their time comparing themselves to others," agrees Shirley Glass, Ph.D., a clinical psychologist practicing in Owings Mills, Maryland,

and a member of the American Association for Marriage and Family Therapy. "And they always find themselves on the short end of the stick. They can become so insecure that they become jealous of the time their husbands spend with a hobby, for example, or jealous of the interest they have in their work. Everything becomes a test of love, a test of loyalty, a test of success."

And if it's an emotion that thrusts between a man and a woman, it can be hard for the one on the receiving end to understand.

That's because men and women experience jealousy for different reasons, according to Dr. Glass. "Primarily, women need to feel secure about being in love. Men need to feel admired. So when a husband says or does something that might be hurtful, his wife's response is, 'Do you love me enough?' Her husband's concern in a similar situation might be, 'Why are you putting me down? Don't you respect me? Don't you admire me enough?' "

REFRAME YOUR PERSPECTIVE

Jealous people are often very sour. They have been robbed of their self-esteem, and it shows in their relationships. "When a woman comes into a marriage feeling worthless and depends on her husband to repair the damage from the past," says Dr. Glass, "any rejection or crisis in the marriage would be perceived as a terrible blow, just devastating."

"It's also difficult for these women to establish or maintain friendships," adds Dr. Norton. "When you have an intimate relationship it requires feeling and expressing joy for the other person's successes. The chronically jealous person is unable to experience that kind of joy. Her jealous comparisons to the other person are likely to leave her feeling resentful and bitter. It's as if your friend, by having more, somehow renders you less; if she succeeds, then you're a failure."

How can you stop such destructive feelings? Well, you can't just tell someone not to feel jealous, says Dr. Norton. "It's a bit like telling someone not to be upset when they're upset. A feeling is a feeling, and it's almost impossible to turn one off, especially when it's jealousy. We can help people step back from hurt, anger, depression and frustration. But jealousy seems to be so internalized. Instead, what we try to do is help the woman reframe what it is she's experiencing."

One woman Dr. Norton worked with, for example, expressed a great deal of jealousy for a neighbor. "In my patient's view, this woman has perfect kids. They're getting all A's in school, they always say the right thing, do the right thing, make their parents so proud. My patient's children don't seem to measure up," she says.

"I helped her look at the situation from a different perspective. I asked her, 'Tell me what you like about your children.' And she promptly listed a few wonderful traits. Then I asked her, 'Could things be worse for them than they are now?' Of course, she immediately realized what I was getting at. They could have a terminal illness or be on drugs."

Reframing also helps you adopt a more empathetic look at the person you are jealous of, continues Dr. Norton. "I asked my patient, 'Do you think your neighbor experiences her life as perfect as you think it is? Do you think she is ever envious of others?' The idea is that you can always find somebody who has more than you do. So what?"

FOCUS ON YOURSELF

"People often have an awareness that a jealous reaction is too great for a particular event. It's important to recognize an inappropriate response and to put it into perspective," says Dr. Glass. Suppose two people tried out for the lead in a show. If you didn't get it, it would be normal to be somewhat jealous. After all, you wanted it a great deal; you're disappointed because it meant a lot to you. An abnormal reaction would be to feel hatred for the other person or to be self-abasing.

"People need to find something about themselves that makes them feel good, to find their own strengths," says Dr. Norton. "In therapy we help people change their locus of control from external to internal. In other words," she explains, "jealous people are swayed by things outside of themselves—things over which they have no control. And it haunts them. As a normal part of the therapeutic process, we teach patients to reclaim control over themselves. When people become more internally controlled, they are not focused on others and what those others have. They are focused instead on themselves. They're moving toward self-actualization, to satisfy themselves so they no longer feel in a terrible state of deprivation."

ASK YOURSELF QUESTIONS

Putting this idea into practice is actually pretty easy, says Dr. Norton. The first thing you need to do is realize that most of us grew up believing we had no choices. That meant that we were *ex*ternally controlled. Your mother ordered you to clean up your room, your father ordered you to take out the trash, your teachers ordered you to do your homework—everyone was in control of your life except you. There were no choices.

Now, the way that lack of control manifests itself in your adult life is that you still feel as though you have no choices. Intellectually you may tell yourself that you do. But deep within your gut, you really don't *believe* it!

Yet the key to overcoming jealousy is to get your gut in tune with your head and actually make choices rather than feeling compelled to do what other people want you to do.

How? Whenever you feel compelled to do something, says Dr. Norton, stop and ask yourself three key questions. "Do I have to feel guilty if I don't do this?" "Do I have a choice?" and "Why do I feel that I don't have a choice?"

That feeling of compulsion you experience should be a red flag warning you that the questions are necessary, she adds. Once you begin to consciously raise questions about a particular course of action, you begin to understand—in your gut as well as your head—that you *do* have a choice and you *are* in control of your life. That fixes your locus of control exactly where it belongs, says Dr. Norton: right inside *you*.

After that, says Dr. Norton, there's no reason to be jealous of anyone. How could you be jealous of someone else when you've actually *chosen* to be who and what you are?

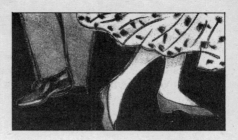

MARRIAGE

A NEW SHIFT IN EXPECTATIONS

*A*nd they lived happily ever after."

Yeah, sure. In fairy tales maybe. Or in your dreams. Almost without exception, women marrying for the first time expect their future to match the fairy-tale ending they grew up hearing. Real life often offers something less, however. At least it does for 50 percent of couples—that's the current divorce rate.

Women still carry the fantasy that a knight in shining armor—the perfect mate—will come along and they will live a life of bliss forever, says Constance Ahrons, Ph.D., professor of sociology at the University of Southern California in Los Angeles and associate director of the university's Marriage and Family Therapy Program. "It's a myth that's sure to cause some major disappointments for many."

"In the past, most women expected to get married, be housewives and mothers and be supported financially by their husbands," says Michele Weiner-Davis, a marriage and family therapist in Woodstock, Illinois, and author of *Divorce Busting: A Revolutionary and Rapid Program for Staying Together.* "And their husbands' expectations went along those same lines.

"But since the women's movement of the 1960s and 1970s, expectations of marriage have shifted somewhat. Women may still want their husbands to be financial successes, but now they are also hoping for men who can be more feeling, more sensitive, more open—in fact, more like women."

Many experts believe that unrealistic expectations—both women's *and* men's—account for many of the problems experienced in new marriages.

GREAT EXPECTATIONS

Women think that when they get married they're going to have a best friend, someone they can really open up to, who will understand them and be their staunchest ally, says Dr. Ahrons, who is also the coauthor of *Divorced Families: Meeting the Challenge of Divorce and Remarriage*. Meanwhile, men's expectations revolve around their wives' "being there" for them, nurturing them during their stressful times, being a support and a helpmate. "When those expectations are not met, a great deal of discontent is sure to follow," says Dr. Ahrons.

With all of these different expectations, it's no wonder that couples who expected to make beautiful music together often strike some sour notes right from the start.

" 'My husband can't communicate,' is probably the number one complaint that I hear in my practice," says Weiner-Davis. "What's really happening, though, is that he's communicating in a form she doesn't understand. It's not the stereotypical female style of communicating that she's used to; it's the male style."

Women tend to meet their intimacy needs through verbal communication, says Dr. Ahrons, whereas men are more likely to feel connected through actions. In other words, men and women have different emotional intimacy requirements and communicate those needs quite differently. "A man might feel particularly close with his wife, for example, if she's just sat through a football game with him, whether it was on TV or they went to the stadium," says Dr. Ahrons. "She was there for him. Women, on the other hand, feel close to their husband if the two of them just sit and talk for hours."

"It helps if each spouse can translate the other's language," says Weiner-Davis. "One woman complained to me that her husband buys her roses all the time, but he doesn't say he loves her. What she needed to understand was that for some men, roses are the equivalent of a verbal, 'I love you.' "

WHAT YOU SEE IS WHAT YOU GET

It's a big mistake to think that once you marry someone, you'll be able to change any behavior that displeased you before the wedding, says Dr. Ahrons. "People rarely change their basic nature," she says. "So she spends her time trying to change him, and he spends his time trying to change her, and neither one of them is facing the reality that they are not going to meet each other's needs in quite the way they had anticipated."

INGREDIENTS OF A HAPPY MARRIAGE

Believe it or not, there hasn't been much research devoted to what makes a *happy* marriage. Much of what there is, though, has been done by Florence Kaslow, Ph.D., director of the Florida Couples and Family Institute in West Palm Beach. Her research revealed a group of factors that highly satisfied couples seem to have in common.

- Open expression of love and affection
- Mutual trust and respect
- Shared interests and values
- Shared love for and interest in their children
- The ability to give and take
- Sensitivity to each other's needs and wishes
- An egalitarian relationship in which power issues are not a battleground
- Playfulness and having fun together
- A good sense of humor

One woman admits that she played along with her fiancé's bar-hopping behavior even though she hated that scene. "I just thought that after we got married I'd be able to change him, so that he'd want to stay at home every night with me." Instead, her husband continued his pub crawling and complained that his wife had changed after they got married from a fun-loving woman to a stick-in-the-mud.

"Women often try harder to please their men during the courtship time," admits Dr. Ahrons. But it's also true that during the rush of a new romance, people are often blinded to a person's real nature. Then after the marriage, when the initial passion cools down, they see each other more clearly—and not as generously.

That's often when the squabbling begins.

FIGHTING FAIR OR OTHERWISE

Money, sex, communication, infidelity, parenting, household responsibilities—these are what couples argue about most often, say the experts. But it's not *what* you argue about but *how* you go about it that can strengthen or weaken a marriage. "There are different styles in fighting and expressing anger," says Dr. Ahrons. "One person might withdraw and one person might continue to pursue, for example." Marriage counselors find themselves teaching the one who withdraws to withdraw less, and the one who pursues to pursue less. "It gives the couple some balance in the way they handle an argument," explains Dr. Ahrons.

A certain amount of arguing is inevitable, the experts say. Just about all marriages have their ups and downs, and that's life. "We all complain from time to time about our spouses," says Weiner-Davis. "But complaining indicates to me that a person is still trying to mend her relationship. She still cares. The biggest hint of major trouble is when the person who's been complaining suddenly stops. That's usually a sign that things have gone downhill drastically, and she's given up hope."

Dr. Ahrons says that there are other warning signs.

- You are constantly fighting with each other.
- Your marriage is bringing you more misery than satisfaction.
- You are withdrawing from each other.
- You've had a good sex life in the past and now you don't.
- You have started deceiving each other.
- It becomes very uncomfortable to be around each other.

HOW TO MAKE IT BETTER

If you suspect your relationship may be in trouble but you're not ready to throw in the towel, is there anything you can do to make it work?

It can be done, says Weiner-Davis. "I have two simple formulas that I recommend to couples. The first is: If it works, don't fix it, do more of it. I ask couples to examine those times in their relationship when they didn't fight and to look at what each one did to contribute to those peaceful times. They ask each other, 'What do we do when we feel loving toward each other?' 'Where do we go?' 'How do we talk to each other?' 'Who else is around at those times?' 'When are these good times most likely to occur; least likely?'

"Couples can usually implement those positive strategies—whatever they are—even in the midst of heated discussions, although people sometimes slip back into old patterns from time to time," she says.

Weiner-Davis also asks the couples she works with to identify what she refers to as their more-of-the-same behavior. That's the second simple formula. "Think about it," she says. "Most people have a way of responding to certain issues, and they'll respond that way over and over again in spite of the fact *it never works*. I help couples free themselves from those self-defeating rituals and try a new approach."

The point is, if what you're doing isn't getting you the desired result, try something completely different, even if it's weird.

MARRYING FOR MONEY

Ever dream of putting an end to all your financial woes with two little words? Say "I do" to the right guy and you could trade in that stack of unpaid bills for charge accounts at all the right stores. What a fantasy!

Actually, marrying for money is done, and it's not necessarily a recipe for failure, says California marital therapist Constance Ahrons, Ph.D. "Any marriage can work out—even one like this," she says. "But each person must understand and agree to the ground rules and that there are certain trade-offs being made. Love, perhaps, being the biggest."

A woman who marries for money is frequently insecure, says Dr. Ahron. "She often feels that the only way to gain access to money, and the power that goes along with it, is through marriage," she says. "She has probably learned to like the materialistic things in life more than anything else and feels incapable of earning them on her own."

But while she may be marrying a man for his money, and he is quite aware of it, he can accept it because he feels he's getting something in return. "She may be very young and beautiful, a trophy to show off," explains Dr. Ahrons. "Or perhaps she has agreed to take total care of his life, to manage the whole home scene, be a good hostess and not make any other demands on his time.

"How often do you see a young, beautiful woman on the arm of an older, rather plain man, unless he's fabulously wealthy, too? Out here in Los Angeles, it's quite common. But here's a twist. As women become economically successful in their own right, they have started to have relationships with younger men," she says.

"I heard a wonderful example of breaking this kind of robotic behavior on a radio talk show," says Weiner-Davis. "A woman had begged her husband for their 55 years of marriage not to come to the breakfast table without his shirt on. It didn't bother her so much when he was younger, she admitted, but now that he was old it wasn't very appetizing to see that flabby body while she was eating. Yet, no matter how many times she repeated her request, it fell on deaf ears.

"One morning," recounts Weiner-Davis, "the woman had prepared an elaborate breakfast for her husband, and once again he came to the table naked from the waist up. Suddenly she got an idea and left the table in a flash. She went to her room and stripped from her waist up, then quietly returned to the table. Her husband literally started choking at the sight. Apparently he immediately left the table, got dressed, and according to the woman, never came to the table again without clothes on."

The point is, says Weiner-Davis, you need to break the cycle, the repetitive request that ultimately gets ignored. It makes the other person take a fresh look at the relationship and can do wonders to revive it, she says.

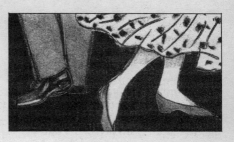

MARRIED MEN

FALLING IN LOVE WITH MR. WRONG

*T*he Other Woman. It's a provocative label that conjures up diverse images of negligee-decked mistresses, scheming femme fatales, pathetic, lonely women waiting beside silent telephones. They're the images of sad movies, Jackie Collins novels and country music. But their link to reality is tenuous.

"Most 'other women' are just like you and me," says San Diego psychotherapist JoAnne Bitner, Ph.D., who should know. Dr. Bitner is herself a former "other woman" whose life and group therapy sessions for women involved with married men became the subject of a made-for-TV movie several years ago.

In fact, in the future, says one expert, it will be the rare woman who hasn't been involved with a married man.

According to one source, between 15 and 20 percent of all single women over 35 in the United States will have an ongoing relationship with a married man—that's roughly 11 million American women dancing the "cheater's waltz" with someone else's husband. While these figures may include some "kept" women, purely sexual liaisons and women with a destructive streak that makes them specialize in snaring other women's men, they aren't the norm.

In fact, the norm is far more normal than most people think. More often, says Dr. Bitner, "these are women who meet and have long-lasting friendships that develop into love, just like any other relationship happens."

WHAT'S A NICE GIRL
LIKE YOU . . .

Sometimes, she says, love just happens, marital status and morals notwithstanding. As too many women discover, sometimes the man of your dreams is already taken, but the strength of the attraction overshadows age-old constraints against getting involved. "Your drive for being loved is sometimes more powerful than that particular taboo," Dr. Bitner says. "And that drive, like the taboo, goes all the way back to forever."

There are other, very pragmatic reasons why these relationships "just happen." In her book, *The New Other Woman*, Ohio State University sociology professor Laurel Richardson, Ph.D., points out that current demographics as well as cultural trends and realities help lead to illicit relationships. Statistically, and for a variety of reasons, the available pool of single men has diminished to puddle size, creating, according to Dr. Richardson, "a striking shortage of men for single women older than 27 in the United States." At the same time, she notes, society still requires women who wish to be considered "normal" to be part of a heterosexual couple. "Given the demographic constraints," she writes, "many single women who accept the goal of heterosexual couplehood will have to turn to socially disapproved ways to achieve it."

For practical purposes, two particular groups of women, Dr. Richardson notes, are more likely to seek "heterosexual couplehood" in the arms of another's husband: older women, for whom "the good ones" are quite likely to be married (among single women over 55 who are sexually active, about 45 percent are involved with married men), and women who are so busy career building they decide "half a loaf" is all they have time for.

SWEET TO BITTER

Although some love affairs may last a lifetime, these relationships are seldom permanent. Only about 25 percent result in marriage. "Most love affairs last about two years," says Dr. Bitner. "There's a process you go through. First the attraction, then the hopeful period when you think that maybe this is going to work out some way, followed by the realization that it is not going to work out, that he is not going to leave his wife. You ask yourself, 'Can I live this way?' Most women can't, and then it's over with."

While the clandestine aspect of the relationship may be titillating at first, the sex wonderful, the romance captivating, the love sweet, after a few months a woman may find her self-esteem slowly being eroded. Gradually, what was sweet becomes bitter, what was captivating becomes galling. Living her secret life, she runs the risk of becoming socially isolated, tethered to a phone that "might" ring, lying to those closest to her, unable to share her happiness or sadness with anyone. She may come to dread weekends and holidays when she may not only not see her lover but be totally unable to reach him. It is he who controls their relationship, not she, which may throw her "psychologically off-balance," according to Dr. Richardson. Giving up control of her time—indeed, her life—can lead to anger, resentment and depression.

"Sundays were always the worst because I knew I couldn't get hold of him in any way, short of calling him at home," says Sherri Chadwick, a 28-year-old journalist who became involved with a local politician. "Sometimes I would get so panicked—I mean, he could have *died* and I wouldn't have known until I read his obituary in the paper—that I would take a few drinks to calm me down. When it got to be my Sunday ritual, I knew it was time to bolt."

ONCE IN A WHILE IS NOT ENOUGH

Although she may fight it, at some point the other woman must face the fact that she is indeed the "other" woman in her man's life. Someone else always comes first. The realization, however slowly it dawns, can be quite painful.

"I felt really bad almost all the time," says Linda Friel,

32, who ended her 2½-year relationship with a married man 15 years her senior. "It took me more than a year to realize why. The bottom line of this relationship was that every day he spent with his wife in that other life was a rejection of me. I was sitting around waiting for him to choose when, of course, he already had. He had chosen her. I was at the end of the line, behind her, the kids, his job and the community. I got what was left over after they got their due. I was the secret he was too ashamed to tell. I had to face the fact that I felt bad because I was being rejected *on a daily basis*. No one's self-esteem can survive that."

The irony, she says in retrospect, was that she believes that, like most other women in a similar situation, she played a vital part in keeping his marriage together. "For more than two years, *I* was what made his married life bearable."

But what makes the other woman's life bearable? She accommodates. For those who choose to stay, an unusually strong sense of self-esteem helps, says Dr. Bitner. "And a nice network of friends. You need to get a very busy, very fulfilling life outside of the relationship with him. You need a career to keep you busy and that keeps your self-esteem up in other ways. He is not necessary to your self-esteem. You make sure you have something to do on Christmas, Easter, other holidays. You have your own financial system. You have a life of your own and he is an adjunct to it. That's the only way it works."

Cindy Merrill lives 300 miles away from her lover, whom she sees only one or two weekends a month. "Because we live in different cities, I'm able to keep control over it. If I were seeing him all the time, I would fall in and drown," she says.

But she doesn't simply count the days until they're together. Along with a successful career, she collects antiques, raises and shows Persian cats and teaches horseback riding. "I have a really busy, and committed life, a happy life," she says. "I fixed it so the relationship has to revolve around my other life. I had to. I simply couldn't be treated like that on a regular basis and still feel good about myself."

Linda Friel leads an active life, too, but she found it wasn't enough. "I probably spent more time with my lover than most women in this situation do. We worked together and he had no trouble getting away nights, weekends and holidays, even if only for an hour. Although I loved him with all my heart—still do, I guess—it wasn't enough. I want him all to myself. I wanted a husband and kids, just like his wife had. He kept telling me he was going to leave her, but after 2½ years, he was no closer to leaving than he was when I met him."

WHAT'S YOUR CHOICE?

What makes Cindy stay and what forced Linda to leave? "Whether you stay or leave has more to do with where you are in life and what your expectations and promises are than anything else," says Dr. Bitner. "If you're over 35 or 40 and you've been married, you realize the odds aren't very good that there will be another person in your life. It makes it a lot easier to say this is a really great person that I have half a relationship with, but that's better than nothing at all. If you're young, have never been married and want marriage and kids, the relationship is less attractive and harder to bear. You think there must be something better for you out there."

Linda also found herself thinking often about her lover's wife and children. "I think I felt a little guilty, even though I knew I wasn't breaking up a happy marriage and his kids were teenagers. But it's tough to live with anyway."

When it comes to wives, Dr. Bitner says, in her experience "other women" either rationalize that they "are not the ones being unfaithful and aren't responsible in any way" or feel conversely, "that some sort of sisterhood thing has been violated."

GETTING OUT

Whether your lover is married or single, breaking up, as the old song goes, is hard to do. How do you know when it's time? "If you've been in this for more than two years and you haven't come to grips with why you are there, you're still trying to get him to change and you're still miserable, it might be time to go," says Dr. Bitner. "If there is some kind of addictive quality to the relationship, that should put up some warning flags for you. If you are selling your soul, your morale or your self-esteem for the relationship, it's probably not a healthy thing. You leave when it becomes too painful and you want the pain to stop."

A support group would help. In Dr. Bitner's group, 90 percent of the women eventually left their lovers (including Dr. Bitner herself). "They heard each other talk, they had advice for each other and they started to see their own relationships in a different light," she says.

But there are few support groups for "other women." Supportive and empathetic friends may be able to help. "I had two friends who were also involved to varying degrees with married men and we helped each other," says Linda. "I was the first to leave, and the two others followed shortly afterward. We sort of talked each other out."

What is most helpful, though, says Dr. Bitner, is to get angry. "If you store up enough anger and resentment, you can coast on out of it," she says. "You have to have something to use to solidify your resolve. Remember what it would be like if you stayed in. Then you have to take your anger and turn it into energy, until you have enough anger you can't take it any more."

That's what ultimately gave Linda the strength to walk away from the man she loves. "Eventually, the pain of being with him was stronger than the pain of being without him."

CHAPTER 49

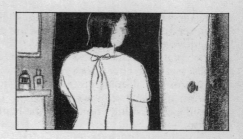

MEDICAL CARE

THE SPECIAL NEEDS IN WOMEN'S HEALTH

*B*esides your loved ones, who else is as familiar with your body as your doctor? Who else has seen you in compromising positions, half-naked, feverish and in pain? It's an unusual relationship, to say the least, to have with a person who's not a close family member. Yet you entrust your very life to this person. You drop your pants, bare your breasts and spill your guts to him or her. And in return you expect this person to listen to you, comfort you, teach you about your body and your health and maybe even heal you.

As one woman aptly stated, "When the doctor/patient relationship is good, it's very, very good, and when it's bad, it's horrid."

WOMEN ARE HUMAN, TOO

For women it's an especially tricky relationship. "Historically, women have not been treated kindly by the established medical profession, neither as health care consumers nor as health care providers nor as subjects of medical research," notes Lila A. Wallis, M.D., clinical professor of medicine at Cornell University Medical College in New York City, and Perri Klass, M.D., research fellow in pediatric infectious diseases at Boston City Hospital. "Women have repeatedly complained that their doctors don't take them seriously, that their symptoms are cast aside as being imaginary or 'psychosomatic.' "

Dr. Wallis and Dr. Klass point out that when it comes to diseases that affect both men and women, studies are often done on all-male groups and the results generalized to women, "as if men were truly the generic humans." Consider these studies funded by the National Institutes of Health.

- Research on the prevention of heart disease (including the use of low doses of aspirin) involved the long-term monitoring of 40,000 men, even though heart disease is the number one killer of women, too.
- A report called *Normal Human Aging* was based entirely on men.
- The famous concept of the Type-A personality (the ambitious, aggressive workaholic) was developed from a study of 4,000 California business*men*.

Maybe even worse is the dearth of research money devoted to the study of women's health issues. According to the federal General Accounting Office, the National Institutes of Health spends less than 13 percent on women's health issues, less than 2 percent on obstetrics and gynecology and less than 0.5 percent on basic breast cancer research.

TREATING THE BODY

"Women want and deserve to have a doctor who is clinically competent to treat their own particular health care concerns," says Karen Johnson, M.D., assistant clinical professor of psychiatry at the University of California, San Francisco, and a co-sponsor of a movement to develop a women's health specialty in medical education. "And that's no small matter considering how much of our medical knowledge has actually been based upon the research and understanding of the adult *male* body. It's a fundamental flaw in medical education, and one that doctors need to be aware of when treating their women patients."

The fact is, women need physicians who incorporate an understanding of complex female hormonal functioning along with other aspects of health and disease. Many "routine" medical conditions in women require special attention in diagnosis and treatment because of potential hormonal interactions.

"It helps that women are joining the medical profession at all levels," contends Dr. Johnson. "Attention has now been drawn to the fact that there are holes in medical education, and those holes must be filled in with appropriate research. The findings will eventually filter down to the physicians in clinical practice, and that will make for better medical care for women. But it could take years."

TREATING THE PERSON

Yet, if women have complaints about their medical care, those complaints center more around the doctor/patient relationship than the level of clinical competence displayed, says Linda Mangels, Ph.D., a behavioral psychologist and president of the American Academy of Risk Management in Longwood, Florida.

"Everyone's looking for a Marcus Welby," she says. "They want their doctors to be caring, compassionate *and* competent. When you're sick, you're in a vulnerable position. You're frightened of what might be wrong, there's the fear of the unknown hanging over you and you long for your doctor to simply take the time to explain what's happening, to show how much he cares and to listen to your concerns. The doctors who can fill that prescription rarely get sued, because the relationship they've developed with their patients is based on genuine respect and friendship."

Compassion can come from anyone, but it's expected more from a woman doctor. "When a woman finds a male doctor who's compassionate she'll talk about him as an *exception* to the rule, and he earns extra points in her book," says Dr. Johnson. "On the other hand, we expect women doctors to be compassionate, and when they're not, it makes us very angry and disappointed."

Still, patients often prefer to be treated by a doctor of their own sex. Dr. Mangels says based on her research, she has found that women generally prefer pediatricians and gynecologists to be women.

"Women doctors can identify with their women patients on a level that male physicians rarely can," adds Dr. Johnson. "Similarly, there may be health problems that men have that women doctors can't identify with."

Indeed, in one study of 185 adults, 43 percent of the women and 12 percent of the men preferred a female physician, while 31 percent of the men and 9 percent of the women preferred a male physician. Interestingly, women who preferred women doctors perceived them to be more humane, while men who preferred men doctors believed that they were more technically competent.

IN SEARCH OF DR. PERFECT

There's no doubt that modern medicine shines in many areas of acute care, says Alexandra Todd, Ph.D., author of *Intimate Adversaries: Cultural Conflict between Doctors and Women Patients*. "Yet patients complain of impersonal, overly technical treatment by uncaring doctors," she notes. Dr. Todd, who spent 2½ years observing communications between gynecologists and women patients, reports that the majority of women she talked with had a low opinion of their medical care. "Although they often cited positive experiences with individual doctors and staff, they had had enough negative interactions and results to foster feelings of discontent," she notes.

Not that great doctors don't exist. To find out what qualities go into making the ideal physician, Dr. Mangels surveyed more than 200 doctors who had practiced medicine for more than 20 years without being sued. And in another survey she interviewed more than 250 patient families to find out what turned them off so much about their physicians that they wanted to sue them. Her results add up to a recipe for the perfect doctor. Besides compassion and competence, she found that women wanted physicians who treat them with basic courtesy and take the time to answer their questions.

Today's women want to be treated as intellectual equals, says Dr. Johnson. "They're saying to their doctors, 'It's my body, I'm a knowledgeable person, I read, I listen, I inquire, I'm curious, and I'm here to get your advice.'"

There's nothing worse than having a doctor act as though he can't believe you asked *that* question, says Dr. Mangels. "Nobody likes to feel stupid."

It's part of every doctor's responsibility to educate patients so they can participate in treatment decisions, insists Dr. Johnson. And the doctors shouldn't use medical jargon, either, adds Dr. Mangels. "In any situation, but especially in life-threatening conditions, doctors need to educate you about your illness, the treatment options available and the consequences of those treatments," she says.

Adds Dr. Johnson, "Women don't want to be told by their doctors, 'Don't you worry about that. Let me do the worrying.' Today's patients want to be educated and informed so that they can be part of any health care decisions."

How does this work in practice?

One young mother says that her child's pediatrician always includes her in his diagnosing. "He'll say, 'Look in this ear. See how nice and pink it is? Now look in this one. See how red it is by comparison?' Or he'll show me the spots in my daughter's throat," she says. "I feel like I get a health lesson every time I go there, and I'm delighted to be the student."

Patients need to know that if they call their doctors, those calls will be returned. It shows that the doctor is genuinely concerned. One woman says that when her daughter had hepatitis, the doctor actually called *her* every day to see how her child's recovery was progressing. "I was truly touched by that extra effort," she says.

Women also value doctors who don't keep them waiting. Patient surveys consistently show that many simply will not tolerate long hours in the waiting room. One study by Dearing and Associates, a Spokane, Washington, organiza-

TREATING THE WHOLE WOMAN

Imagine going to just one doctor for *all* your particular health needs—from head to toe, from cradle to grave. It's a vision that's just beginning to take shape—women's health as a new medical specialty. That's the brainchild and dream of a number of women doctors who believe that physicians specializing in women's health should have expertise with primary care, obstetrics and gynecology and psychiatry. Women's health, after all, isn't only about reproduction.

The obstetricians/gynecologists have by default been viewed as women's health physicians because they are currently in the only field of medicine where the clientele is exclusively women, says University of California professor Karen Johnson, M.D., who is actively involved in the development of the new specialty.

"You have to remember that obstetrics and gynecology is primarily a surgical specialty," she says. "Only a limited number have comprehensive training in the nonreproductive health care needs of women. Your average obstetrician/gynecologist doesn't know a great deal about hypertension, heart disease, thyroid disease, gallbladder problems, depression or sexuality, for that matter. Consequently, they don't have the clinical competence to present themselves as women's health specialists.

"That's why the American Medical Women's Association is developing a core curriculum in women's health that would become a base against which medical education programs and residency programs could measure themselves," she says.

Dr. Johnson, along with Laurel Dawson, M.D., a physician with the Bay Spring Women's Medical Group in San Francisco, detailed the idea of a women's health specialty in the November/December 1990 issue of the *Journal of the American Medical Women's Association*.

Currently, they say, a woman who is suffering from premenstrual syndrome might have to see three different doctors to treat the symptoms. She might see an internist for the headaches, anxiety, weight gain or other nonspecific symptoms. She might be consulting a psychiatrist for depression, irritability, episodes of rage or other psychological problems. Meanwhile, a gynecologist might be treating her with birth control pills or progesterone. "Each physician is treating symptoms that appear to be part of a premenstrual symptom complex," they note. "However, they are working in isolation when a coordinated effort would be more sensible." Indeed, many women see several specialists before being accurately diagnosed and treated.

Not surprisingly, the very idea of a specialty in women's health has met with more than a little resistance from the established medical community, admits Dr. Johnson. "Any time you propose a change in the status quo, people will resist," she says. "What's more, some physicians who already take care of women feel hurt or insulted by our proposal, as if we're insinuating that the care they give is inferior, which isn't necessarily so. And a part of the resistance is economic—plain old dollars and cents. If we develop a specialty in women's health, whom do you think women patients will choose to see?"

tion that gather health statistics on women, found that women comfortably wait only about 20 minutes past their appointment time. If they wait longer than that, they wait mad.

One woman says she changed gynecologists because the typical wait in his office was 45 minutes. "I probably would have stayed with him, however, if I thought his examinations were through," she points out. "But he'd press each breast twice, do an internal in a few minutes, and then be on his way. I could sense his impatience if I had any questions that needed answering."

WHAT YOU NEED TO KNOW

But women, too, have a responsibility to communicate honestly with their doctors. "Women need to be less submissive in medical interactions, asking questions that ensure their understanding and their informed agreement in medical decision making," notes Dr. Todd. "They need to learn to push for the right to tell their stories. Doctors need to reassess their long-held, often unexamined attitudes toward women and patients, learning a new language to discuss health issues."

As Dr. Mangels puts it: "I don't see a lot of bad medicine being practiced out there. I see a lot of bad interpersonal skills. In many ways, it's up to the patient to communicate to her doctor what she expects from their relationship. It needs to be stated clearly that she wants to be an active part of the doctor/patient relationship and to share in the responsibilities of treatment."

"To ensure that you get the kind of relationship that's right for you, you need to interview prospective doctors. And do it when you're well, not sick," stresses Dr. Johnson. "Find out what the doctor's values are, what his or her background is, what it's like to be in contact with him or her, whether you share similar expectations from the relationship and how well he or she communicates with you."

See also Gynecologists

CHAPTER 50

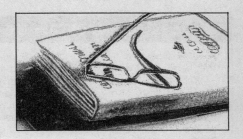

MENOPAUSE

NEW ATTITUDES ERASE OLD NOTIONS

Women—famous or otherwise, on national talk shows or in their own living rooms—will talk about their marriages, their divorces, their face-lifts, tummy tucks and breast implants. They'll discuss their cancers and their mastectomies, their sexual persuasions and their drug addictions. They'll even talk about their weight gains, graying hair and their ages. But whether they're 46, 52, 60 or 70, seldom do you hear them talk about menopause. Why is that?

"Menopause is an undeniable marker of aging," says Kathleen MacPherson, R.N., Ph.D., professor of nursing at the University of Southern Maine School of Nursing in Portland. Although nutrition, exercise or good genes can keep you looking healthy and attractive as you grow older, becoming menopausal is likely to make you all too aware of the many negative myths associated with this normal stage of life.

Attitudes toward older women—which leave a lot to be desired in our youth-worshipping society—may also lead us to view menopause in a negative way, adds Linda Gannon, Ph.D., professor of psychology at Southern Illinois University at Carbondale. And our own mothers may contribute to a negative view of menopause as well.

For generations, women anticipated the "change of life" as they would an impending storm. They braced themselves,

PUTTING OUT THE FIRE

For those whose hot flashes are intense, frequent and disruptive, here's what doctors say you can do to help.

Keep a log. Note the date, time, intensity and duration of the hot flash. Also, record the circumstances preceding it: what you ate or drank and how you felt. Women report hot flashes become worse and more frequent during times of stress. Drinking caffeinated coffee also can promote a hot flash.

Consider biofeedback. This technique, which uses electronic sensors to detect changes in body temperature and muscle tension, has helped many women stifle headaches. It has also been shown to be successful in relieving hot flashes.

Don't fight the inevitable. Women who try to control hot flashes can make them more intense. Instead of fighting a hot flash, stop what you're doing, sit down and just let your arms and legs hang loose. Then let the hot flash roll over you like a wave.

Evaluate the possible benefits of vitamin E. According to Lila E. Nachtigall, M.D., a New York University gynecology professor, 400 international units of vitamin E taken twice a day can cut the frequency of hot flashes for some women. Check with your doctor, though, before beginning supplementation. Vitamin E can have a blood-thinning effect.

Consider estrogen replacement therapy (ERT). ERT is considered the most effective treatment against hot flashes. If your hot flashes are so severe that they disrupt your life, discuss hormone replacement therapy with your doctor.

hoped to be spared the worst of it, then sat tight until it passed.

Today that attitude is dissipating. Scientists now know that about 10 percent of all women slip through menopause with hardly a symptom, while 75 percent will have a variety of symptoms ranging from insomnia, hot flashes and irritability to vaginal dryness, mood swings and heart palpitations—all the symptoms that have given menopause a bad name.

WHEN ESTROGEN WANES

Menopause is actually a three-stage process that ends your reproductive life.

The first stage—premenopause—usually begins around age 40, as the amount of estrogen produced by your ovaries begins to decline. Periods gradually become irregular over the next decade, and the consistency of the menstrual flow itself begins to change. One month the flow will be so light you could blot it with a tissue, another month it'll be so heavy you'll wish they'd invented triple-super tampons.

Eventually estrogen levels will drop so low that you won't have enough to trigger a period ever again. This is the actual menopause—a Greek term that means "monthly" and "cease"—which extends from your last period through the 12 months that follow it. It usually occurs somewhere around age 52, depending on when the women in your family stop menstruating. Generally, daughters tend to follow the menstrual patterns established by their mothers and grandmothers.

After you've gone 12 full months without a period, you've reached the third and final stage—postmenopause. Since most women now live until age 78 or so, it's a stage in which you will spend approximately one-third of your life.

VOLCANIC HOT FLASHES

If you're one of the women who'll experience symptoms during menopause, the earliest and most likely symptom you'll experience is a hot flash.

Hot flashes appear to be the result of dropping estrogen levels that alter your brain chemistry significantly enough to jiggle your body's thermostat. Unfortunately, jiggling your body's thermostat—actually a small gland located in the center of your brain—is exactly like jiggling the thermostat in your home. The thermostat incorrectly senses that you're cold and fires up the furnace. It sends out messages that constrict blood vessels in your skin, which elevates your temperature and makes you feel warm. But—since you weren't really cold to begin with—your body hurriedly reopens the blood vessels in an attempt to cool itself down. The result is a rush of blood to your upper body and face—which is why you appear flushed—and a torrent of sweat.

How bad is a hot flash? Many women feel only a slight flush with a few beads of sweat. Others feel overwhelmed.

Flight attendant Clarice Harrell, 46, describes her hot flashes as "a volcano coming out the top of my head." As for the sweat, she says, "I'd wake up soaking wet two, three times a night. Looking back, it's no wonder I was testy during the day."

THE MYTH OF MADNESS

Night sweats and the loss of sleep that goes along with them are certainly to blame for some of the irritability that many women feel just before and during menopause. But the real culprit behind irritability, forgetfulness, mood swings and what some women characterize as the blues is not so much the flashing or sweating evidence that estrogen levels are dropping—it's the low level of estrogen itself.

"Estrogen naturally enhances mood," explains researcher Barbara B. Sherwin, Ph.D., an associate professor of psychology, obstetrics and gynecology at McGill University in Montreal. That's why some women feel blue or irritable when estrogen levels drop.

Actually, "I thought I was going crazy," says Clarice. "I'd be walking around in a black cloud one week and happy the next. If something was sad, it became a tragedy. If it was funny, it became hysterical. My emotional balance seemed to be out of whack. It was like having PMS times 50, but it never went away," she adds. "All I did was snap at my friends. It just seemed too hard for me to be nice—even to the people I cared about most."

The moodiness that Clarice describes is unpleasant at best, but it is not the kind of major depression that requires heavy drugs to treat. The idea that menopause causes major depression or major personality changes in otherwise healthy women is a myth, says Dr. Sherwin. A study at the University of Pittsburgh, for example, found that women who had recently gone through menopause did not have higher levels of anxiety, stress, anger, nervousness or depression than a similar group of women who were still menstruating.

Furthermore, population studies indicate that there is no increase in major depression among normal, healthy women, says Dr. Sherwin. When clinical depression occurs during menopause, it usually occurs among women who are already having fairly significant problems.

Fortunately, when dropping estrogen levels do cause mood swings, irritability or the blues among normal women, it's usually a relatively short-term problem that is easily handled. (See "Swinging Along with Your Moods" on page 334.)

WHO FARES BEST?

Not everyone experiences mood swings and other "emotional" problems during menopause. But does that mean there's a particular kind of woman who is immune to the psychological effects of declining estrogen?

Very likely. In a study of 500 menopausal women, Ann J. Clark, R.N., Ph.D., director of the University of Alabama at Birmingham Center for Nursing Research, found that women who are assertive, independent and authoritative experience fewer symptoms and distress during menopause than women who are more likely to characterize themselves as deferent, traditionally feminine and emotional. She also found that women with a strong purpose in life are less likely to report distressing symptoms than those who lack such a purpose.

Having a purpose seems particularly important, agrees Dr. MacPherson, who returned to school for a Ph.D. when she was in her late forties. "My concern was getting through graduate school," she notes. "I was so excited about all the things I was learning, I just didn't think much about menopause."

Susan Lassiter, a 55-year-old copy editor, feels the same way. "I think because I was so caught up in my work, I didn't have time to think about my plumbing," says Susan.

SWINGING ALONG WITH YOUR MOODS

Just because menopause puts hormones in a decline doesn't mean your whole life should go downhill.

Surround yourself with women your own age. Psychology professor Linda Gannon, Ph.D., says any activity—from church socials to political fund-raising events—that brings you together with other women your age will help you cope with your own menopause. "When people are isolated, they tend to feel their problems are unique," says Dr. Gannon. "It's a relief to find out that other women feel the same way they do."

Nursing professor Kathleen MacPherson, R.N., Ph.D., agrees. She's led self-help groups for women going through or about to face menopause. "There's nothing like being part of a group to find a wide variety of views about menopause and learn from them," she says. "There have even been a few young women who joined because they wanted to know and understand what their mothers were experiencing."

Put your body on a schedule. Research has shown that when certain rhythms in our bodies are disrupted, it tends to have a negative impact on our psychological functioning, says Dr. Gannon. And during menopause your menstrual cycle, which is one of your body's natural rhythms, is likely to be erratic. Consequently, it might help to make your body's other rhythms as predictable as possible. In other words, eat on a regular schedule, exercise on a regular schedule and sleep on a regular schedule.

Discover the joys of exercise. Evidence suggests that regular energetic exercise may improve your mood when it drifts toward the blues. A brisk walk, for example, can raise levels of endorphins—good-humor hormones that are known to drop during menopause.

"I can remember how my mother always talked in hushed tones about 'the change.' She'd say, 'You have to take special care of yourself at this time.' But I don't know what she was talking about. Menopause barely made a ripple in my life."

Why such disparate attitudes? Women facing menopause today were raised to be more than baby producers and baby tenders, explains Dr. Gannon. So losing the ability to have children is not as big a deal to them as it was to their mothers, who frequently had more limited options for self-fulfillment.

PERMANENT CHANGES

One group of menopausal changes that does not disappear along with monthly periods are those that affect your vagina, bones and heart.

In all three cases, estrogen has done an important job

SOOTHING THE WAY

If your vagina is a casualty of the dryness that comes with menopause, here's what you can do about it.

Keep sex alive. Regular sexual activity helps keep natural moisture flowing and maintains pelvic muscle tone.

Replace lost lubrication. If dryness becomes a problem, you may want to try a nonprescription lubricant. One called Replens comes in single-dose tamponlike dispensers and seems to stay in place better than standard water-soluble lubricants.

Choose personal hygiene products with care. Use mild (nondeodorant and fragrance-free) soap or cleansing bars. Avoid personal hygiene sprays, which can irritate dry, sensitive vaginal tissues.

Think twice about using antihistamines. These drugs don't discriminate; they dry mucous membranes in the nose *and* in the vagina.

Consider estrogen. Even the most severe vaginal symptoms can be reversed with estrogen replacement therapy, say the experts. And the dose is lower than that used to resolve hot flashes. You may also want to try an estrogen cream applied directly to the vagina. It can instantly relieve the itching and dryness that comes with a drop in your body's estrogen production.

over the years. It has maintained the thickness and moisture content of vaginal walls, maintained the thickness and strength of bones and apparently contributed to maintaining a healthy cardiovascular system by boosting levels of the "good" kind of cholesterol and reducing levels of the "bad."

Yet studies indicate that too much of the bad cholesterol and not enough of the good leads to clogged arteries, heart attacks and death. Too little bone density and bones become brittle and break. Too thin and dry a vaginal wall and infections become likely and intercourse painful.

Fortunately, doctors say, estrogen replacement therapy can prevent all these potential problems and leave you free to enjoy your menopause.

Enjoy menopause?

Absolutely. One of the best-kept secrets in medical science (and something your mother was probably too shy to mention) is the fact that menopause brings with it higher levels of androgens—marvelously aggressive hormones secreted by the adrenal glands—that ignite your sex drive in a way that you haven't experienced since adolescence.

Is it any wonder a major study found that 96 percent of those women who had initially viewed menopause with regret actually felt good about it once they got to it?

See also Estrogen Replacement Therapy, Heart Disease, Osteoporosis

CHAPTER 51

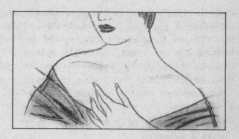

MENSTRUAL PROBLEMS

THE MESSAGE BEHIND THOSE MONTHLY MISERIES

*K*aren Arlen was on a business trip to New York when she suddenly began experiencing midcycle bleeding. "At first I thought it was just spotting, which I've had before, but it went from spotting to really flowing, like a period," she says. "I was scared. I'm 48, so it crossed my mind it could be the beginning of menopause, but I wanted to be sure."

When she returned home, Karen made an appointment with her gynecologist. "I was a little apologetic about it," she confesses. "I told her it was probably nothing but menopause and she agreed, but she told me not to apologize. Any midcycle bleeding could be the symptom of something far more serious, like cancer. She told me I was right to come in for a checkup. She said at 28, you wouldn't expect to find uterine cancer. At 48, you might."

In Karen's case, a few tests assured her that she didn't have cancer and that her irregular bleeding was, indeed, the first symptom of menopause. But her experience is illustrative of what every woman should do about any irregularity in her menstrual cycle, from bleeding to cramps: See a doctor. While in most cases the cause is going to be something simple, it's not wise to take chances, warns Jill Maura Rabin, M.D., assistant professor of obstetrics and gynecology in the Division of Urogynecology at Long Island Jewish Medical Center in New Hyde Park, New York.

"If you haven't already, establish a relationship with a physician you trust," says Dr. Rabin. "Taking care of an out-of-the ordinary symptom sooner rather than later is better because if you ignore it, it won't go away, and you may worsen your prognosis."

DON'T TAKE PAIN FOR GRANTED

Don't even take cramps as a given. Although they're rarely anything serious, they can be a symptom of endometriosis or fibroid tumors or infection, which could threaten your fertility. And in most cases cramps, even severe, debilitating ones, are "curable."

As Mimi Cohen found out. From the time she got her period as a young teenager, Mimi suffered from severe cramping two or three days before her menstrual flow started and during the first few days of her period. "I remember at 15, going down to the nurse's office and her looking at me and saying, 'My God, you're green,' " Mimi recalls. "I was really miserable. I've missed whole nights' sleep because of the pain."

For most women, over-the-counter medication such as ibuprofen, a nonsteroidal anti-inflammatory drug, work like a miracle, says Penny Wise Budoff, M.D., author of *No More Menstrual Cramps and Other Good News*. "But there are all degrees of menstrual pain. For some women, they're fleeting. If they get up and move around, they will feel better. There are other people who feel like they're going to die and may need a doctor's prescription of nonsteroidal anti-inflammatory drugs, like Anaprox, Ponstel or Motrol."

Your doctor will want to rule out fibroid tumors, which are nonmalignant-growths in the uterus, and endometriosis, a condition in which parts of the endometrium (uterine lining) break away and implant in the lower abdomen. These misplaced tissues respond the way the endometrium does during your menstrual cycle. That is, they bleed and cause cramping, and therefore irritate the lining of the abdomen, causing pain.

THE PROSTAGLANDIN CONNECTION

In most cases, however, menstrual cramping is caused by hormonelike chemicals in the body called prostaglandins. Prostaglandins cause uterine contractions, not only during menstruation but also during labor. The contractions, which you experience as cramps, serve an important purpose, says Dr. Rabin. "During your period, a portion of the lining of the uterus cleaves off. What makes it shear off is vessel spasm, which is caused by prostaglandins. Blood vessels in the uterus contract and expand, and as they do, they produce more and more prostaglandins. What the prostaglandins do is keep the process going. Ultimately, all this expanding causes the blood vessels to leak, and this leads to the shearing off of the surface layer of the uterine lining."

Their work doesn't stop there. "During the first day when the blood flow is heavy, the cramping serves to seal off the blood vessels at the level where the lining was sheared off to prevent hemorrhaging," says Dr. Rabin. "As the uterus contracts, it moves the blood and lining out."

Everyone produces prostaglandins. Why do some women have more pain than others? "Everybody gets cramps," says Dr. Rabin. "Some people may just have a different pain threshold. Some people may not consider them anything. They're at such a low level they don't even feel them. But some women may produce more prostaglandins or they may have receptors in their bodies that bind prostaglandins in a way that allows them to continue to work more strongly."

Normally, drugs like ibuprofen and Anaprox eliminate pain from cramping because they're known as antiprostaglandins—drugs that block the body's production of prostaglandins or that prevent the chemical from landing on its receptor. They can also help relieve the diarrhea and nausea—and occasionally, hot flashes—some women experience, which is caused by prostaglandins landing on receptors in the bowel and colon.

Your doctor may need to experiment to find the right drug for you. Mimi Cohen tried over-the-counter ibuprofen and prescription Anaprox and got little relief. Then, when her doctor prescribed another antiprostaglandin drug for neck pain, Mimi discovered it eliminated her cramps, too. "So he just continued prescribing it for my cramps," she says.

Some women find exercise helps, says Dr. Rabin. "Exercise helps oxygenate the tissues better so that the body's toxins and the waste products that are being formed get whisked away faster," she says.

There are some other "natural" methods that work for some women, such as meditation, drinking eight to ten glasses of water a day and switching to a low-fat, low-sugar diet, with very little alcohol and no caffeine, a regimen that some clinicians find also works for premenstrual syndrome.

SO MANY CAUSES

There are two groups of women who can almost expect to experience irregular periods—young girls who are just starting to menstruate and women approaching menopause. In both cases, the menstrual irregularities are usually related to ovulation, which may itself be irregular. "These are women at opposite ends of the spectrum of reproductive life," says Dr. Rabin. "A young girl's ovaries are just starting to produce a mature egg each month. At that time, you may not ovulate every month so you may not have a period (ovulatory cycle) every month, or they may be irregular. You may not have regular periods when you don't have regular ovulation, which is true in the beginning and at the end of reproductive life."

It's important, however, to see your doctor if your periods are irregular in any way—absent, infrequent, particularly painful or accompanied by excessive bleeding. "Irregular periods or abnormal vaginal bleeding can be a sign of cancer of the lining of the uterus or the ovaries, and this becomes more worrisome as the woman gets older because the incidence of cancer increases with age," says Dr. Rabin.

There are other causes of abnormal bleeding as well. Fibroid tumors can cause abnormal vaginal bleeding—particularly excessive bleeding—as can benign ovarian masses or other benign problems in the lining of the uterus. Adenomyosis, which is the growth of endometrial tissue into the uterine wall, can cause excessive bleeding and is most often seen in women in their forties. Endometriosis can cause heavy bleeding as well as bleeding between ovulation and menstruation. You can have abnormal bleeding if you have a polyp in the uterus or cervix. Those are all functional problems, says Dr. Rabin.

You also can have dysfunctional bleeding and irregular ovulation due to a problem that's not related to the reproductive system, says Dr. Rabin. Thyroid problems, diabetes and blood ailments such as sickle-cell anemia and hemophilia can cause irregular menstrual bleeding. Hormone imbalances, which can have many causes, including pituitary tumors, can interfere with ovulation and cause excessive or irregular bleeding.

Treatment varies according to the problem. There are a number of drugs—including hormone-based drugs such as oral contraceptives and antiprostaglandins—that can cut down on excessive blood flow. Oral contraceptives are often prescribed to regulate the menstrual cycle. Drugs that shrink fibroid tumors or surgery that either removes the tumors or the uterus (hysterectomy) will also relieve heavy menstrual bleeding if it's caused by uterine growths.

One of the things your doctor will want to rule out— especially if you have missed one period or more or have irregular ones—is pregnancy, especially ectopic pregnancy, in which a fertilized egg implants outside the uterus, a condition that can threaten both your fertility and your life. Abdominal pain is one of the early signs of ectopic pregnancy and should receive medical attention.

OVARIES ON THE FRITZ

Once it's certain that you're not pregnant, your physician will want to know if you are ovulating. Women who ovulate tend to have irregular periods. Women who don't may have no periods at all—a condition called amenorrhea—or may have irregular periods or experience spotting. (Some women experience midcycle pain as a sign of ovulation. This is perfectly normal and is usually a good sign that you're ovulating.)

If your doctor suspects your menstrual irregularities are caused by lack of ovulation, he or she may ask you to monitor your basal body temperature daily. At ovulation, your body temperature rises about 0.5 degrees and stays elevated until you menstruate. That reflects the effect the hormone progesterone has on your hypothalamus, the section of the brain that regulates temperature. There are a number of other tests that measure ovulation, including endometrial biopsy, an office procedure in which the doctor removes a small piece of endometrial tissue that can be analyzed for everything from hormone levels and signs of ovulation to precancerous and cancerous conditions.

Failure to ovulate can have many causes. Stress can stifle ovulation, as can excessive exercise and eating disorders. A condition known as polycystic ovaries, in which the ovaries become enlarged because they contain a number of partially matured but unexpelled eggs, is caused by a hormone imbalance. It is often corrected by fertility drugs, such as clomiphene citrate (Clomid). Thyroid problems and tumors of the ovary and adrenal gland can also interfere with ovulation and thus cause menstrual irregularities.

THE OVERWEIGHT FACTOR

Women who are 20 percent or more over their ideal weight may fail to ovulate because they have excess estrogen, which is stored in body fat. In those larger amounts, the estrogen acts in much the same way supplemental estrogen does, by interfering with the normal estrogen/progesterone fluctuations that trigger ovulation, prepare the uterus for pregnancy and, if no pregnancy develops, cause the endometrial lining to shed. "The excess estrogen in the overweight woman's body effectively shuts off the ovulation center in the brain," says Dr. Rabin. "This condition is often reversible. She needs to lose weight."

And not simply because her fertility is affected. In obese women—indeed, in any woman who does not ovulate for any length of time—the excess estrogen can cause the endometrial lining to build up, but without progesterone to counteract the estrogen, the lining isn't completely shed. Not only does the woman not have a normal period, but the buildup of endometrial tissue can cause hyperplasia, a precancerous condition that, if not corrected, can become malignant.

THE PROBLEM OF BEING TOO THIN

At the other end of the spectrum, a woman who is very thin may stop menstruating because her body fat has dropped below the level needed to support the menstrual cycle. Amenorrhea, as the condition is known, is seen frequently in women with eating disorders and in athletes. Recent studies have also shown that otherwise normal women who lose weight on calorie-restricted vegetarian diets may also have amenorrhea.

Recently, researchers have begun looking at the menstrual histories of female athletes, especially runners and those in endurance training, who often fail to menstruate. Once thought to be a benign, even welcome side effect of exercise, amenorrhea is now being linked to osteoporosis and, in some cases, irreversible bone loss. In some studies, in fact, about half of all runners with amenorrhea came down with hairline fractures known as stress fractures, compared with about 30 percent of runners who have normal menstrual cycles. Studies also show the longer the menstrual irregularity exists, the greater the injury and bone loss risk.

One reason athletes face these unwelcome side effects may be that without sufficient body fat, in which estrogen is stored, they simply do not have enough estrogen to support menstruation or to maintain proper calcium balance. Calcium is a key mineral for healthy bones.

If you are very active and you aren't getting a period, you're better off not considering it a "perk" of being an athlete. Studies show that if you restore your normal menstrual cycle, either by cutting back on your activity or through estrogen replacement therapy (usually oral contraceptives), and increase your intake of calcium, you may be able to restore the bone you lost.

But don't delay. Some studies suggest that bone loss associated with long-term amenorrhea (three or four years) isn't reversible with estrogen or calcium.

See also Premenstrual Syndrome

CHAPTER 52

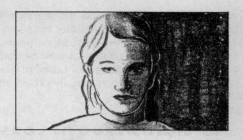

MISCARRIAGE AND STILLBIRTH

WHEN PREGNANCY GOES WRONG

*L*oretta Andrews already had two children and was expecting her third when suddenly, without warning, she miscarried in her third month.

"Afterward," says Loretta, now the mother of four, "I kept thinking about a woman who lived in our old neighborhood. She had had a miscarriage and I remember trying to console her by saying, 'It's okay, it's Mother Nature's way of keeping you from having a deformed baby.' After I lost my baby I wanted to call her and apologize because what I said to her meant *nothing*. *Nothing*. I knew, because it meant nothing when people said it to me."

Judith Lasker sailed through an easy first pregnancy. She went into labor on a sunny summer day, working in the garden with her husband until she felt it was time to go to the hospital. When she arrived, her doctor examined her and told her the baby was in a breech position and that she might require a cesarean. After taking an x-ray, her doctor decided against the operation and a few hours later wheeled her into the delivery room where her daughter was stillborn.

"The first thing the nurse said was, 'It would have been worse if she had been 5,'" recalls Judith, who is now the mother of two healthy girls. "She was probably right, but that wasn't the choice I was considering: Do I want a baby that dies at birth or one that dies at 5? I had expected a live baby and mine was born dead. Her attitude—the attitude of many people—is 'You don't know this baby, it's not a big deal, just get pregnant again.' I used to think that, too. But I can tell you, I still occasionally cry for my baby, and it's been 12½ years."

UNACKNOWLEDGED LOSS

The loss of a child through miscarriage or stillbirth is often an unacknowledged loss, felt profoundly by parents and misunderstood by those around them.

For Judith Lasker, Ph.D., the loss of her child affected her so deeply that she, along with Susan Borg, a childhood friend who had also lost a baby shortly after birth, wrote one of the first mass-market books on pregnancy loss, called *When Pregnancy Fails*, which explores what they call "incomprehensible" grief. Dr. Lasker, a sociology professor at Lehigh University in Bethlehem, Pennsylvania, has become an expert on the subject.

No one really knows how many parents face the loss of a child each year, but based on figures kept by the National Center for Health Statistics, Dr. Lasker estimates 800,000 families a year mourn a child lost through miscarriage or stillbirth.

Prenatal tests may warn of a genetic condition that will take the life of a newborn. Stillbirth and miscarriage may be preceded by symptoms—bleeding or lack of fetal movement or pain. But they may also happen without warning, and there frequently is no explainable cause. Because this is often a couple's first experience with death, suddenly bereaved parents or "almost" parents may not know how they're "supposed" to feel and may be bewildered by the sadness that overwhelms them, says Dr. Lasker.

Those around the bereaved couple—family, friends, even medical personnel—will urge them to put it behind them, to move on—something they may want to do but find they can't. People will try to "cheer you up," but that's not going to happen.

"People try to say things to be helpful," says Dr. Lasker. "They look for ways to diminish the loss to make you feel better. 'You'll have another one and it'll be all better.' It may never be *all* better. The loss you feel is real. It's part of who you are. Although you might never feel *all* better, most people feel a lot better with time."

MISCARRIAGE: A COMMON EVENT

Although most experts estimate that 14 to 18 percent of all pregnancies end in miscarriage, the number is probably much higher. According to U.S. government figures, only one-quarter to one-third of all embryos conceived become live infants. The remainder are lost at some stage between fertilization and birth, but particularly during the early stages, usually before the woman even knows she is pregnant.

About three-quarters of all miscarriages occur in the first 12 weeks and, according to laboratory tests, about 60 percent are due to some abnormality of the embryo—a genetic problem or a random mutation. The rest usually happen because the embryo failed to implant properly.

Miscarriage is more common in women who have had several previous miscarriages, in very young (under 18) and older women and in those with endometriosis, a condition in which uterine tissue implants elsewhere in the abdominal cavity. Late miscarriages, those occurring between 13 and 20 weeks, are usually caused by implantation problems, although the fetus may be normal. About 35 percent are caused by chromosomal defects.

If a cervix is abnormally weak, as it often is in women whose mothers took the synthetic hormone diethylstilbestrol (DES) during pregnancy, it may dilate too early and the baby can be lost. Uterine abnormalities, such as a double uterus, may also cause miscarriage. Uterine infections (including sexually transmitted diseases), fibroid tumors and other growths such as scar tissue, malnutrition or exposure to radiation or toxic chemicals by either parent are also linked to miscarriage, as are smoking, excessive use of alcohol and certain drugs, including birth control pills. In some cases of habitual miscarriage, there may be a hormone problem or an immunological factor.

Sometimes miscarriages can be prevented, but few can be stopped once they start. As Dr. Lasker notes, some doctors will recommend bed rest at the first sign of danger. It may help. Sometimes, even when there is bleeding, the cervix stays closed. In about half the cases of early bleeding, women do not miscarry. But the doctor's bed rest prescription may be made to "allay potential feelings of guilt" if a miscarriage does occur.

NO EASY ANSWERS

Your first reaction to a miscarriage—indeed, any pregnancy loss—may be "What went wrong?" While it may help if your physician is able to pinpoint the cause of your loss, especially if there is a lifestyle factor that could be altered, "many times there is no answer," says Dr. Lasker. "So people come up with their own answers. They blame themselves. 'What went wrong?' becomes 'What did I do wrong?'"

With the barrage of prenatal advice a pregnant woman receives, it may be tempting to make some sense out of a pregnancy loss by blaming yourself. Some couples even see their loss as a punishment for something they did in the past—using birth control or premarital sex. "Our friends help us with this. They ask, 'What could it have been? Was it this you did, was it that you did?' says Dr. Lasker. "Many people come up with an explanation that focuses on their own behavior, even when the doctor says it is clearly not."

But, she says, guilt is not necessarily a bad feeling at a time like this. Like the shock and disbelief that often accompany a trauma, it's a way to help us come to terms gradually with the loss. "Guilt is a piece of grief," says Dr. Lasker. "It's part of making sense of it. It allows you to believe that you have control over the outcome. If you have no control, it could be worse psychologically because it means you can't control it the next time. You can't prevent it from happening again, which may very well be true but which can add to your bad feelings. But as your grief diminishes, your sense of responsibility diminishes. You'll recognize your guilt as irrational."

MOST MISUNDERSTOOD FEELINGS

The grief that follows miscarriage may be baffling both to the couple and to those around them because of the assumption that the parents are not "attached" to the lost fetus—which, studies have shown, is not true. Mothers especially form a strong emotional attachment to their babies early in pregnancy. Dr. Lasker's research, involving hundreds of couples who suffered a pregnancy loss, found that a mother's grief was usually more intense the later in pregnancy she suffered her loss, but other studies indicate that the length of the pregnancy is not as significant as how emotionally linked a woman feels to her baby. A woman who feels her child to be "real" even in early pregnancy may suffer as much grief over a miscarriage as she would if the child were a newborn.

Those around her, including medical personnel, however, may attempt to minimize her loss. In one study, hospital personnel said they recognized miscarriage as a tragedy, but the authors of the study referred to their recognition as "the silent sympathy" because it was so rarely expressed.

Efforts of family, friends and medical personnel to be helpful often backfire, says Dr. Lasker. You may hear, "Oh, you can always have another baby," although you yourself may not be so sure.

Dr. Lasker found that many women who miscarry suffer from a host of physical and psychological symptoms. You may have trouble sleeping and eating. You may become preoccupied with your loss and have trouble concentrating on anything else. A miscarriage can arouse feelings of guilt, helplessness and self-doubt and fears about future fertility. You may feel like a failure as a woman because you were unable to do what others do so easily. You may become hostile, angry and depressed. Even if you feel you are "over it" within a few months, you may feel sad when your due

WARNING SIGNS

Contact your doctor if you experience any of these conditions, which doctors say can be warning signs of an impending pregnancy loss or a medical emergency that could be threatening to you or your baby.

- Spotting or bleeding (through some slight spotting can be normal in early pregnancy and a small amount of discharge can occur in late pregnancy as the cervix starts to open)
- Passing clots or tissue
- Cramping or abdominal pain
- A fever over 100°F
- Fainting
- Puffiness of the face and eyes, especially if it occurs suddenly
- A burning sensation when you urinate and discomfort afterward
- A severe headache in the forehead or behind the eyes late in pregnancy that doesn't respond to medication
- Leakage of fluid from the vagina, which could mean your membranes have ruptured
- A diminishing of pregnancy symptoms
- An absence of fetal movement for 8 to 10 hours, particularly if the fetus is normally active

date arrives or during a holiday that you expected to celebrate with your child.

While Dr. Lasker says that couples find the most comfort and solace in each other, there is a limit to how much you and your spouse can help one another. Grieving, as Dr. Lasker points out, is a lonely process. Not even the most loving spouse can take all your pain away. There may also be a difference between your grief and your spouse's. Dr. Lasker's research, like many other studies, indicates that a father may not feel the same kind of attachment a mother feels toward her unborn child because the child has not become a physical reality to him. He may also have different ways of expressing his deepest feelings.

FROM THOSE WHO HAVE BEEN THERE

When sociology professor Judith Lasker, Ph.D., of Lehigh University in Pennsylvania, and her colleagues surveyed hundreds of men and women who had experienced pregnancy losses, they asked them what advice they would offer others going through the same experience. Here's what they had to say.

- Rely on and talk to others.
- Be positive.
- Put it in perspective.
- Go on with your life.
- Hang in there; you'll survive.
- Accept grieving.
- Know your needs.
- It will get better.
- Everyone grieves in her own way.
- You're not alone.
- Don't blame yourself.
- Try again.
- Rely on faith.
- Get good medical care and an understanding doctor.

You may become angry at your spouse for not feeling about the loss the way you do. He may feel helpless and frustrated because he is not able to comfort you. You may want to talk—many women find "talking it out" helpful—and he may find those discussions unbearably painful. "Part of the difference may be the different ways men and women express grief," suggests Dr. Lasker. "Men and women are raised in different ways. Men are told they have to be strong and take care of their wives, and as a result much of their own grief is neglected."

TIME HEALS

Getting over a pregnancy loss takes time. In one study, it took parents six months to two years to resolve their feelings. Though there are a number of ways to mourn and survive your loss, Dr. Lasker says, "probably the thing that truly diminishes grief is time." There are other things Dr. Lasker says you can do.

Give meaning to your loss. You need to make some sense of something that seems so senseless. If possible, find out what caused your pregnancy loss, says Dr. Lasker. Almost all of the couples in her study thought it was essential to have the cause of their losses explained.

"For some people, the only way to give what happened some meaning is by talking to others," says Dr. Lasker. "For other people, their religious faith helps. In our study, among people who considered themselves religious, those with the strongest sense of faith did better."

Perform a ritual. Even for a miscarriage, some kind of ritual that acknowledges your loss may be helpful, even if it's planting a tree in memory of your lost child.

Get help. Getting over your loss may not be easy. Having a supportive spouse, family and friends is very important. But because the grief that accompanies pregnancy loss is so misunderstood, you may need to seek comfort elsewhere. Your religious adviser, a psychologist, social worker, counselor or support group such as Share, Amend or Compassionate Friends may be able to help.

"We have found that support groups can help some people but not others," says Dr. Lasker. "For some people to go to a group of strangers and talk about their pain is difficult. But it may be worth it, because these are the people who will understand your pain."

Although fathers may benefit less than mothers from a support group, it can be helpful for your spouse to attend one or two sessions with you, if only to help him understand your feelings, says Dr. Lasker. "It may help him to see that you're not the only woman who is crying all the time."

CHAPTER 53

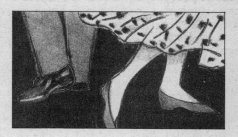

MONEY

PRIME PLAYER IN THE BATTLES
OF THE SEXES

*T*here is no commodity on Earth as emotionally explosive as money. It causes the most arguments, breeds the strongest resentments, creates the most jealousy and is the number one cause of marital problems.

Think about it for a moment. What does money mean to you? Independence? Control? Self-esteem? Power? Security? Happiness?

Psychologists say these are among the most common attitudes of individuals who fight about money.

Where do we get our ideas—our feelings and anxieties—about money? It's pretty much based in our childhood experiences, says Victoria Felton-Collins, Ph.D., psychologist and certified financial planner.

Think back: How did your parents handle money? What role did your mother have in financial decisions? Were you rich, poor or middle class? All these things have some influence over your attitude about money today.

But there's one other thing that plays into the equation here: your sex, says Dr. Felton-Collins. By virtue of being female, your feeling toward money is likely to be very different than your brother's—and possibly even your husband's. And difference of opinion in and of itself breeds conflict.

HE MAKES, SHE SPENDS

Money wars probably have been going on since the day the first coin was minted. And, at least where men and women are concerned, a lot of arguments are based on the question of who holds the purse strings.

Even with more than 69 percent of women in the work force, society today still views the man as the primary breadwinner and assumes he takes the major responsibility for financial decisions, says Judith Siegel, Ph.D., associate professor in the School of Social Work at New York University in New York City and a practicing marital therapist in Westchester County. Women, on the other hand, have been brought up to be the bread bakers and the family caretakers, even if they have full-time jobs as well.

Consequently, women typically measure success and fulfillment by how well their marriage and family are doing and men by how much money they have in the bank, says Dr. Felton-Collins, who is also author of *Couples and Money: Why Money Interferes with Love and What to Do about It.*

Men and women also have different fears about *not* having money, she says. Because they aren't as well-anchored in the work force, many women are possessed with "bag-lady fear"—an insecure feeling of ending up penniless and roaming the streets with their small possessions in a shopping cart. Men's fears revolve around "losing face," when he can't meet the mortgage or send the kids off to camp. He worries about letting down friends and family.

It's a divergent viewpoint that keeps alive the old cliché of the man as the sole breadwinner: She spends it as fast as he makes it. "Unfortunately, it's a stereotype based in reality," admits Rosemarie Schultz, Ph.D., a clinical psychologist in Chicago who specializes in issues of women and money. "After all, when a husband was the only wage earner in the family, it was his money and only his money that a wife *could* use to shop or run the house. Yet today, even with more than 50 percent of married women out in the work force—spending a good deal of their own money—the old reputation persists."

Dr. Schultz attributes it to the male ego. "Perhaps to protect their egos in the face of losing the sole money-earner role, men need to keep that old stereotype alive, even though it isn't appropriate anymore," she says.

WOMEN AND MONEY

Historically, women having control over money, their *own* money, is a relatively new phenomenon. "In the last 10 to 20 years, women have come to see money as a way to enhance themselves, to further themselves and to give themselves comforts—without having to depend on a man to do it," says Dr. Schultz.

But there still is a big difference between what men and women have to spend. Women only earn approximately 73 cents of every dollar earned by men—an average of $20,204.94 a year compared to a man's $27,678. "When push comes to shove," says Dr. Felton-Collins in her book, "men and women use money differently because they possess different amounts of it. Three thousand years ago, according to the Bible, when the value of a human being's work was priced, men were worth 50 shekels of silver, women 30 shekels." It's not much different today.

There's no question that this pay disparity is harmful to a woman's security about money and her economic life, says Dr. Schultz. Even her emotional life. Some women, for example, find it easier to stay in an unhappy marriage than try to "make do" on their smaller incomes.

LOVE AND MONEY

But many women today *are* financially successful. They compete head-to-head with men for power *and* money. They marry later, live alone, take responsibility for themselves and their money. And they do it well.

If money caused marital strife in the days of one wage earner, it has the potential to cause double trouble in a relationship where two people are calling the shots.

"Financial decisions are difficult enough when only one

person is involved," says Dr. Judith Siegel. "When two individuals share financial decisions, conflict is almost inevitable." Each is forced to defend values, wants and needs that are not completely understood by the other. "Many arguments over money are created by a partner's frustration and resentment at a spouse who wishes to use the money in a different way," she points out. "You want to spend, he wants to save, or vice versa."

Money problems really boil down to power, says Dr. Siegel. "For most couples money is a finite commodity, and spending in one area prohibits spending in another. This creates competition between the individual needs of each spouse and leads to feelings of deprivation in the 'loser.' " In healthy relationships, she says, couples are able to share power in ways that are flexible and cooperative.

Couples also have the tendency to use money as a tool or a weapon, says Dr. Schultz. "If you use money to entice, impress, win the approval of others or subdue or entrap others, you're using it as a weapon, and it becomes destructive to yourself and your relationship. When it's used for your own general welfare or the welfare of others, to better yourself and enhance yourself and others, then it's used as a tool, and it's constructive."

CALLING THE POT BLACK

But, say the experts, it really doesn't matter who handles the money in a marriage as long as both are in agreement. It can even be both of you, says Dr. Siegel. "It could be that every Thursday night you take out the bills and start writing checks together or discuss the payment schedules. Or perhaps one week you do the bills, the next week your spouse does them."

But before you get to those kinds of specifics, the experts recommend that you get a meeting of the minds on your basic money-handling philosophy. "How a wife and husband set up their finances is an interesting reflection of what I call couple versus individual commitments," says Dr. Siegel.

There are three possible scenarios. There's the one-pot

system in which all the money is pooled and drawn from a joint account. "This is putting your strongest emphasis on *we*," says Dr. Siegel. The second is the two-pot system in which each has a separate checking account and savings account and is accountable for his or her own expenses. "This system is bringing a very strong individual emphasis to the relationship," she says. And the other option is the three-pot family in which each of you has individual accounts plus a joint account for household expenses. "This is saying that we have both individual and shared identities," she explains.

No one system is better than another, she says. "The important thing is that you communicate with each other before the decision is made and feel comfortable with your choice."

And it works. Carol Regan, 44, is an architect who makes considerably more than her professor husband. "He's a traditional kind of guy and never thought he could bear up in a marriage in which he was outearned by his wife," she says. "But he doesn't feel that way at all because of the way we control our finances." The Regans use the three-pot system. They each have their own savings and checking accounts and make their own personal purchases. "Every week we each put an equal amount of money in the household account to pay those expenses. Big purchases we share 50-50. When we bought furniture, we split the bill. When we go on vacation and go out to dinner, it's the same deal. It doesn't bother him that I have more money to spend on myself because he feels that he's carrying his fair share of what's really important."

Margo Armstrong, a 47-year-old pharmacist, says that she and her husband have somewhere between a one-pot and a three-pot system. "Almost everything we earn goes into our joint checking account," she explains. "But we each maintain individual checking accounts as well. In that way, we can purchase presents without the other one knowing what it cost. Even though we each have children from a previous marriage, we believe that all the money we earn is for everyone. I don't resent the money he sends his ex-wife for child support, for example, and when it came time to put my daughters through college, the money came from both of us. We operate as a team."

And teamwork is what it is all about, says Dr. Siegel. "It is easy to see how tightly woven love and money can be," she says. "Esteem, commitment, closeness and affection are expressed through the giving and taking of money." And the decisions on how money is spent are based on power, mutual respect and trust. "Unresolved problems in any one of these areas could make mutually satisfactory spending impossible."

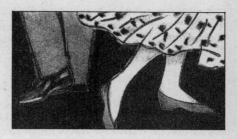

MONOGAMY

A FOUNDATION BUILT ON TRUST

*Y*ou're not alone if you sometimes suspect that the only men who are always faithful are the Marines. Although their motto *Semper fidelis* is simply the Latin version of a wedding vow, it sometimes seems that all's fair only in war, not love.

Study after study seems to bear that out. Various polls have found that somewhere between 40 and 50 percent of married men have extramarital affairs, as do about a third of all married women. What's more, nearly 70 percent of married men under 40 who haven't already strayed say they expect they will, according to another survey. Although there is a common perception that more men than women are unfaithful, some experts who investigate the social morality of other societies say that where there is no double standard for adultery, wives philander just as much as their husbands. At least one study found that women account for most of the increase in extramarital affairs.

Of course, there are some who regard fidelity as an unnatural state, as uncomfortable as a shoe on the wrong foot, a sociological aberration constantly at war with human biology. Although there's abundant evidence that we're naturally monogamous—most people prefer to marry one person at a time—there seems to be no biological imperative for remaining faithful to one person *forever*. In fact, suggests anthropologist Helen Fisher, Ph.D., for some of us there may even be an innate urge in quite the opposite direction—an urge we will risk anything to fulfill. Even death.

NATURALLY UNFAITHFUL?

"I've looked at adultery in 42 societies and it occurs in every one," says Dr. Fisher, author of *The Sex Contract: The Evolution of Human Behavior* and a research associate in the Department of Anthropology at the American Museum of Natural History in New York City. "Historically, it occurred even if you could lose your head for it. Today we have a society with people dying because of sexually transmitted AIDS and people are *still* adulterous. In America, if somebody said you could die from eating broccoli, you can be positive that no two people in America would eat it again. Yet we continue to be adulterous, which argues for the fact that there is some biological component to it."

Why would we be biologically wired to be unfaithful? The evolutionary explanation is quite simple, as Dr. Fisher explains. "On the grasslands of Africa four million years ago, early men gained a genetic advantage by fathering children by as many women as they could. By having children with more than one woman, a man insured himself a larger genetic leverage in the future. A woman could not bear more than one child a year (and probably only every three or four years, because ovulation was often inhibited by nursing). So adultery could not give her more children, but it would give her extra resources and more protection. So philandering was useful to both sexes. Consequently, those with an adulterous nature had a greater chance of surviving down the ages."

Although the theory makes evolutionary sense, the question remains: Is biology destiny? Don't we have some choice in the matter? After all, at least half of us remain *semper fi* in wedlock. Yes, says Dr. Fisher, we certainly have a choice. But for some of us, fidelity may be a struggle.

TRUTH AND LOVE

Fortunately, in reality, we are more than prisoners of our biology, says Jeanette Lauer, Ph.D., dean of the College of Liberal Studies at the United States International University in San Diego.

We are also emotional creatures who value love, trust, friendship and commitment, all hallmarks of the 300 long and happy marriages Dr. Lauer and her husband, Robert, studied several years ago and wrote about in their book *Til Death Do Us Part*. Although the Lauers didn't ask about fidelity directly, Dr. Lauer says those qualities are "incongruous with infidelity."

"The qualities they valued—and both men and women mentioned the same ones in virtually the same order—are vital to a relationship," she says. "They keep people from straying."

In fact, fidelity is the linchpin of marriage, says Florence Kaslow, Ph.D., director of the Florida Couples and Family Institute in West Palm Beach and past president of the International Family Therapy Association. "It is one of the cornerstones of marriage, part of the foundation. If you tamper with the foundation, it quickly crumbles."

Fidelity—with its implication of loyalty and commitment—is an integral part of any intimate relationship, one in which you bare your heart and soul to another person. "Usually, no one knows you as well as your spouse does," says Dr. Lauer. "This unpeeling of yourself, allowing another person to get in and know you as you are, leaves you vulnerable, which is why trust is such an important element of marriage." In fact, says Dr. Lauer, one of the reasons infidelity cuts so deeply is that it is a betrayal of that trust, "a virtual act of treason."

We also recognize infidelity for what it is—a red flag. In a survey done in 1990 by a Canadian magazine, 87 percent of the respondents said that extramarital affairs are a signal that a marriage is foundering.

"It was in my case," says Trudy Meyers, a 47-year-old horse trainer who was repeatedly unfaithful in her first marriage and has always been faithful in her second. "If I were to be unfaithful now, it would destroy my marriage and me. In my first marriage, I felt that if my husband found out, so what? The marriage wasn't that valuable to me. I wouldn't do anything to risk this marriage. I don't even have the desire to cheat."

FAITHFULLY YOURS

If your marriage or committed relationship is important to you, you realize that faithfulness isn't something you can take—or leave—lightly.

"Any relationship takes work," says Dr. Lauer. Some men and women stray because they have unrealistic expectations. When the physical excitement and intensity begins to cool, they also feel the relationship is changing, too. And it may, but not necessarily for the worse.

Most relationships first go through an infatuation phase, a physical change that is literally, says Dr. Fisher, "a brain bath of chemicals" that are nature's own amphetamines. Like any drug, they wear off and we move into the attachment phase, a calmer, more secure and, in time, deeper love. "But a lot of people go into marriage being in love with love," says Dr. Lauer. "They have the notion that this goofy, feel-good time is the most important time. Then the first difficulty comes along and they realize, hey, this is work. Affairs seem like such an easy answer because they bring back the excitement of the early part of the marriage and help you ignore the problem."

Couples who are committed to one another put all their energy into working things out instead of into extramarital affairs, which help them avoid rather than resolve the issues plaguing their marriage, she says.

"When we asked the couples we interviewed to plot their ups and downs, their charts looked like roller coasters," says Dr. Lauer. "But through it all they remained committed to their marriages, to the institution of marriage and, most important, to the person they saw as their best friend. Because of their commitment, over time they developed good communication skills and learned how to handle conflict, which made their marriages even better."

She suggests that couples always make time for one another. "In today's busy lifestyles, it's easy to become two ships that pass in the night. If someone is your best friend, by definition it means you spend time together. Examine your priorities and rearrange them if you have to. Instead of dividing up the household chores, do them together. It takes more time, but it's more fun. Take control of your calendar and make your relationship a high-priority item. Schedule sex. It sounds terrible, but anticipation can be part of the fun."

HIDDEN TEMPTATION

A threat to your relationship can sneak up on you when you least expect it—even when you're happy and aren't looking. Even a relationship that is not sexual—"we're just work buddies"—can upstage your marriage, warns Dr. Kaslow.

"I've seen this with people who are learning to be co-therapists," she says. "They're together all the time, constantly talking and processing their relationship, which deepens into a very rich friendship. They often wind up talking more in depth with their co-therapists than they do with their spouses. Even if it doesn't become sexualized, even if it's not an 'affair,' it gives each of them a sense of what's possible and may damage their marriage. The other spouse senses the closeness and may become jealous and antagonistic."

If you begin to feel an attraction for someone that goes beyond being safe, says Dr. Kaslow, "you need to define your parameters and not go outside them. If you feel it could go over the line and jeopardize your marriage—and you want the marriage to last—you have to pull back."

That doesn't mean you should drop all of your deep friendships. Friendships are very important. But you need to be careful that they don't compete with your relationship with your spouse or significant other.

To keep a relationship honest and true, you can't let little things build up into big ones, cautions Dr. Lauer. "When you have a problem, talk about it," she says. "Check in regularly with one another. Yours is an important relationship. Watch over it."

See also Infidelity, Marriage

CHAPTER
55

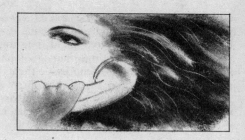

MOTHER

A RELATIONSHIP LIKE NO OTHER

A grown woman feels a lot of emotion when it comes to her mother. It's a relationship that can be harmonious or hostile. Sweet or contentious. Loving or malevolent.

"One thing it almost never is is neutral," says Karen Johnson, M.D., assistant clinical professor of psychiatry at the University of California, San Francisco, and a psychiatrist in private practice who specializes in the psychological care of women. Consider these two very diverse but very real disclosures.

"My mother is probably my best friend," says Dina Farber, a 27-year-old newspaper reporter. "She accepts me for who I am, even if I mess up. I go to her for advice and help, but also just for good conversation. Sure, we've had some fights over the years, but there's never been a problem so large that it's challenged the basic nature of our relationship."

Sharon Cook's experience is entirely different. "My mother drives me crazy and has for years," says the 41-year-old lawyer in total frustration. "Nothing I do ever pleases her. When I buy her a present, she'll accuse me of buying something *I* like because I know I'll inherit it. One year for her birthday, I took her to an elegant French restaurant—something she loves but never gets to do because it's something my father hates. She told me when I paid the bill that it really wasn't a present to her because I enjoyed it, too. And she said I only did it because I couldn't find the time to buy her a present. I find her so difficult sometimes I want to kick and scream."

But Sharon also has learned to laugh about what she calls her predicament. "My mother's skewed view of the way I treat her has taught me something. When I buy her presents these days, I *do* buy what *I* like. There's an off chance she will leave it to me!"

Mother/daughter relationships are sometimes idealized, sometimes maligned. "But there is little doubt that women's preoccupation with their mothers borders on obsession," says Dr. Johnson.

DOUBLE TROUBLE

"Not *all* mothers and daughters have trouble, but nearly all have trouble sometimes," says Paula J. Caplan, Ph.D., author of *Don't Blame Mother*.

After all, who is more like you than your own mother? There's a "natural" identification, a shared female identity that sustains the mother/daughter attachment, explains Dr. Johnson.

"Because mother/daughter relationships tend to be very close, they combine the potential for much joy as well as much pain," adds Dr. Caplan. "Part of the special pain between mother and daughter comes about because they feel that anger and alienation are *not* supposed to be part of the mother/daughter relationship." So when it happens, the sting is severe.

According to our cultural ideals, she explains, a mother is supposed to be gentle and loving—and so is her daughter. But because of the instinctive skill a woman has for understanding other people's emotions, many mothers and daughters can both wound and heal, both hurt and delight each other better than anyone else.

PLEASING MAMA

Dina says that her mother's approval means a lot to her, even though she's an adult living hundreds of miles away. "I value my mother's opinions because although she's made mistakes in her life, she's been able to fix them successfully. I could easily marry a man my father didn't approve of, but I'd have a hard time settling down with a man my mother didn't like.

"When my mother questions or disagrees outright with a choice I've made, I can easily feel crushed," continues Dina. "The funny thing is, once my mother realizes how upset I get, she falls all over herself apologizing and softening her message."

But too much approval seeking can also cause problems, stresses Rosalind C. Barnett, Ph.D., a clinical and research psychologist at the Center for Research on Women at Wellesley College in Massachusetts. "Approval seeking leads to constant struggle," she says. "A problem increasing numbers of today's young women face is pressure from their mothers to be the achieving, successful women their mothers never were." Whether the daughter gives in or rebels, the result is a no-win situation. "It rarely leads to a satisfying life," says Dr. Barnett.

Daughters may find it hard to distinguish between choices they are making for themselves and those they are making to please their mothers. "In either case," says Dr. Barnett, "unresolved issues with one's mother can color and distort a daughter's successes or failures."

THE GENERATION GAP

A major source of misunderstanding between mothers and daughters is the enormous difference in their lives. This is especially true of women in their forties and fifties who have mothers in their late sixties, seventies or eighties. In fact, the idea of an adult daughter with a living mother is somewhat new. As recently as 1963, less than 25 percent of women over 45 had a surviving parent—usually the mother.

"Compared to our mothers, we are considerably better educated, are engaged in a wider range of career options and activities, are able to shape our reproductive lives both in terms of the number and timing of our children and are much freer to end destructive marriages," says Dr. Barnett. "In short, we have far more options than did our mothers." All the makings for a volatile relationship.

Dr. Barnett says that in one study of recently divorced middle-aged daughters, about one-quarter of the women had *never* discussed their marital situation with their mothers, typically because they expected disapproval or lack of understanding. "Some women admitted delaying their divorces because of the anticipated negative reaction from their mothers."

One woman says that her mother gave her a hard time for a year after learning that she was seeking a divorce. "She insisted that I hadn't tried hard enough to change him," she says. "I had tried for 17 years. I thought that that was enough, but my mother insisted that I could have made it work if I had persisted. She eventually accepted my divorce, but it took several years before she could admit that I was better off."

Fortunately for today's younger women, says Dr. Barnett, the generation gap is not so pronounced. A woman in her twenties has a lot more in common with a mother in her forties or fifties than her mother does with her grandmother. Which, in part, may be why Dina and Sharon's relationships with their mothers are poles apart.

GREAT EXPECTATIONS

It would be unrealistic to hope that mothers don't have *some* expectations for their daughters, says Dr. Johnson. "As long as a mother recognizes that her expectations are not necessarily those her daughter holds for herself—and she accepts that—the relationship should be all right. In a healthy relationship, a mother will understand that her daughter may not look at the world in the same way she does or even share the same values or interests. It can be extremely disruptive to the mother/daughter relationship if they can't appreciate that in each other," she states.

Sharon says that she actually had an excellent relationship with her mother during her teenage years. "I was very popular in high school and had lots of boyfriends. That pleased her. She put very few restrictions on my activities. I was allowed to go to parties and had late curfews, much later than my friends had. She basically trusted me.

"In looking back I would say our relationship started to turn when I chose my career, which was to her a man's job," says Sharon, who is still single but happy and content in a long-standing monogamous relationship. "She wanted grandchildren. She still can't forgive me for breaking up with a man who was going to be a doctor and came from a rich family. According to her, I blew it, and she has never let me forget it, even to this day. And we're talking 20 years ago."

It's true that an adult daughter's way of life affects the quality of her relationship with her mother, says Dr. Johnson. But she needs to see it in the proper perspective. "One of the most important factors to a mother may be whether or not her daughter is 'settled.' Being settled means having a sense of doing and having done what she wants, having concrete plans for the future and being able to imagine what her life will be like. In a healthy relationship the mother may not agree with her daughter's choices, but she recognizes that her daughter has a right to them because she's a separate person who has developed in her own unique way."

MOMMY BASHING: A BAD REPORT

And it's good to know that this is the way it usually is. Despite our culture's tendency to blame Mom for her daughter's troubles, says Dr. Barnett, "we found that, in general, daughters have positive relationships with their mothers."

According to a survey of 238 middle-aged women, Dr.

UNDERSTANDING MOM

Does your relationship with your mother drive you crazy? Do you wish you'd wake up some morning and find out that you were, maybe, adopted? Do you shudder thinking that *you* have the potential to be this exasperating individual someday?

Mother/daughter relationships do not have to be this way, emphasizes psychiatrist Karen Johnson, M.D., who specializes in women's relationships. You as a daughter can take the first big step in smoothing out a difficult relationship. And it starts by looking at mom as a human being— not just as a mother. From there, you need to consider the following:

Try to understand your mother's motives. "It's important for you to appreciate how external factors influenced your mother's life, and consequently your own," says Dr. Johnson. "A mother who becomes incredibly anxious and controlling when her daughter reaches puberty, for example, might be reacting to the fact that she was sexually abused when she was her daughter's age. By controlling all her activities, she's simply trying to protect her daughter from suffering the same fate that she did. Meanwhile, her daughter believes her mother is just being nasty and wants to ruin her life."

Learn your mother's history. The more you know about your mother, the more you can see her as someone other than your mother. Try to recall what you know about your mother's childhood, suggests Paula J. Caplan, Ph.D., author of *Don't Blame Mother.* "Since children seem very human to most of us, we are less likely either to worship or condemn them than adults."

For instance, you should know the following: How old were your grandparents when your mother was born? What was her life like with them? What was life like economically, politically and socially as your mother was growing up?

Look for similarities between you and your mother. "Ask yourself which of the following you share with her," says Dr. Caplan, "values, fears, political attitudes, types of friends, religious beliefs, favorite food, sources of joy and frustrations, mannerisms, gestures, physical features, sense of style, etc."

(continued on page 370)

Ask your mother about her experience with you from the very beginning. Dr. Caplan suggests asking: "What kind of pregnancy did she have? What were you like in the womb? Did you kick or were you quiet? What was your birth like? How did she feel the first time she saw you? What did she enjoy about you as a baby? And what drove her crazy about taking care of you? How scared was she? Did she think she was a bad mother or an inadequate one?"

Let her know, says Dr. Caplan, that you realize and understand how hard being a mother can be, and you'd like to know what it was like for her—from her point of view.

Consider your mother's responsibilities. "Mothers tend to be overburdened with the responsibilities of raising children," claims Dr. Johnson. "And I don't just mean the practical day-to-day tasks, which are in and of themselves daunting. But there are the bigger issues. Mothers tend to be held responsible for the psychological well-being of their children, too. They are often the first ones blamed if their kids don't 'turn out well.' "

Don't assume your mother was invulnerable or all-powerful. The more you know about the difficulties your mother experienced in raising you, the more charitable you can be in your feelings toward her, says Dr. Caplan. In other words, think about how the problems she faced might have affected her treatment of you. "Do you remember times she seemed too tired to play with you or exceedingly irritable or very emotionally needy? Could those have been the times her burdens were heaviest?"

As one woman pointed out, she never realized how unhappy her mother's marriage to her father had been until her mother got divorced. "When I saw how calm and cheerful she became after her divorce and remarriage, I finally understood that her short temper had very little to do with me."

Put yourself in her shoes. No matter how different you are from your mother, try to imagine what it would have been like if you had to live your mother's life, says Dr. Johnson. "I did that recently, and I decided that my mother did the best job she could under the circumstances."

Barnett found that by the time a woman reaches age 35, she has "come to terms" with her mother.

She also found a correlation between the quality of the mother/daughter relationship and the daughter's psychological health. "Most daughters who experienced their relationship with their mothers as positive overall also reported higher self-esteem, overall life satisfaction, happiness and optimism than daughters whose relationships were more troubled," she says.

And when a relationship is bad, she says, daughters who are younger, single or have no children of their own seem to suffer the most. "In other words," she says, "the fewer roles we as adult daughters occupy, the more central to our mental health is our relationship to our mothers."

THE REFLECTING POOL

In fact, having a child of your own can help mend a difficult relationship, says Dr. Johnson. "There's a dynamic shift that goes on once the daughter has had a child of her own. For the first time, you really share the same role with your own mother," she explains. "Many women find that when they become a parent, they can empathize with their mothers in a way they never could before."

Charlotte Campbell couldn't agree more. "When my daughter turned 18 and went away to college, I thought my job was over and I could relax," says the 47-year-old financial planner. "It came as a complete surprise to me that when my daughter had problems at school, I reacted the same way I had when she was 7 or 12. I now understood why my mother always frets when I go on a business trip alone or when I have a setback at work."

After all, she says, "once a mother, always a mother."

CHAPTER 56

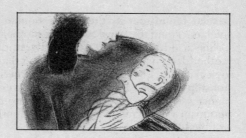

MOTHERHOOD

THE MYTHS, THE MYSTERIES, THE MAGIC

*M*any of today's mothers were raised and nurtured on the image of Donna Reed and June Cleaver, those miraculous moms of the small screen who raised wonderful children and had squeaky clean houses without raising their voices or lifting their fingers. Today's young girls learned the trade from Clair Huxtable of "The Cosby Show," who was only different from her predecessors because she added a law career to her résumé.

To whom can we turn for a dose of reality?

Perhaps the closest you can come to getting a better understanding of what motherhood is all about is talking to other mothers who, usually with little prodding, will reveal the "warts and all" of what is truly the world's oldest profession. That's what researches Eva Margolies and Louis Genevie, Ph.D., did when they interviewed 1,100 mothers of all ages and published the results in their book *The Motherhood Report: How Women Feel about Being Mothers*.

Their findings? Only one in four mothers has very positive feelings about motherhood and one in five views it in very negative terms. The majority of mothers have mixed feelings. But there's an up side to this decidedly gloomy view of motherhood. Although for most mothers the bad times outnumber the good ones, ultimately the good times *outweigh* the bad, an important distinction. As the research-ers put it, "a little joy goes a long way"—because it has to.

A DIFFERENT KIND OF LOVE

Becoming a mother is perhaps the most significant change a woman ever makes in her life, far greater than choosing an occupation or marrying. Regarded in most cultures as an initiation into adulthood, motherhood may be the most intimate connection one human being has to another. It is a relationship that usually begins with symbiosis—preg-nancy—and is forever colored by the woman's first sense of "oneness" with her child. The feeling during pregnancy of "whatever happens to the baby happens to me" persists well beyond childbirth.

"Your heart gets split open in a way that you had never expected," says Christiane Northrup, M.D., a clinical assis-tant professor of obstetrics and gynecology at the University of Vermont College of Medicine, co-president of the Ameri-can Holistic Medical Association and the mother of two. "You know what falling in love is like, but until you've had a child, you don't have a clue what it means to love someone for whom you'd be willing to lay down your life."

In fact, many women are surprised by the intensity of the feelings they have for their children, which, in some ways, are deeper than in other love relationships.

"For the first time in your life, you can't imagine losing someone; it's unacceptable to you and you don't think you could survive it if you did lose them," says psychologist Ellen McGrath, Ph.D., executive director of the Psychology Center in Laguna Beach, California, herself the mother of two. "In our culture, most women are prepared for the eventuality of losing their husbands because that's how it is. If you lose a husband, you can more easily find another. But a child is irreplaceable."

One mother says she feels she became "a hostage to fortune" with the birth of her only child. "He is so precious to me that I feel horribly vulnerable," she admits. "I'm so afraid something will happen to him that I'm obsessed with having a second child. But I know that's not the answer."

But mother love is not purely the province of the woman who gives birth. The mother/child bond is no less strong for most adoptive mothers.

Rachel McGinnis is a 36-year-old former financial analyst who found herself unmarried at 30 but yearning for children. Through a friend, she learned that an agency in the state where she lives was looking for foster parents for children born to mothers with AIDS. She took in her first infant, Peter, a blond, curly-haired charmer. The experience was so rewarding, she eventually adopted three more children. All but one are free of the disease. One, 3-year-old Joey, has AIDS and has been in and out of hospitals for a year with a variety of AIDS-related ailments.

"When Joey came into my home it was with the knowledge that he was going to die," says Rachel. "When he got sick, most people thought I was going to be able to handle it. I was not. It was like a part of me was dying with him and was rebirthed when he got better. People tend to think, 'Oh, they're adopted, if something happens you can get another one.' But adopting a child and giving birth to one is virtually the same. The adopted child simply grows in a different part of your body—your heart."

THE TWO FACES OF MOM

And then there is motherhood's flip side. In the Margolies/Genevie study, 45 percent of all mothers said the day-to-day responsibilities of raising children were more drudgery than pleasure. More than a third said they lacked adequate patience and nearly half said they didn't control their tempers very well with their children. Some even admitted to having revenge fantasies—a "safe" outlet for the furies of motherhood that could well serve to alert mothers to their frustration before it gets out of hand. What creates these ambivalent, sometimes negative, feelings?

Part of the ambivalence you may feel as a mother will be your perhaps unconscious sense that life as you know it is over—which it is. The changes children can make in your life are dramatic and sweeping. Everything is different, from the time you get up in the morning to the kinds of relationships you have with important people in your life.

To help some of her clients get a perspective on the realities of motherhood, Suzanne Pope, Ph.D., director of the Colorado Institute for Marriage and the Family in Boulder, has them perform a telling little exercise. She asks them to make a list of everything they do in their lives "from small to large, from when they get up in the morning to their relationships and what they're doing in their careers." Then, she says, "I tell them to imagine that every single one of those things changes. I want them to feel the overwhelming frustration that mounts when they imagine every single thing in their life being different. Then I tell them to imagine being so exhausted they can't deal with it. That's loss, and we live in a culture that doesn't support the fact that this is a loss. If there is any one word I would talk about in connection with motherhood it's 'surrender.' You're asked to surrender your control over your life."

Not even your time is your own anymore. With children, you can't easily get away for a romantic weekend. You can't dash out to the store for a quart of milk without making arrangements. You may find it difficult to do the simplest things.

Kids wake you up out of a sound sleep, throw tantrums in the supermarket, won't eat what you cook them, change their minds 15 times a second, are defiant, rebellious and illogical—sometimes right up through the teen years. "Sometimes I feel like I'm raising Sybil," says one mother of two toddlers, referring to the pseudonym of a woman with multiple personalities who was the focus of a book and movie. "It's like, who are you today?"

But there's more to the ambivalence than the sense of loss and the often trying aspects of child rearing. You are beginning a relationship that may be the "most poignant and intense one of your life," says Dr. Pope. "A relationship this empowering will possess you. You're not just losing part of your life, you're entering into a relationship that will at times own you. What you ought to be thinking is, 'No wonder I feel the way I do!'"

GET REAL

Unfortunately many women—perhaps most women—come to motherhood unprepared for these realities. In fact, many women approach motherhood with illusions of becoming the "perfect" mother.

The study by Margolies and Dr. Genevie found that among the mothers they surveyed, only one in four was realistic about motherhood. Seventy percent were mired in their misty sense of motherhood as a kind of perpetual rerun of "The Donna Reed Show," in which children were always sweet and loving and well-behaved and parents were always even-tempered and understanding. For many, their only exposure to children was through babysitting or caring for nieces and nephews who tended to be on their best behavior. Consequently, they saw all the joys and none of the responsibilities. Many, whose experiences should have made them more realistic, wanted to be "perfect" mothers to make up for their own imperfect childhood. Yet, say the researchers, those with realistic attitudes had an easier time coping with the vicissitudes of motherhood.

WILL I LOVE MY BABY?

Few, if any, women are really prepared for new motherhood. "When my friends ask me what their lives are going to be like after the baby arrives, I always say, 'You know how your life is now? It's not going to be anything like that anymore,'" says one mother.

During pregnancy, many women think only as far ahead as childbirth. But as the birth of a new baby nears many find themselves asking themselves: Will I love my baby?

Don't expect love at first sight, warn psychologists. Numerous studies have found that while most women feel very positively about their new babies, a significant number feel indifferent or negative. Even among those who feel positively, not everyone calls those feelings love. Even in the mother/child relationship, love is something that grows. For some women, it grows over a matter of minutes, while for others it takes days, weeks or months.

In recent years, many researchers have called into question the idea that there is a "critical period" for bonding. Previously it was thought that skin-to-skin contact was necessary within the first 24 hours to assure normal bonding. Today, the experts recognize that contact with the baby is only one of the many factors that influence the affection of a mother for her child. In one study, however, mothers who fell in love with their infants after the first day said it happened during a quiet private time.

But don't be alarmed if you find you have ambivalent feelings about your new baby. You're in good company. In *The Motherhood Report,* by researchers Eva Margolies and Louis Genevie, Ph.D., many mothers with children under 12 said infancy was their least favorite stage of childhood. One study found that it was common for mothers to express both positive and negative emotions about their new babies simultaneously. Some mothers claim to resent the time their children demand at the same time they admit they love taking care of them.

Generally, the first three months of your baby's life will be the hardest for you because he or she may not be sleeping (and neither are you) or may be fussing frequently, and you may be having trouble with nursing. During that time, your bad feelings may seem to outnumber the good ones, but most women find their affection growing as their children do. Once you begin to understand your new baby—who is, after all, a stranger—and he starts to smile and coo at you, the love affair will almost surely take off.

NO "REAL" ROLE MODEL

How do you get a realistic attitude when it's virtually anathema to say a bad word about motherhood? Our mothers—our first role models—may be of little help. Caring for a home and children was the sole source of their self-esteem. Most mothers today work in addition to shouldering most of the responsibility for children and the household. "Our mothers can't teach us because they didn't live the way we do," says Dr. McGrath.

There's often a "reality" gap between today's mothers and their mothers. "I remember trying to talk to my mother about how I felt," says Lydia Carroll, a photo stylist and mother of two daughters now in their twenties. "There were many times I hated being a mother. I felt guilty because I hated playing with my kids. I felt that anything that interested a 3-year-old would be boring to me. I asked my mother if she had ever felt this way and she was aghast. 'Oh, no,' she said. 'I loved being a mother.' The implication, of course, was that there was something wrong with me. Even I thought there was."

The lack of good role models for motherhood puts today's mothers at a disadvantage and may contribute to the mythmaking. "I think that most of us have pretty unrealistic pictures because there are so few role models, so we construct our own pictures of what motherhood is supposed to be," says Dr. McGrath. "A lot of us deny our fears by constructing something that is much more positive than could ever exist."

Turning to other mothers—through parent support groups or neighborhood mother/baby groups—can be helpful in shattering the mother myths we hold, as long as everyone regards the group as a way to share experiences rather than as an opportunity for a brag session. But if everyone is honest—and most will be—you'll be able to see that your negative and ambivalent feelings are normal.

STRESS: THE OCCUPATIONAL HAZARD

You'll also find that most mothers consider motherhood stressful. In fact, one researcher calls stress a time-limited occupational hazard of young mothers. Any woman can empathize with the mother who ranked as "very stressful" the day her son, seatbelted in a running car, managed to put the car in drive and send it rolling down a 60-foot ravine. Neither child nor car was harmed, but the researcher added no such damage report on the mother.

So how do you deal with these kinds of stresses?

Take time out, just for you, advises Abby King, Ph.D., senior research scientist at the Stanford University School of Medicine's Center for Research in Disease Prevention.

"In one of the studies we did with working women—many of them were moms—we encouraged them to spend a half-hour once a day doing something they enjoyed. Some of them had trouble identifying what they enjoyed, it had been so long. Others felt guilty taking time for themselves. Taking care of yourself will have benefits for your family. It's not just you who will feel better. You need to get comfortable with making yourself a priority."

One pleasurable activity Dr. King suggests is exercise. Several studies she and her colleagues have done indicate that something as simple as a half-hour walk is a double-duty antidote to stress. "First, it gives you time away from your stress. Second, through some physical or psychological mechanism, being in the fresh air, breathing, socializing, seems to have additive benefits," she says.

A daily walk could also help "with postpartum downs, weight gain and fatigue," suggests Dr. King. "In terms of body image and self-esteem, we have found that exercise has good effects. Women who exercise feel more in control of their lives, which has been shown to be a good stress reducer."

THE GUILT TRIP

It's no wonder so many mothers feel stressed, especially when you consider their susceptibility to guilt. It's easy to feel guilty that you're not doing enough for your children, or feel you're not doing the right thing.

In one small study done in California several years ago, researchers found that the college students they surveyed were more inclined to blame their mothers than their fathers for their emotional problems. (On the positive side, the students tended to blame themselves and society for their problems more often than their moms.)

While no one can diminish the importance of a loving, responsive mother to a child's emotional development, a child is far more than who his mother made him, say psychologists. He is influenced by his genes and the other people in his life, and studies suggest that the child may take a hand in his own upbringing. His temperament may actually influence how he is "mothered." In fact, Margolies and Dr. Geneive concluded from their study that "better children produce better mothers."

"If you join a mother/baby group, you'll get to look at all the optional ways of mothering and you'll see there's no perfect way," says Dr. Pope. "You get a sense of your unique way and you also get a sense of your child's uniqueness."

Once you see that other mothers have the same struggles, it might give you the impetus to go a little easier on yourself. No one can expect to be—or should be expected to be—the perfect mother.

GOOD ENOUGH IS GOOD ENOUGH

The term *good-enough mother* was coined in 1965, and the concept may serve as an antidote for the need, if you have it, to be "the perfect mother."

The good-enough mother does her best, recognizing she's going to make mistakes sometimes but that she'll do right often enough to raise "good-enough" kids. She also learns to trust her own judgment. After all, she knows her child better than anyone, including the experts. She needs to trust her ability to do "the right thing," even if it flies in the face of other opinions.

"The good-enough mother has a sense that there really is no perfect way," says Dr. Pope. "She knows there's no manual anywhere. She's knows she's going to make mistakes. She operates from her own connection to herself and her child, to what she knows about herself and what she knows about her child. She honors her relationship with her children more than everyone else's opinion."

Which, as a mother, you're certain to hear, whether it's words of wisdom from your own mother, from the latest parenting book or from the stranger in the street who wonders if your little one "shouldn't be bundled up a little more." It's often hard to hear your own voice raised above this chorus. But that's what you need to do. "But first you need to be committed to the idea that you have some wisdom inside you," says Dr. Pope.

Sometimes, she says, she suggests that mothers keep journals to help them get back in tune with their own mothering skills and knowledge. She also recommends that women read and listen to as much advice as they can. "You then realize how contradictory it all is, which can force you to claim your own wisdom about your child, to claim your position as mother," she says. "You need to realize that you're blazing your own personal path with your child, which is frightening, but exciting, too. You're the best expert you've got."

Diane Mayer says she learned everything she knows about child rearing from her children. "When I brought my oldest son, Jason, home from the hospital, I was still going back and forth in my mind about how to respond to his crying. One book I read said it's best to pick him up; another said the opposite. Then, there was my mother telling me what to do and my mother-in-law telling me what she did. So what did I do? When Jason cried, I had the irresistible urge to pick him up and comfort him. So I did. It felt wonderful and right. I never questioned myself after that."

THE MARRIAGE GOES ROUND

Your marriage is the foundation on which you've built your family, and your mate is what psychologists call a psychosocial asset—your best hedge against stress.

Yet, Margolies and Dr. Genevie report that twice as many women said their marriages took a turn for the worse after they had children as said their marriages improved.

"Other studies also show that marital relationships do go down, take a real dip and stay down until the last child leaves home," says Dr. Pope. "This casts a shadow on the idea that you can have a good marriage and a child, too."

Hopeless? No, says Dr. Pope, just challenging. "When you have children, you can't just hope that it all works out. There's a fairly high divorce rate when children leave home.

Couples discover they're strangers when they do turn back to each other. They either find there's not much left or that they grew in very different ways. What that says is that people need to make a commitment to get back to their relationships."

By the time your child is 18 months to 2 years old, when he's less demanding and you're a little more rested, you really need to "reconnect," says Dr. Pope. Your marriage needs to take a front seat again.

"During the first two years, it's okay to put the relationship aside for awhile, for the couple to orient themselves around the child, but even during that period, it's important to 'check in' with each other regularly," she says.

Keep in touch with each other's feelings. As the mother, you may be feeling exhausted, not only because of the hours you're putting in or the sleep you're missing, but because you feel you're mothering the world. Your husband may feel like he's the house custodian, a functionary who does odd jobs but has no clear-cut role in the family anymore. "Don't expect within three weeks of having a baby you'll be out dancing," says Dr. Pope. "But be gentle with one another and know what the issues are you're both facing. Don't take anything personally and talk about that day when you're going to have your time again. Keep the light at the end of the tunnel lit."

CHAPTER 57

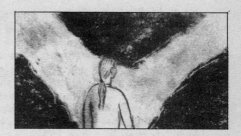

MOTHERHOOD
VERSUS CAREER

WHY SOME ARE RIDING
THE MOMMY TRACK

*I*n the late 1980s, at the height of the new Baby Boomlet, a magazine called *Parenting* was launched. Its target: the upscale modern parent with lots of disposable income and, if the advertising was any indication, a need for disposable diapers. In other words, the two-paycheck couple who parked two cars in the garage and their kids in day care.

But in May 1988, the magazine ran an out-of-character cover story on what it saw as a new phenomenon. "Stay-at-Home Moms," the cover lines trumpeted. "A Choice That's Working."

For most of *Parenting*'s Baby Boom readers, that statement must have come as a surprise. Raised on images of housewives wearing pearls as they dusted, they had had their consciousness raised in the 1960s and 1970s, when the women's movement assured them that a woman's place was anyplace but home. Most women had taken that counsel to heart. In a study done at the University of Southern California, only 3 percent of female high school seniors in 1986 expected to be full-time homemakers by the time they were 30, compared to 12 percent of high school seniors in 1976. Apparently, young men's consciousness was raised, too, although not as high. A third of the male class of 1986 thought mothers should stay home with their kids, compared to half of the class of 1976.

Without any comparative statistics, the *Parenting* article implied that many women, while not returning home in droves, are opting for home and kids instead of career. According to Labor Department statistics, in 1990 there were slightly more than 11 million American women—33.3 percent of all mothers—who chose to stay home. While that number is less than it was in 1988—when 35 percent of all mothers, or 11.6 million women picked motherhood over career—it indicates that women's desire to leave their children in the care of others is slowing down.

WHO'S HOMEWARD BOUND?

If there is a new stay-at-home mother, it's the woman who has discovered that motherhood offers an undreamed-of emotional fulfillment that even the most lucrative and prestigious job can't, the woman who thought her dreams were wrapped up in a career—until a baby came along. A woman like Carol Marden.

If someone had told Carol she would be the full-time mother of two at 36, she would have laughed. "I had an MBA. I wasn't about to waste that at home," she says. "I wanted to be president of a company in my thirties. I had always wanted *more*."

But in 1986, after her first son was born, Carol found herself faced by a surprisingly tough choice. While on maternity leave, the division of the Fortune 500 company where she worked offered her the president's job. "Even though it was what I'd always wanted, I really had to think about it," says Carol. "I felt very clingy to my son and I didn't want to leave him."

Her husband convinced her to "go for her dream" and she did, although it meant a commuter marriage and a grueling schedule. But after the birth of their second son three years later, Carol went home. No hesitation. No regrets. "In a couple of years, I'd like to start a home-based company," Carol says. "But right now, I'm happier than

I've ever been. I don't feel the need for more. I have everything I need."

A happy ending? For many women, it is. But is it the choice for you? Alluring though it may be at times, being a full-time mother is certainly no easy job. "I see career women in my practice and every time they have a child, they wonder whether they would like to stay home," says Gisela Booth, Ph.D., a clinical psychologist and assistant clinical professor of psychology at Northwestern University in Chicago. "They go through a kind of wistful fantasy of how nice it would be to stay home, at least for a few years. After a few months, most decide no."

NO EASY JOB

Why do more women than not turn down what looks like the good life? Finances probably play a role for many. Today, the one-paycheck family is an economic anomaly. But there may be something more. Perhaps it's also because these women intuitively sense that new stay-at-home mothers are blazing trails through a mine field.

Once pressured to stay home, women are now pressured to go to work. Women who make the brave choice to stay home are risking having their self-esteem detonate in a job that, at least according to one study, many of us think is more stressful than a career. In fact, quite a number of studies have found that homemakers actually are less healthy and more prone to depression than working women.

"Everybody somehow thinks that if a woman stays home she has the best of all worlds," says Matti Gershenfeld, Ph.D., director of the Couples Learning Center in Jenkintown, Pennsylvania, and a frequent lecturer on stay-at-home mothers and self-esteem. "The truth is, absolutely nobody understands her—often including her husband. Women who stay home feel like they are antediluvian. Nobody understands why they are doing this. People say things like, 'Oh, you like doing diapers' or 'You like doing the kitchen floor.' There is an attitude that other people are using their minds and you are sitting at home rotting."

MOM, LET KIDS BE KIDS

When your job is raising kids, it's tempting to use them to fulfill your needs for self-esteem, says Gisela Booth, Ph.D., professor at Northwestern University in Chicago. That places a terrible burden on kids. If you expect them to be perfect, you're setting them—and yourself—up for failure.

In fact, some women assume that because they stay home, their kids are bound to turn out better than the kids next door, whose mother and father both work. But children don't come with a foolproof instruction manual, nor any guarantees.

"The woman who stays home all the time may in fact be too controlling and not let her kids be independent enough," says psychologist Matti Gershenfeld, Ph.D., of Couples Learning Center in Pennsylvania. "If you've given up your career for your kids because you want them to be perfect, you've just got to tell yourself, 'Well, they're not going to be. I'm doing this because I consider children very, very important and worth my time and energy, and I want to give it my best shot.' That's all you can rightly expect."

Here's some other advice psychologists offer for staying sane while staying home.

Take some time off. When you decide to stay home with your children, you're signing up for a job that runs 24 hours a day. Even more than the working mother, you'll need a break. If possible, hire a babysitter once a week and go out with your husband or some friends. If you can't afford it, barter babysitting services with your neighbors or friends.

Get help from your husband. If you and your husband mutually decide that you're going to stay home and care for your family, then you have the right to ask him to be fully supportive. That means helping out with the job that never ends. "If the baby cries at 2:00 in the morning, I would certainly get up and feed the baby, because you can take a nap during the day and he can't," says Dr. Gershenfeld. "But he should certainly be helping out with bathing the kids, doing the laundry, going food shopping or just taking the kids off your hands for a while."

Find a support group. If you're the only stay-at-home mom in your neighborhood, things can get mighty lonely. In fact, a researcher studying the effects of multiple roles on women found that women who had few friends—working-class women in this case—suffered from a host of physical problems and were more prone to depression.

Along with the companionship and rescue from isolation friends represent, you need to feel "that you're not the only one who made this decision or that not everybody looks down on you," says Dr. Gershenfeld. "You need support for a value system. This is very important."

Nancy Gaither, a former book production editor, says she approached her decision about whether to stay home with her two girls, ages 5 and 3, with much trepidation. She had her own notions of what stay-at-home moms were like—and it didn't sound much like her. "I knew what work involved, I felt secure there. I didn't know what it was like to be a full-time mom," she admits. "I had fear of the unknown, a fear of turning into that monster we all know, the woman eating bon-bons and watching 'General Hospital.'"

A working woman who retreats home may also find that all the self-esteem she earned in the work world crumbles when she's faced with the struggles of raising kids. Several years ago, Carolyn Kessell gave up her executive job with a computer software company to stay home with her two children. Her new job was a rude awakening. Writing "Welcome Home," a monthly newsletter for stay-at-home mothers, Carolyn says during her first few months she felt "utterly helpless, exasperated, humiliated and confounded by the likes of two people who are not a chairman of the board and a new president, but instead are a 3-year-old girl and a 22-month-old boy.

"How can a person who got a start-up company off the ground and built a customer service division that became the industry standard be perplexed at getting two children to nap at the same time?" she asks helplessly.

It's stressful to work in isolation, as many full-time mothers do. It's also stressful to have only one arena in which to find fulfillment. When a working mother has a bad day at home, she can at least hope for a good day at the office, and vice versa. A full-time mother never even gets to leave work.

A MATTER OF CHOICE

Still, plenty of women are doing it—and doing it success-fully. One of the reasons stay-at-home motherhood is, as *Parenting* noted, "a choice that's working" is that for 1990s homemakers, many of whom have already made their mark in the work place, home *is* a choice.

The results of a nationwide survey of over 1,000 Ameri-can mothers showed that women who chose to stay home and raise their children because they wanted to were quite happy. But the women who stayed home because they thought they had no other options or who felt they had to follow in their mother's footsteps were miserable. Other studies linking homemaking to poor health also note that dissatisfaction with the role may be the determining factor.

"The new stay-at-home mother has proved to herself she can do it, so now she can make a choice not to," says Suzanne Pope, Ph.D., director of the Colorado Institute for Marriage and the Family in Boulder. "But what if a woman hasn't proved it to herself? She'll always have that lingering doubt—is it that I didn't want to or is it that I couldn't?"

You need to choose full-time motherhood the way you do any career. It also helps to be convinced that the decision you've made is the best one for you and your family. No matter what others may think, you really are performing an important role. You are, after all, staying home to raise and nurture your children, not to keep your no-wax floor shiny.

"There is a lot of satisfaction in this job," says Nancy Gaither. "I'm the one helping my kids navigate their way through life, sort out the issues of right and wrong. I'm the one helping them decide who they're going to be, bandaging their emotional and physical wounds. I have chosen what I want most in life, and I'm going after it. If I achieve it, I'll have achieved the most important goal in my life. But I'd be lying if I said I never miss my paying job. There's something very tangible about being rewarded with a pay-check."

THE QUESTION OF MONEY

In fact, money is an issue in more ways than one. Getting by on one pay instead of two is certainly a big adjustment. But so is living on someone else's money. "There is a feeling of loss of independence," says Nancy. "A paycheck is also a very tangible symbol of one's significance. When it was taken away, I felt a sense of loss."

For some women, bringing in some money helps assuage the guilt they feel for, as they see it, "forcing" their husbands to shoulder the entire financial burden of the family. For others, a paycheck represents some financial independence, which, for most working women, may be the hardest thing to give up.

Nancy deals with those feelings by taking over the family finances. She budgets the household expenses "and I take care of our investments, meager though they may be."

Some women do in essense become the family comptroller, and they do some very creative economizing if money is tight. Some haunt thrift shops and auctions for clothing and furniture that may need only minimum refurbishing. Others throw themselves into couponing and refunding. One young mother took to couponing with a vengeance, occasionally walking out of the supermarket wheeling a basketful of free groceries. It was a skill that came in handy when her husband was briefly laid off from his job. "We never had to worry about eating," she says proudly.

ONE YEAR AT A TIME

If you had a career before, you can have a career again, although in some cases you might find you've fallen down the career ladder somewhat or may need a refresher course in your field of interest. The important thing to remember is that staying at home was a choice you made from the vast array of options you had—and probably still have.

"I don't think anybody should make the commitment to be at home more than year by year," says Nancy Gaither. "It's been nice for me to know I had the option to go back to work. It gives me a sense of control, that I didn't give myself a life sentence."

You may also find that your experience at home translates into improved job skills. Nine months after the birth of her third child, Carolyn Kessell had to return to work for financial reasons. She found a nice job in the marketing department of a small technology firm. She also found that her years at home, far from diminishing her work skills, had enhanced them.

"When I went back to work, I found I was much more secure and confident, and I can attribute that directly to staying home," says Carolyn. "It comes from having to deal with who I was as a person and finding out I liked who I was. There were no titles behind my name that proved to me I was a quality person. That was something I learned because of my years of staying home with the kids and being a nobody."

CHAPTER 58

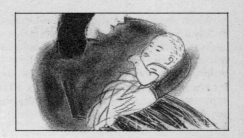

MOTHERHOOD
MINUS MARRIAGE

SOME CHOOSE TO GO IT ALONE

*A*t 36, Jane Mattes found herself in the same dilemma as the modern woman in the comic strip that made its way to a popular T-shirt a few years ago. "Oh, no," the woman is shown crying in dismay, "I forgot to have children!"

"I was very involved in my career," says Mattes, a New York City psychotherapist, explaining her own "oversight."

Not only didn't she notice that "everyone who wanted to get married was getting married," she didn't hear the ticking of her own biological clock until it began sounding like a time bomb. "I was very naive in thinking that everything was always going to be possible. I didn't realize that options do change and close. I suddenly realized one was closing very quickly and I would have to hurry up if I wanted to have children. I could accept that marriage might be late or never, but to not have a child was unthinkable."

Today, Mattes is the mother of a teenage son, fathered by a man who is no longer part of her life. She is also the founder of a 1,000-member national support group for those women daring enough to scale formidable social, legal and emotional obstacles to choose deliberately what others have had thrust on them: single motherhood.

When she founded the New York-based Single Mothers by Choice shortly after the birth of her son, Mattes was unaware that it was an idea whose time had come. Although still small, the numbers of the modern "unmarried with children" are growing. The National Center for Health Statistics reports that from 1980 to 1988 the birth rate jumped 69 percent for unmarried white women, the largest increases occurring among women over 25 years of age.

PROFILE OF MS. MOM

Who are these women who choose to parent solo? Like Mattes, most of them are older, financially secure career women who "forgot" to get married, never found Mr. Right or never looked for him, but who want to be mothers before the door to that option closes forever. Some psychological studies reveal a sketchy picture of a woman who may be isolated and narcissistic, choosing motherhood to battle her loneliness or fear of intimacy (or of men) or to compensate for rejecting parents. On the other hand, other studies find very little difference between single-by-choice mothers and other mothers. In fact, in those studies another picture emerges: that of an ego-strong, emotionally healthy woman for whom motherhood, not necessarily marriage, is an integral part of her identity and whose life is enriched by her child.

Andrea Cowley is an amagalm of those various psychological profiles. Andrea, a graphic designer, left a passionless, childless marriage in her thirties to have a baby with an 18-year-old construction worker who had a crush on her. "I had everything—a good marriage, a good career, lots of money and awards, but I was empty," says Cowley. "Today, I am blessed."

Cowley's relationship with her daughter, now 12, is the antithesis of her relationship with her own parents, who, she said, made her feel unloved. "Through my daughter, I felt love for the first time in my life," says Cowley. "For me that's the best part of being a mother. I'm looking at love all the time."

For Sally Hemphill, adopting her Korean daughter was

the culmination of a lifelong dream that, she concedes, never really included marriage. "Even as a child I wanted to be a mother," says Sally, a music teacher. "I decided if I wasn't married by the time I was 30, I would adopt. Of the two things, marriage and motherhood, having a child was my first choice, not my second. I always thought I'd make a good mother but a lousy wife."

"WHO'S DADDY?"

Once a woman makes the decision to become a single mother, she has various means to motherhood, each with its own advantages and pitfalls. When she first started her organization, Mattes says, a large number of women were choosing donor insemination, but lately more are adopting or using a partner. "More and more doctors are using frozen sperm, which is much less successful for conception than fresh sperm or intercourse," she says.

Donor insemination offers several important advantages over a partner: There's minimal risk of any later legal wrangles over custody or acrimonious conflicts over the child's upbringing. Andrea's worst times over the last 12 years have involved her daughter's father. "He's angry that he can't live with us. He wants us to be a family and it's not going to happen. Once, the woman he was seeing tried to convince him to sue for custody. Fortunately, he didn't, but the thought of it was terrifying."

But choosing a daddy from a sperm bank also raises some *Brave New World* issues: How do you explain to your child that her father is a number on a sealed file? It's commonplace for sperm banks to collect detailed medical histories of sperm donors but so far, only one, The Sperm Bank of California in Oakland, allows a child access to her father's name once she reaches 18—providing that the donor has consented.

"Among our members, the biggest issue is 'What are we going to tell the child?'" says Mattes. Experts agree it's vital for children to know the truth about their parentage, which, for some, becomes an important part of the quest for identity during adolescence. For adoptive mothers of

WHAT KIND OF KID WILL SHE BE?

One of the unknowns of single-by-choice motherhood is how this unconventional arrangement will affect your child. New York psychotherapist Jane Mattes and a colleague have undertaken a ten-year study to determine, in part, just how children of solo mothers turn out. But from her experience with members of Single Mothers by Choice, she says she can make some preliminary educated guesses at what her research will uncover.

"My guess is we're going to find children who are brighter than average because research has found that that's true of children of older mothers," she says. Emotionally, single-by-choice mothers are a lot like older mothers.

"Another thing I've noticed from our meetings is they are all very strong children," she says. "These are children who have a presence, who are used to being important in somebody's life, who are expecting to be heard. These children are not afterthoughts. They are of primary importance to their mothers."

While this undiluted attention may give these children "personal dynamism," says Mattes, it may also make them "hell on wheels."

Discipline may be harder for the single parent. In fact, says Virginia psychologist Maria Mancusi, Ph.D., "research shows that children in single-parent families are less compliant than children in two-parent families. For one thing, the single parent can't double-team a child, which is a powerful tool, so she needs to be very consistent in her discipline."

One thing you probably won't have to worry about is you or your child being stigmatized. For many people, the term *unwed mother* these days conjures up the image of a teenager, not a career woman. There are also plenty of single-parent families around, the only difference being that most of them exist because of misfortune, not choice. And, says Mattes from her own experience, "for every person who thinks this is terrible, there's someone else who thinks it's just wonderful."

American children, the task is sometimes easy. For those who used donor insemination or a partner, it's a more delicate issue because the explanation is complicated by the child's understanding of sex and reproduction and, in the case of absentee fathers, some strong emotions. Also, when the time comes, some women find themselves struggling with an unexpected sense of guilt.

"Although you know that feeling guilty can be damaging to your child and to you, often you can't help thinking that you brought a child into the world knowing he would not have a father," says Mattes. "You've made an unusual choice that has a lot of unknowns attached to it, but you're also offering your child a lot of really important, positive things."

And those, she says, are the things you should stress. For one thing, the child of a single mother is usually loved and wanted. "The single mother is thrilled to have a child," says Mattes, "perhaps even more than the happily married couple, because she didn't think she was going to have a family. She's happier, more content. Her child is to her a gift from Heaven in many ways and she has nobody else on which to spend her time, energy and commitment. With that in mind, you have to say to your child, 'I really wanted to be a mother. I really wanted a child enough that I was willing to take on the responsibility by myself.' Don't put it in the negative: I couldn't find a man, nobody wanted to be a daddy. The important thing to stress is there are different kinds of families and this is our family."

THE REAL WORLD

Clearly, single motherhood is not a choice to be taken lightly. "It's practically certain that it's going to be a lot harder than you think," says Maria Mancusi, Ph.D., a psychologist in Springfield, Virginia, who specializes in parent/child relationships. "You have a lot of fantasies as all parents do about what it's going to be like, and I think you're going to be as shocked as double-parent families are when they realize how awfully hard it is to raise a child. The reality is going to be much harder for the single parent who's going to be going through it all alone."

The first fact of life to dawn on the solo mother is that she is "it." She bears the entire burden of child rearing, from answering the 2:00 A.M. cries to filling up the rainy afternoons to riding out the stormy adolescence. Almost always a working parent, the single mother arranges for and worries over child care all alone. When the child is sick, she stays home from work. When she is sick, she must arrange for someone to care for her child. She has no "backup system," says Dr. Mancusi, no partner with whom to share parenting's trials and joys. The stress can weigh heavily on her.

"I don't think you can do it alone," says Mattes. "You need people to be there emotionally. No one cares as much as you—and that's a poignant, lonely feeling. When your baby takes his first step and says 'Mama' for the first time, nobody will be as thrilled as you."

But you need to have others who care, too, she advises. She stresses the importance of building a support group of family and friends who can help out when you need it. "You have to know there are people you can call in the middle of the night who will come and be with your child," she says.

THE FATHER FIGURE

Mattes recommends that single mothers try to arrange for an important male figure in their child's life, whether it's the child's own father, a grandfather, uncle, friend, teacher or Big Brother. In Mattes's case, the husband of her best friend—her son's godfather—volunteered to be his "father figure."

"It's my feeling that unless the child has some intimate contact with both sexes, he's really not equipped to relate to both sexes in the real world when he grows up," she says. "These kids have to have not just a Santa Claus figure, but someone who's involved with them on a real level, who really cares about them, who they can get into arguments with and work it out with—a relationship that grows."

Another adult in a child's life can also help "dilute" the solo parent's more negative qualities. Sally Hemphill says there have been times she's wished she had a partner to "hold me back when I overreact. It would have been very helpful, for instance, during homework, if I had had someone else who could come in and say, 'Here, I'll handle math.' It would have saved me and the child a lot of stress."

DON'T FORGET YOURSELF

Adult companionship is just as important to you. You need to have interests and relationships beyond your children. It's easy to settle into the cozy, contented life of the loved and loving parent, but you run the risk of depriving yourself of other satisfying adult relationships and of overburdening your child with the responsibility of meeting all your emotional needs.

"Kids are going to want to be the center of your life no matter who you are," says Dr. Mancusi. "Single parents particularly want to give in because they really are the center of the child's life, and that's very gratifying. But you may tend to overparentify a child, especially a child of the opposite sex. A boy can become a little Dad. I think you can unconsciously put a lot more responsibility on a child than he can really handle."

Allowing your child other adult relationships can break up the intense and exclusive twosome you're likely to become. As a single mother you can become too wrapped up in your child, who is likely to be an "only."

Dr. Mancusi warns against trying to be both mother and father to your child. "You may find yourself going overboard in meeting your child's needs out of guilt that you've deprived him of a so-called normal family," she says. "It's a fallacy that you have to be both mother and father to this child. Just being one good parent is all you really need to do."

THE SECRET OF SUCCESS

Single parenthood, in fact, has more going for it than against it. The ideal solo mother? She's a coper, says Mattes, someone with a sense of adventure.

"You have to know you're the kind of person who can ask for help when you need it, who can be creative about finding solutions to cope with problems and not passively let life act upon you, who can feel comfortable making a choice with some unknown ramifications, who can live with the uncertainty," says Mattes. "After all, this is an adventure, and adventures always have their share of unknowns."

Says Dr. Mancusi: "If you're a healthy individual, you're not using your child to meet your needs, you have a healthy balance between being able to give love to your child and also able to love yourself, you can develop a child who's independent and loving and you can do great. In fact, you can do better than if you were a single parent because of a bitter divorce. No question about it, you can do quite well."

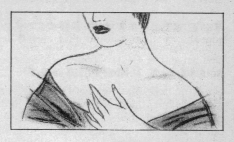

NUTRITION

WOMEN HAVE SPECIAL NEEDS

*I*f nutritionists were to issue a report card for all Americans today, women might get a solid B in nutrition, particularly if we were marked on a curve. That's because most surveys have found that women regularly outscore men in nutrition knowledge and practice.

But don't think you can rest on your laurels. What we *don't* know about nutrition literally fills volumes. According to one survey, 55 percent of the women polled had no idea how much milk they'd have to drink to meet the Recommended Dietary Allowance (RDA) for calcium, a mineral of vital importance to women because of their risk of postmenopausal bone loss.

With more and more evidence mounting that what we eat has a direct link to our risk of killer diseases such as cancer and heart disease, now is not the time to settle for a B in nutrition. And it's not the time to fly by the seat of your pants.

"Plain old common sense may not always work when it comes to nutrition," says registered dietitian Marsha Hudnell, a nutritional consultant for Green Mountain at Fox Run, a weight-management facility for women in Ludlow, Vermont. "It might have when we didn't have a large variety of foods to choose from. But today, I question whether there's an innate wisdom in the body that lets us choose the foods we need. Too many other attractive foods

are vying for our attention. You need to be more knowledgeable than you would have even a decade ago."

A LITTLE KNOWLEDGE . . .

Unfortunately, the surveys that give such high marks to
women's nutritional know-how also find that we're likely
to make food choices based on our weight rather than
our health; go for "quick fixes" and fads over good, solid
nutritional meal planning; and eliminate foods—and
meals—rather than practice moderation.

It takes some expertise to know how to get enough
calcium in your diet without going overboard on fat. It
takes some knowledge to design a low-calorie diet that
doesn't shortchange you on nutrients. You also need to
know that there are special times in a woman's life when
she has special nutritional needs. Our nutrient requirements
are affected not only by our age but also by our lifestyles
and attitudes. The nutritional needs of a teenager, a pregnant woman, a dieter, a working mother and a retiree are
all different.

For example, teenagers are not known for their good
eating habits. In fact, says Hudnell, teens may be at higher
risk than most women of suffering nutritional deficiency
"because they have higher needs, are probably less concerned about long-term effects of diet and are more interested in looking good at the moment. So if it means skipping
meals or not eating a well-balanced diet to keep their weight
down, that's what they do."

EVERY WOMAN'S NEEDS

No matter what her age, a woman's biggest dietary challenge will be getting enough iron, zinc and calcium.

With menstruation there is blood loss and, depending
on menstrual flow, there can be significant loss of iron
and zinc, both of which are found mainly in meat. Iron is
particularly hard to get in sufficient amounts in the diet,
especially for women, whose requirement for the mineral—
15 milligrams a day—is higher than men's. It's in many

foods but abundant only in foods such as liver, fortified cereals and prune juice. With the possible exception of the cereal, these are hardly staples of the typical woman's diet.

But the iron needs of some young women may not be critical, particularly for those with minimal menstrual loss, according to Bonnie Worthington-Roberts, Ph.D., director of the Nutritional Sciences Program at the University of Washington. "Their iron needs are not going to be as sizable as they might be otherwise."

There is also some controversy over the RDA for iron. "It's very hard to reach 15 milligrams even when you're eating a well-balanced diet," Hudnell points out. "A lot of people will argue it's unrealistically high."

Most women also have a tough time getting enough zinc in their diets. According to one study, only about 8 percent of all women consume the RDA of this mineral, abundant in meat but present also in grains, legumes, nuts, seeds and milk and other dairy products.

THE CALCIUM CONCERN

But the biggest concern for most women is calcium, says Dr. Worthington-Roberts. And for teens it's especially crucial. "There's continued substantial growth after the onset of menstruation and that period of time, from about age 11 to 24, is when bone development is most significant," she says. "So calcium intake is particularly important."

Calcium continues to be an important nutrient through your adult years. "Take care of your bones while you're young," says Dr. Worthington-Roberts. "Eat a quality diet, with lots of calcium and vitamin D in the years between 11 and 30, because all of us are going to lose bone starting at 35 and the rate of loss increases after that."

Your best bet for meeting your calcium needs is to eat low-fat dairy products, green leafy vegetables and calcium-fortified cereals. "For young girls worried about their figures, this can be a real challenge," cautions Dr. Worthington-Roberts.

Salmon with bones, sardines, collards and tofu treated with calcium sulfate are relatively good sources of calcium.

But again, these foods are not a staple of the typical female diet.

What to do? Supplementation can help. "The supplement with the greatest amount of calcium per tablet is calcium carbonate, which is 40 percent elemental (pure) calcium," says Dr. Worthington-Roberts. "Calcium gluconate is about 10 percent calcium, so you have to take a lot more to get the same amount." For women who suffer from constipation and gas from taking calcium carbonate, the alternative is calcium citrate, which is better tolerated even though it has less calcium.

EAT-AND-RUN SYNDROME

While studies show more men are now cooking, there are still more women in the kitchen. According to one Gallup poll, nearly three-quarters of the women interviewed say they do most of the shopping and cooking. Too busy to make meals from scratch, many cooks turn to frozen or prepackaged food or take-out restaurants.

And, says Dr. Worthington-Roberts, that doesn't have to be a bad thing. Good, nutritious, low-fat, low-sodium meals can be had in the frozen food section or, these days, even from the Golden Arches.

"The commercial food industry has responded quite well to people asking for nutritious options that are fast," she says.

Among all those greasy burgers at your local fast-food restaurant, you're just as likely to find low-fat alternatives, salads, even carrot sticks. In the supermarket get into the habit of reading labels. Look for low-fat, well-balanced prepackaged meals. Learn the various names fat and sugar go by on food labels. For example, says Hudnell, surveys have shown that we've cut out some of the obvious fats from our diets—heavily marbled red meats, for example—but replaced them with cheese, desserts and some mixed-grain dishes that can be just as high in fat.

Busy or not, the one best nutritional gift you can give yourself is to lower fat in your diet, which isn't always easy to do when you're busy. "For most women, this is going to make the most difference," says Dr. Worthington-Roberts. "It will help with calories. It will help with blood cholesterol. It will probably decrease risk of breast cancer. It will make weight control easier."

So, even if you don't have time to whip up a meal from scratch every night, don't avoid the fruit and vegetable section of the supermarket, says Dr. Worthington-Roberts. Fruits and vegetables are a low-fat alternative that ought to be on your table, and they're not all that tough to prepare. You can steam vegetables in the microwave, and there's no preparation time at all for putting out a bowl of fruit for dessert. "Also, fruits and vegetables are in the spotlight now because they are believed to have cancer-preventing qualities," says Dr. Worthington-Roberts. "Plus they're low-calorie."

THE SKIMPY DIETER

When a national magazine polled its readers about sex in 1991, it discovered that at least some of the health-conscious respondents didn't consider cheating on their mates nearly as sinful as cheating on their diets. For the weight conscious, the new morality focuses on our relationship to food, not each other.

Studies have pointed to two common traits among women and their relationship with food: Most women are or have been on a diet, and many of the food choices they make revolve around weight, not health. Sometimes those choices are good ones—cutting back on fatty red meat, eating more salads, paying more attention to the fiber in their diets. But many times, when motivated by weight-loss goals, they're unwise.

For example, says Hudnell, many women do apply the moral concepts of "good" and "bad" to food. Good is seen as "low-calorie," and bad as "high-calorie," which leads to a lot of meal skipping and food phobias, which can quickly unbalance an otherwise carefully considered diet, she says.

For example, she points out, "a lot of women cut back on bread. Even though there has been a turnaround among many people on their perception of bread as fattening, the misperception still persists among the dieting public. We see a tremendous number of women who resist eating four servings of bread a day when the recommendation now is six."

Foods that are dropped from the diet because they're perceived as "bad" take on the aura of "forbidden fruit," says Hudnell. "If you try to prohibit them, you will probably end up bingeing on them. Something that is prohibited is more attractive. This kind of dieting promotes weight gain. We see it all the time."

Another unwise choice many women have made is to stop drinking milk, one of the richest sources of calcium there is and, because it's thought to be relatively high in calories, one of the "bad" foods dieters spurn. "They've even stopped drinking skim milk, in the interest of saving calories," says Hudnell. But this doesn't mean some women are ignoring the cry for calcium-rich foods. "Since 1980, cheese overtook milk in food consumption, so the problem isn't calcium, it's fat," says Hudnell. "Even low-fat cheeses have more fat than skim milk. Many women need to be more moderate in their consumption of cheese."

If a dieter is skipping meat and milk, she might also be missing out on riboflavin, one of the energy-releasing B vitamins. Riboflavin deficiency is rare, but studies have shown that highly active women increase their need for riboflavin. "Dieting women who are exercising heavily might find it a problem," suggests Hudnell.

ADVICE FOR MOMS-TO-BE

A woman's needs for nutrients—and calories—will never be higher than when she's pregnant or breastfeeding. Pregnancy is also a time when the appetite goes through some dramatic changes. You may have morning sickness, which can make eating a revolting thought, followed by months when you have an appetite rivaling that of Homer Simpson. You may also have food cravings, a well-documented and little understood phenomenon of pregnancy that may or may not have any physiological base.

Along with getting enough calories, you need to pay particular attention to your consumption of foods rich in calcium, iron and folate. And in some cases, you may need to start paying attention to your nutritional needs *before* you're pregnant.

In all likelihood, your doctor will prescribe a vitamin supplement during your pregnancy. It will likely contain a good dose of iron, since iron deficiency is the most common nutrient deficiency found among pregnant women in the United States. It's tough to get enough iron in your diet when you're not pregnant, and it's even harder when your need for it increases.

However, says Dr. Bonnie Worthington-Roberts, although prescribing vitamin supplements is a long-standing practice among obstetricians, many women do not need them. "There's no evidence they have any particularly beneficial effect," she says. "You need to be careful about your use of vitamins during pregnancy." And you shouldn't take *any* supplements without approval from your obstetrician.

Once your baby is born, your calorie requirements will go up if you are breastfeeding, says Dr. Worthington-Roberts. You may need anywhere from an additional 300 to 500 calories a day, although there is some controversy over the exact amount. "There is some evidence that during lactation women are a bit more efficient at using calories," she says. "But on the other hand, most women are quite inactive after birth so their calorie expenditure goes down. They also have a pregnancy fat pad left and some of that fat pad is used for the calories needed for lactation."

She says that your need for extra calories most likely will be dictated by your lifestyle and your activity level. "It's just going to vary from woman to woman." For example, a study of women training for marathons found that the breastfeeding runners who ate over 3,000 calories a day still lost weight.

Your best bet is to eat as well as you can to protect both yourself and your baby. If you're not getting enough vitamins, neither is your baby. And dieting during lactation can affect both the nutrient quality and eventually the quantity of breast milk you make, says Dr. Worthington-Roberts. If you aren't eating well, your stores of nutrients eventually will be drained and will put you at risk of nutrient deficiency.

MENOPAUSE AND AFTER

This is the time that calcium intake becomes of vital importance to women—but this shouldn't be the first time in your life you pay attention to how much you're getting in your diet.

Your risk of osteoporosis goes up after menopause, although you've experienced some bone loss since your midthirties. If you were smart, you regarded your calcium intake throughout your life as an individualized retirement account, putting a little in each day as a kind of nest egg for the future.

At menopause, the only sure way to markedly slow down bone loss is estrogen, says Dr. Worthington-Roberts. But not every woman is a candidate for estrogen replacement therapy. Will calcium help?

"Calcium can help slow bone loss, but it doesn't prevent it," says Dr. Worthington-Roberts. "Estrogen is the best. Taking nothing is the worst. So, yes, nutrition does make some difference."

If you opt for calcium, how much should you be taking? Assuming your diet has at least 500 milligrams—the average for an American woman—an additional 800 to 1,000 milligrams is needed, she says. "But if you've been calcium conscious and drinking nonfat milk, you could be getting 800 to 1,000 milligrams."

As a woman gets older she also has to pay more attention to her caloric intake, especially if she's sedentary. And this can impact the vitamins and minerals in the diet. The loss of muscle mass in old age means you burn fewer calories. This means you need less food to maintain the same weight.

With the decrease in food intake comes a corresponding decrease in the number of vitamins and minerals in the diet. "At this point in your life it becomes even more important to choose foods wisely," says Marsha Hudnell.

Choose foods of high nutrient density, she suggests.

NUTRITION FOR ONE

A Gallup survey found that on any given weeknight, two out of ten adults eat alone. Chances are most of those solitary diners are single, perhaps living alone. Eating is such a social event in our culture, it loses some of its appeal when there's no one sitting across the table. So there isn't a whole lot of motivation to cook.

"Rather than going for what's nutritious, singles may go for what's quick, and that means they will often come up short on the nutrition end," says nutrition expert Bonnie Worthington-Roberts, Ph.D., of the University of Washington.

But being single is such a national trend that the food industry, even supermarkets themselves, are making it easier for singles to eat well. "You never used to be able to buy anything in a package that would just serve one or two. Now those options are available," says Dr. Worthington-Roberts. "Even in the meat section, you can buy little roasts. That was never the case ten years ago."

If you're looking for a quick take-home supper, many supermarkets have salad bars and hot meals to go. There are some entrepreneurs who cater strictly to the busy career person, providing a week's menu of delicious, healthful meals that can be ordered ahead and picked up. Frozen dinners—many of them low-fat, low-sodium and low-calorie—cook up in 6 or 7 minutes in the microwave.

But there are other options, too. Some supermarkets sell cut-up vegetables for stir-fry, an easy and simple meal that cooks up in a few minutes. For singles who enjoy cooking but don't have the time, they simply need to stop shopping and cooking for one. Instead, they can prepare several portions at once and freeze the extras to be microwaved later in the week as needed.

Those are foods that have a high ratio of nutrients to calories. For example, a cup of skim milk contains 30 percent of the RDA for calcium and 90 calories. A cup of whole milk has the same amount of calcium but contains 150 calories, so the more nutrient-dense product is skim milk.

"A piece of carrot cake may have a lot of vitamin A in

NUTRITION, THE PILL AND THE IUD

It wasn't all that long ago that doctors gave out vitamin pills along with a prescription for oral contraceptives. Birth control pills were believed to increase the need for a number of nutrients, including vitamins C, B_6 and folate (a B vitamin).

"The reality today is that birth control pills are so low in hormonal content that the impact on nutritional status is minimal," says nutrition expert Bonnie Worthington-Roberts, Ph.D., of the University of Washington. "Anyone who has been on birth control pills for many years may develop some biochemical evidence of B_6 or folate deficiency, but it is highly unlikely."

If you have an IUD, however, you may be at risk for an iron deficiency. This is because an IUD often increases menstrual flow, and iron is lost through blood. "Many women who get IUDs automatically get an iron supplementation recommendation because of that," she says.

it, but it also has a lot of fat and calories in it compared to a carrot," says Hudnell.

CHAPTER 60

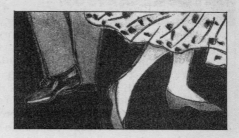

OFFICE ROMANCE

WHOSE BUSINESS IS IT?

The workplace is not designed to accommodate people falling in love.
SPECIAL REPORT, THE BUREAU OF NATIONAL AFFAIRS

*L*ike it or not, the office *is* a place where boy meets girl. In fact, some statistics show that more marriages are made in the office than anywhere else. But then, a lot of marriages are broken in the office, too.

Possibly the most publicly talked about office romance was between William Agee, then chief executive officer of the Bendix Corporation, and his executive assistant, Mary Cunningham. The affair made national headlines because many believed his "favoritism" pushed her up the corporate ladder. Both eventually left the company, married and started their own business together.

Most office affairs don't make national headlines, but they do attract their fair share of in-house interest. The Bureau of National Affairs (BNA) found it such a hot topic that it became the focus of a widespread study in which numerous psychologists, corporate chiefs, middle managers and their employees were interviewed. The BNA found office romances do, indeed, create a lot of uneasy vibrations, from top executives right on down to the rank and file.

UNEQUAL LIAISON

Of course, the Bureau of National Affairs found only certain kinds of office romances make workers nervous. In particular, the kind that involves the boss and a subordinate. The BNA says that this type of affair is the "most disruptive of office routine and most negative in its consequences," especially when one or both of the lovers is married. "These romances cause jealousy and suspicion among coworkers and can result in lowered productivity," says the report. "Such involvements can lead to charges of favoritism." Many workers, according to experts who study office romances, feel abandoned by a boss who obviously sees one of their fellow workers as someone special.

Kathryn Roland, 27, an account executive for a large advertising agency, found this out the hard way. Kathryn says that when her boss, who was married, took a special interest in her, she didn't notice that other people were noticing what was happening. "At first he played my mentor, which was great," she admits, "and so I tried to ignore his marital status. He gave me creative projects to do and took me on power lunches. But to do that he had to go completely around my immediate supervisor, and she resented it. I was too naive to realize that that was unacceptable office protocol."

When Doris Delaney was a 30-year-old reporter and had an affair with her married editor, she knew that everyone felt he was playing her as the favorite, even though their affair was supposed to have been a secret. "The truth was," says Doris, "he was harder on me than anybody. I was never given the advantage."

Actually, the BNA report indicates this is often the prevailing attitude. One expert reported that workers who are dating "will stand on their heads sometimes to be fair." Yet, unequal treatment is still the suspicion in the minds of most coworkers.

Then, of course, there's the even bigger picture. "A relationship between a boss and a subordinate carries another, more obvious risk," says Judith Sills, Ph.D., a clinical psychologist in private practice in Philadelphia. "What happens if—or more likely when—this affair is over? This is a question you can't ignore."

HOW SWEET IT IS

Not all is unfair in love and office romance, however. Some relationships can actually spark up the office atmosphere. One expert called it humanizing. These are, of course, love interests among two single coworkers.

If handled properly, these kinds of love relationships can be "extremely positive," the Bureau of National Affairs reports. "People who are in love are happy to come to work, are willing to work longer hours and are not rushing out the door to get ready for a date."

Sometimes a relationship can create a problem if other employees feel the couple is "looking for excuses to spend time together during work hours and are not pulling their fair share of the work load." Fellow workers resent this.

But any real office problem in this kind of relationship only occurs if the romance comes to an unhappy ending. It creates "an atmosphere of stress not only for the couple but for their coworkers," says the BNA. Workers feel like they have to divide loyalties "like children in a divorce."

OVER AND OUT

What *does* happen when a relationship is over?

Kathryn Roland says when she wanted to end the affair with her boss, he didn't take it well. "Suddenly the special projects stopped. It made me wonder if he had ever recognized me for my intelligence and talent, or if his attention was prompted solely because he was physically attracted to me. It undermined my confidence for months."

But since it was her decision to call off the affair, she didn't experience any real emotional side effects.

Not so for Doris Delaney. She lost it all—her lover, her job, her self-esteem. Often a bitter end is the bitter truth of office affairs. Even the BNA report found that trying to resume a working colleague-only relationship is difficult,

ADVICE FOR CONSENT

Should you or shouldn't you have an office affair? Well, only your conscience really knows for sure. But Lois B. Hart and J. David Dalke, coauthors of the book *The Sexes at Work*, recommend asking yourself the following questions to help you make up your mind.

- How much do I really like this person?
- Have I been seduced into a relationship because it is the thing *not* to do?
- What am I going to gain from this relationship?
- Is my work production suffering because of my interest?
- Am I creating a situation at work that I may regret later?
- Is my willingness to be diverted caused by my low commitment to my job?

Psychologists warn, of course, that finding a rational answer really isn't all that easy. Love is too irrational an emotion.

especially if love, and not just sex, was involved. Often, one or the other winds up leaving the company.

"Staying requires at least some pretense to dignity," says Dr. Sills. "It's not always all that easy to carry off."

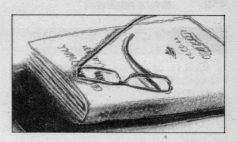

OSTEOPOROSIS

GET AN EARLY START ON PREVENTION

irst she fractured her wrist. Two years later, she broke her ankle. And then, just ten days after that cast came off, she broke her other ankle. Although the broken wrist was the result of a nasty fall, 70-year-old Evelyn Kline did nothing out of the ordinary to cause the other breaks. To make matters worse, healing was slow for this normally active woman and she had to stay on a limited schedule for weeks even after the final cast was removed.

"Although I didn't feel helpless, I must say that having two broken ankles back-to-back affected me tremendously," she says. "My ability to walk—to get around on my own—was threatened. Suddenly I had a sense of my own vulnerability. I was conscious of every step I took, wondering if the next one would cause another bone to break."

For most older women, a broken bone—usually from some minor incident—is often the first indication of osteoporosis, a debilitating condition in which bones become thin, porous and prone to fracture.

And for many, it's a rude declaration that life as they know it is about to change forever. Osteoporosis is a disease with enormous consequences because it can rob a woman of her independence. Weak bones lead to weak constitutions, making a woman fearful to go out and dependent on others both emotionally and physically.

"The fact that I couldn't walk well anymore, that it

could happen again so easily, was paralyzing to me," says Evelyn.

IGNORANCE IS REMISS

When Evelyn's doctor told her she had osteoporosis, he didn't need to explain to her what it was (even though he did). Nor did he have to explain its ramifications. Today, magazine articles and advertisements—mostly for things like milk and vitamins—have made women more aware of osteoporosis than ever before.

But the problem, as some experts see it, is that many women are doing too little about it. In fact, it's not uncommon that until an older woman breaks a bone, she doesn't give her bone health a lot of thought, says Deborah T. Gold, Ph.D., assistant professor of psychiatry and sociology at Duke University Medical Center in Durham, North Carolina. Part of the reason, she says, is lack of knowledge. While most women know what osteoporosis is, many have misconceptions about what causes it and how to prevent it.

STRONG BONES NEED CALCIUM

Bone loss after menopause isn't entirely preventable, but you can slow it down with a diet high in calcium. Some researchers believe the Recommended Dietary Allowance of calcium at 800 milligrams per day isn't enough. Instead, 1,000 milligrams of calcium are recommended for women on estrogen replacement therapy and up to 1,500 milligrams for women who don't take the hormone.

Calcium is most abundant in dairy foods—particularly low-fat dairy products. The lower the fat content, the more calcium it can contain. But dairy foods aren't the only place to turn to meet your calcium requirement. Many other foods, such as dark green leafy vegetables and nuts and seeds, are also good sources of calcium as well as other vitamins and minerals. You should be aware, however, that certain dark greens, most notably spinach and kale, also contain lots of oxalic acid, which binds with calcium and prevents its proper absorption.

Following is a list of the top food sources of calcium.

Food	Serving	Calcium (MG)	% of RDA
Nonfat yogurt	1 cup	448	56
Skim milk	1 cup	352	44
Part-skim ricotta cheese	½ cup	336	42
Low-fat fruit yogurt	1 cup	312	39
Romano cheese	1 oz.	296	37
Whole milk	1 cup	288	36
Swiss cheese	1 oz.	272	34
Provolone cheese	1 oz.	208	26
Cheddar cheese	1 oz.	200	25
Tofu	½ cup	130	13
Almonds, blanched	¼ cup	90	9
Broccoli, cooked	1 spear	83	8
Navy beans, cooked	½ cup	64	6
Sesame butter	1 Tbsp.	63	6
Mustard greens, cooked	½ cup	52	5
Swiss chard, cooked	½ cup	51	5
Kale, cooked	½ cup	47	5
Sunflower seed kernels, raw	¼ cup	42	4
Red kidney beans, cooked	½ cup	39	4
Leek, cooked	1	37	4

"They think, for example, that if they drink a glass of milk every day, they'll be fine," says Dr. Gold, who is also a senior fellow at the university's Center for the Study of Aging and Human development. "Or they believe osteoporosis is completely genetic, so if their mothers didn't have it, then they won't get it, either." Some also think that bone care is something that can be put off until they get older, like after menopause. "But by that age, bone density has already been lost," she says.

The truth is, bone health is something you need to start when you're young, says Dr. Gold. By the age of 30 to 35, the human body reaches what experts call peak bone mass, when bone is strongest and densest. After about age 35, bone loss begins and continues, slowly and gradually—until menopause. At menopause and for several years after that, bone loss accelerates dramatically, as high as 3 percent per year—a loss that's directly related to the absence of the female hormone estrogen. It's the main reason why osteoporosis is considered a woman's disease.

There are also other known factors that can increase your chances of developing the disease. Some you can't change, like early or surgical menopause, a family history of osteoporosis or a small bone structure. But some risk factors you do have control over—a sedentary lifestyle, cigarette smoking and a diet low in calcium all contribute to weakening bones. "The sooner you correct these, the better off you'll be," says Dr. Gold. "If you wait until you're 50, you'll have waited too long."

PREVENTION IS YOUR BEST DEFENSE

Who among you is most likely to get osteoporosis? If you're small, thin, smoke and drink a lot, get too little exercise and have never given birth, the answer is: You are. If you also avoid dairy products, follow a poor diet and have a mother or grandmother who fractured a hip in later life, consider the likelihood even greater.

In fact, if any aspect of this profile fits you, consider yourself at risk, says professor Diane Meier, M.D., of Mount Sinai School of Medicine. But don't consider the disease an inevitability. Osteoporosis *is* preventable.

The secret to maintaining healthy bones for life is to practice a prevention program when you're still young—before bone breakdown begins. But that doesn't mean you shouldn't start now, no matter what your age. A good prevention program is the only break your bones should ever get. Here's what the experts say you should do.

Get plenty of calcium. Bones are composed largely of the mineral calcium. It's also a substance your body needs. When your body can't get it from food—when you're not getting enough calcium in your diet—it steals it from your bones.

Studies have shown that the average woman does not get enough calcium in her diet. Dairy products—low-fat milk, yogurt and cheeses, etc.—are among the best sources of calcium. So, too, are bony fish, such as sardines and salmon. If you suspect your diet is calcium poor, discuss it with your doctor. She may want to recommend a supplement program.

Get adequate vitamin D, too. If you get your calcium from a source other than dairy products, you may be missing out on vitamin D, a nutrient necessary for the absorption of calcium, says Dr. Meier. (Milk is fortified with vitamin D.) She also says that vitamin D absorption can be affected if you don't get out in the sun (which the body needs to make vitamin D) or if you use a sunblock on a daily basis. Vitamin D, however, is toxic in large doses, and you shouldn't take supplements without the supervision of your doctor. It's a subject you can discuss in conjunction with your diet when you see you doctor.

Put exercise into your life. Experts now know that regular exercise can help slow bone loss. In fact, it can even increase bone mass in some postmenopausal women. Weight-bearing exercises—like running, tennis, low-impact aerobics and walking—are the kind that make bones strong. But, note experts, exercise is only beneficial if it is done routinely—at least three to five times a week.

At menopause, assess your need for estrogen. Not everyone needs to take estrogen to protect their bones, says Dr. Meier. If your bone density is high at the time of menopause, then even the rapid loss that occurs during the following few years may leave you with ample bone reserves, she says. A woman whose bone density is low or low-normal at the time of menopause, on the other hand, may be able to prevent future problems from brittle bones by taking estrogen replacement therapy (ERT).

ERT, however, is not risk-free; for one, it's been associated with an increased risk of certain types of cancer. ERT is a decision you need to make in conjunction with your doctor.

FEAR OF FALLING

There's ample reason to take Dr. Gold's advice to heart. Osteoporosis already afflicts 25 million Americans—mostly women—and is responsible for 1.3 million broken bones each year, most commonly in the wrist, hip and spinal column. And it doesn't take much to cause a break. Seemingly mundane activities of everyday life, such as bending over to pet a dog or to pick up a light package, can snap an already brittle bone. Evelyn Kline says that both her broken ankles occurred while she was walking—and she neither fell nor tripped. "I simply noticed a cramping pain in my ankle that wasn't there a moment before."

Hip fractures are the most devastating, says Diane Meier, M.D., co-director of the Osteoporosis and Metabolic Bone Disease Program at the Mount Sinai Medical Center in New York City. About 40 percent of older women who break a hip wind up unable to walk again without assistance. Scarier still, 17 percent of broken hips lead to death, often the result of complications such as pneumonia or blood clots in the lungs.

"The fear of falling and breaking yet another bone can actually cause women to become phobic about going outside," claims Dr. Meier, who is also associate professor of geriatrics and medicine at the Mount Sinai School of Medicine of the City University of New York. "Consequently, they severely limit their physical activities, which in turn can exacerbate the bone-thinning process."

Evelyn says that at one point she was afraid to leave her home, especially after one particularly frightening incident involving an icy sidewalk. "Even though I had my cane with me, I kept slipping. With each step I felt my apprehension grow. I managed by walking on the grass and clutching trees along the way. When I got to the corner I had to step onto the pavement to cross the street. That's when I fell down—hard. When I finally arrived home, I shook and trembled for hours. The thought that I could have broken my back or my leg was terrifying to me. I suddenly felt fragile and old."

FEELING OLD AND HELPLESS

Evelyn's reaction is quite common. When a broken bone leads to a diagnosis of osteoporosis, a woman's self-esteem is broken as well, says Dr. Gold, who studied the psychological and social impact of the disease on a group of women.

Interpersonal relationships can suffer, too. "A woman diagnosed with osteoporosis may look perfectly healthy," says Dr. Gold, "but she's not. When she says to her husband, 'George, I'm not allowed to lift anything heavier than 5 pounds, so you're going to have to carry the laundry downstairs,' George's response is likely to be, 'No way, you look fine to me.' She may be treated like a malingerer, which is the furthest thing from the truth."

Dr. Gold says that her patients often find it difficult to ask for the physical and emotional support they need. As one woman in her group pointed out, "I'm independent and it's hard for me to ask for anything, especially when it's something as little as picking up a package or carrying in the groceries. I've been doing those things all my life. It's hard to accept that you can't any longer."

There are also problems with body image. One mark of osteoporosis is loss of height from the compression of bones in the back. It can leave a woman looking hunched over and oddly proportioned. "Sometimes women become so bent over that their rib cages rest on their hips," says Dr. Meier. "It becomes nearly impossible to find clothes that fit." Some women end up with what's known as a dowager's hump, which is, as Dr. Meier puts it, "like the scarlet letter of old age."

GETTING YOUR LIFE BACK

Osteoporosis requires some adjustments to your life, but it isn't a life sentence, notes Dr. Meier. It starts by learning to put yourself first, which considering the way women are conditioned, is not an easy thing to do.

And if Dr. Gold's study group is any indication, don't expect a lot of unsolicited help. If you need help, you have to learn to ask for it.

Just as important is taking responsibility for your own safety. Most falls occur in the home, so that's the place to make a few simple changes, says Dr. Meier. Remove throw rugs that slip easily. Make sure all electrical wires are tucked away so you can't accidentally trip over them. Replace linoleum or carpeting that may be coming up at the corners. Throw out the high heels and wear stable, flat shoes. Put vanity aside and use a cane or walker if your gait is unsteady. Install grab bars in the bathroom, especially in the tub or shower. Have lots of light, especially in closets, small hallways and stairs.

Dr. Gold adds that bending and stretching can be painful to a person with osteoporosis. For that reason, she recommends that all pots, pans and dishes be placed on the counter in your kitchen. "It may not be as neat as you like," she admits, "but women who follow that advice find a tremendous improvement in how they feel."

See also Estrogen Replacement Therapy

CHAPTER 62

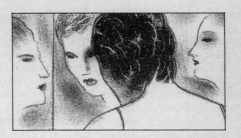

OVERWEIGHT

A PROBLEM TOO BIG TO HIDE

I've been overweight, on and off, since I was a child," says Sara Miller, 39, a teacher now in what she calls one of her thin periods.

"I have been called names, made fun of, harassed, humiliated, shunned and made to feel like a freak of nature. There were many times when I was growing up when I wished I would die. I never went to a school dance. I didn't go to my prom. I can't share in all of that nostalgia people have for their teenage years."

Sara says she was nearly 20—and about 50 pounds lighter—before a boy asked her out. "It took years of therapy to help me repair my self-esteem," she admits. "Even today, with that so far behind me, I can't bring myself to talk about my life in any detail. I'm afraid if I do, what looks like a scar will turn out to be an open wound."

For Sara, as for many overweight women, fat is more than a physical problem, the triumph of appetite over willpower. It can be a painful psychological wound brought on by a sense of alienation and shame.

LOSS OF SELF-ESTEEM

The first casualty of overweight, whether it's from childhood or adulthood, usually is self-esteem, because obesity is so strongly stigmatized in our society. Studies have found that from a very early age, children hold very negative attitudes toward obese people. In one study, children were more rejecting of overweight children than those with facial disfigurements. And children can be cruel. Since our feelings about ourselves are shaped by how others feel about us, women who have been overweight since childhood may learn early to dislike themselves.

"Kids think nothing about calling a fat classmate all sorts of horrible names," says Sara. "When I was in seventh grade, the clique that was the 'in-crowd' at my junior high made me the unofficial class project. I kept a calendar and marked down each day they taunted me. Sometimes, it was every day."

LOSS OF STATUS

There has been some evidence that overweight people—particularly women—are discriminated against both in school and on the job, are less likely to go to college and make less money than others with the same intellect and qualifications but who also happen to be thin. Being fat circumscribes your options. Along with dropping in socio-economic status, an overweight woman may have trouble forming intimate relationships with men and may be deprived of marriage and children.

It's clear that fat is more than the size of the skin you're in. There are moral overtones ascribed to body size. "Fat people are held accountable for their fat—for becoming fat in the first place and for staying that way," according to obesity researchers Janet Polivy, Ph.D. and C.P. Herman. "This is in contrast to thin people, whose thinness is applauded." In studies, fat people are seen as lazy, sloppy, mean and stupid. On the other hand, the prerequisite for beauty is a slim build. The social rewards of thinness are myriad. One study found that attractive people even were acquitted more often or received lighter sentences in simulated court cases than less-attractive defendants.

DIETING DILEMMA

Surprisingly, however, studies have shown that people with weight problems don't have significantly more psychological problems than anyone else. In fact, some experts think dieting, rather than overweight, may hurt your self-esteem more because of the sense of failure that accompanies what is for most dieters the inevitable relapse.

The one sad fact of life about dieting is that most people who diet lose weight but few keep it off. In fact, one researcher pointed out that if a "cure" for overweight is defined as dropping to and maintaining ideal weight for five years, a person is more likely to recover from cancer than from obesity.

Although there are certainly plenty of obese men, fat seems to be more a woman's problem than a man's. Although a quarter of the American population is overweight—defined as 20 percent over ideal weight—35 percent of all women are. That figure doesn't take into account those who feel fat, whose 5 or 10 extra pounds make them feel too self-conscious to tuck their blouses in or too inadequate to go after a good job or leave an unhappy relationship.

FITTING INTO YOUR GENES

Part of the problem is genetics. Many overweight women are battling biology. Numerous studies, including those done on identical twins reared apart, point to a strong genetic contribution to body size. Some people are simply more inclined to be big or to put on weight than others. Some studies have suggested that there are individual differences in how we metabolize and store the food we eat, which is why your friend who thinks ice cream is one of the basic food groups doesn't gain weight on 2,800 calories a day while you will put on a pound after adding a few cookies to your 1,800-calorie-a-day regimen.

Genetics may doom you from the start—in more ways than one. Your self-esteem is almost certain to suffer if your goal is to look model-thin and you've inherited thick ankles or "breeder's" hips. Only about 5 percent of the population is naturally that thin. For the rest, it's a goal attainable only at great price, if at all.

"With society's thin ideal, women have to be practically

anorexic to be beautiful," says Ronette Kolotkin, Ph.D., clinical psychologist at the Duke University Diet and Fitness Center in Durham, North Carolina. "There's so much pressure to be perfect, to have the perfect body, it drives people to feel inadequate. Then they soothe themselves with food. They feel hopeless, saying to themselves: 'It doesn't matter what I do, I still don't have a perfect body. I might as well eat.' "

FAT AS A FEMALE ISSUE

Genetics also explains why men, in general, don't battle the bulge as often as women. In women, milestones such as puberty, pregnancy and menopause are all associated with weight gain. In another of what seems like life's injustices, being born a woman predisposes you to putting on more fat than a man. Even before puberty, girls have 10 to 15 percent more fat than boys. After puberty, they have almost twice as much as boys. Like girls, boys gain weight at puberty, but they put it on in lean muscle tissue and bone. The sex hormones that surge at puberty also seem to encourage fat storage, as does pregnancy, which is nature's way of protecting the mother and fetus from starvation in times of famine. For some reason, as yet unknown, the pounds women put on with pregnancy are particularly hard to lose.

Women also tend to have lower metabolic rates than men. Their stronger-chugging metabolism, in addition to their greater fat-burning musculature, is why men are able to lose weight faster. Chronic dieting, which is epidemic among women, will also make it much harder in the long run for a woman to lose the weight she wants, because in response to the enforced "famine" of a calorie-restricted diet, her metabolism becomes even more efficient at storing fat.

If physical obstacles weren't enough, there are psychological roadblocks as well.

You may sabotage your efforts to lose weight because, like many women, you have no trouble taking care of others but feel selfish or guilty doing things for yourself.

Your loved ones may deliberately or unconsciously discourage you, says Dr. Kolotkin. They may go so far as to eat your favorite foods in front of you or lure you out to dinner to derail your efforts because they feel neglected or are alarmed by the changes—physical and psychological—they see in you. Losing weight successfully can give you a sense of mastery and control that spills into other aspects of your life. "You may have been a doormat and now that you feel more in control, you've gotten assertive," points out Dr. Kolotkin. "It may take them some time to adjust to the new you."

Although a supportive family is one of the factors identified as instrumental in helping dieters keep the weight off, sometimes you "have to teach them how to be supportive," says Dr. Kolotkin. "For example, when they ask if you should be eating something, tell them it's better to praise you for the progress you've made, rather than pointing out your inadequacies."

DEEP-FAT-FRIED COMFORT

There are other traps, too. For most of us, food isn't just food. It's everything from love to medicine. It's stimulating and soothing, comforting and calming. "To say food is just to sustain life," says California psychologist Joyce Nash, Ph.D., author of *Maximize Your Body Potential*, "is like saying sex is only for procreation."

For some women, food satiates many hungers. Recent studies have found that people who have been traumatized as children—who were sexually abused, neglected or lost a parent—may use food for comfort and nurturing. "As children, when they didn't know how to cope with their feelings, they did something that felt good, that helped them cope, and they maintain those bad habits long after," says Dr. Kolotkin.

Food can "provide a distraction from whatever problems really exist," says Dr. Nash. For many women, food serves as an escape, a way to avoid or cope with their problems.

"One of the things that helped me get food in perspective

DIETING: WHAT WORKS

In recent years, research has focused on why some people are successful at losing weight and keeping it off. Professor Rosemary Johnson, Ph.D., of the University of Southern Maine School of Nursing, spent 200 hours observing and interviewing dieters attending a nationally known weight-loss program to learn the secrets of their success.

What she found was that the people who were able to lose weight and keep it off recognized that they were not only changing their shapes, they were changing their lives. Their weight-loss "plan" was more than just a diet, a few hours of exercise and a weekly support group. It was a gradual restructuring of their lives.

The women she interviewed did a great deal of soul-searching and reflection, identifying exactly what they needed to do to achieve their goals. The strategies they chose were different for each of them. "They came up with personalized solutions," she says. "They were finding strategies that fit them, rather than buying into the idea that 'this is what you need to do.' Programs that say 'here's what works' can make you feel like a failure when they don't work for you. Some of the women I interviewed actually dropped out of the program when they realized it wasn't working for them, and they still lost weight."

They became aware of the role of overeating in their lives, delving deeply to determine what other function besides nourishment food served for them. They made themselves a priority, refusing to worry or feel guilty if they did things for themselves first, before they met the needs of those around them. They changed their concept of success and failure, giving up the idea that they had to be perfect to be successful. They applauded themselves for every positive step they took (whether or not it was accompanied by a weight loss) and refused to label a single episode of cheating as failure.

They recognized that the skills they were developing in their weight-loss effort were going to have to last a lifetime, because weight maintenance would be, for them, a matter of lifelong vigilance. "They were establishing new identities for themselves as thin people," says Dr. Johnson.

was going to a weight-loss support group," says Cassie Herold, who is in the process of shedding the 60 excess pounds she put on over the last eight years and one pregnancy. "The moderator asked everyone in the group to tell why they ate. As we went around the table people were saying they ate because they were stressed, because they were anxious, because they were depressed, because they were sad, and I realized *nobody* was saying they ate because they were *hungry*. We were all using food like a universal antidote to everything that was bothering us."

Dr. Nash calls this the law of the hammer.

"The law of the hammer means once we find a solution or coping mechanism, we use it on everything, even if it's not appropriate. We don't realize that we need different tools for different problems."

In fact, in a study by registered dietitian Susan Kayman, Dr. P.H., and her colleagues while at the University of California, Berkeley, women who were successful at keeping off the weight they lost were less likely to use food as an escape and more likely to meet their problems head-on. For example, they didn't eat when facing marital or family problems. They realized that a cookie would not care for their kid's problems nor would apple pie fix a broken marriage, so they looked for real solutions. "Regainers, on the other hand, thought they couldn't deal with problem situations so they went back to their old coping strategy—they eat to feel better," says Dr. Kayman, now a weight-maintenance specialist for Kaiser Permanente Medical Group.

WINNING AT LOSING

"The keystone of a successful weight-loss program has to be a real switch in the head in terms of self-definition," says Dr. Nash. "You need to stop struggling. It's not unlike the person who is struggling with a cigarette habit. As long as the cigarette smoker is saying to himself, 'Oh, I really want a cigarette,' that struggle becomes the focus of her life and sooner or later she is going to capitulate and have a cigarette. She has to throw a switch in her head that says,

'I am not a smoker.' Believing you are a smoker who is quitting is different from believing you are not a smoker. The same is true with the dieter. The dieter has to get beyond, 'I'm a dieter, I have a weight problem, I'm a chocoholic.' If that's how you feel, that's who you are. You need to throw that switch in your head that says, 'I don't struggle with chocolate anymore, because that's not who I am. I'm a person who eats healthy food in moderation.' "

In recent years researchers have learned a great deal about weight loss by looking at the lives and efforts of the "big losers." Out of that research come a few other tips that seem to spell success for millions of overweight people.

Exercise. It's the consistent factor in most studies of successful losers. In her study of dieters who kept their weight off for at least a year, Dr. Kolotkin found that almost all of them exercised. And they weren't training for the Ironman competition, either. "We were so relieved to see that they didn't knock themselves out seven days a week. They were only exercising three or four days a week and the typical person was walking. This is proof you don't need to make heroic changes, but consistent and moderate changes."

There has also been some scientific evidence that exercise can improve your mood, a boon to those who turn to food in times of upset and stress.

Keep a food diary. In Dr. Kolotkin's study and in others, including one done at the Kaiser Permanente Center for Health Research in Portland, Oregon, keeping a food diary was associated with permanent weight loss. By writing down all the food you eat and counting calories, you can easily adhere to your new sensible eating habits. Some experts recommend that you also chronicle your moods, which will help you identify what situations and feelings send you scurrying for jelly doughnuts or candy bars. You can also keep track of how often and how long you exercised. Many successful dieters say a food diary helps them feel in control of their eating.

Take your time. Give yourself a reasonable amount of time in which to lose the weight you want. You don't want to set yourself up for failure by expecting to lose 60 pounds in a few months. It will also help to not think of yourself as having to lose 60 pounds. Break your weight loss into smaller, more manageable bites, say a pound a week. You'll also give yourself time to get used to the new you. "Weight loss takes time," says Rosemary Johnson, Ph.D., assistant professor at the University of Southern Maine School of Nursing in Portland. "Someone who has had a lifetime battle with weight may have more emotional undergrowth to cut through than someone who put on weight more recently."

Develop new coping skills. Another thing time will give you is a chance to replace old bad habits with some new skills. You *know* chocolate doesn't really make everything all better. When you've finished that candy bar, the problem is still there. But you have it within your power to find what will make things better. Learning how to cope with your problems, whether it's managing stress or controlling your urge for a cookie, will give you a sense of self-mastery that chocolate never could.

Forgive, forget and fix it. You are bound to have a few slipups, a chocolate truffle here and there, a belt-busting meal once in a while. Remember, one slipup does not a failure make. "People who are successful at managing their weight are more flexible in their thinking and approach," says Dr. Nash. "They don't have that 'all or nothing' attitude. They can accept a little indiscretion tonight, knowing they're going to manage it by getting a little more exercise this evening or doing better tomorrow."

See also Dieting, Exercise

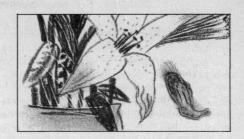

PELVIC INFLAMMATORY DISEASE

THE ONE PEOPLE AREN'T TALKING ABOUT

*F*act: More than half of all cases of pelvic inflammatory disease (PID) are caused by sexually transmitted disease. Did you know that?

If you're a white, middle-class woman with PID, your answer probably is no. Why? "Most likely because your doctor didn't want to bring it up in front of you," says Dr. Penny Hitchcock, an epidemiologist and program officer in the Sexually Transmitted Diseases Branch of the National Institute of Allergy and Infectious Diseases in Bethesda, Maryland. "And having a sexually transmitted disease still carries a stigma in our society."

Fact: About one million cases of PID occur yearly, 200,000 of them among teenagers. And each year, PID leaves as many as half of these women and girls infertile. Did you know that?

If not, you should. Because PID is a potentially devastating disease, both physically and emotionally. It is also almost always preventable.

PID is an inflammation of the reproductive system that begins as a bacterial infection in the vagina and cervix and travels to the uterus, fallopian tubes and ovaries. It's a serious infection, often requiring hospitalization and intravenous antibiotics. Symptoms can be severe, too—pain or cramps in the pelvic region, pain during urination, fever, nausea and abnormal discharge from the vagina are all common.

But for about half the infected women, PID doesn't cause any symptoms at all, or only minor ones, says Dr. Hitchcock. Such was the case with Annette Dwyer, a 33-year-old bank teller, who got the disease as a teenager as a result of a chlamydial infection, a common sexually transmitted disease "that was going around at the time."

"When I first got sick, my symptoms were bad—some cramping and discharge—but I didn't do anything about it for a month or so," she recalls. "Besides, I was kind of scared. But then the pain in my stomach got worse, and I thought maybe I had appendicitis."

Annette went to her doctor, who suspected PID. "When he told me what I had and explained how serious it was, I got really scared," she says. "I told the boy I was seeing because he had to get treated, too, for chlamydia. But I never told any of my friends and I didn't want my parents to know. I was too embarrassed." Unfortunately for Annette, the scar it left is permanent: She's infertile.

With PID, the emotional baggage is heavy. "In addition to having to deal with a sexually transmitted disease, you must be concerned with the most fundamental of feminine biological activities—the ability to bear children," Dr. Hitchcock says. "A woman may not even be aware that she has had a pelvic inflammatory disease in her youth until she finds herself unable to have children. It can be emotionally devastating."

PID AND THE IUD

A sexually transmitted disease may be the most common cause of PID, but it's not the *only* cause. An intrauterine device (IUD), a coil or object inserted through the cervix into the uterus for birth control, is also associated with PID.

The risk of developing PID is highest for the first three months after insertion, according to Dr. Hitchcock. During this time your body is making changes and adjustments to accommodate a foreign object. The process can create a change in the normal vaginal environment, leaving defenses down and your reproductive system open to infection. However, if the IUD is inserted properly and both partners are monogamous, the risk of PID with an IUD is no greater than without one.

Douching is also being investigated as another possible cause. In studies at the University of Washington and the University of California, San Francisco, researchers found that women who douched three or more times per month were at least three times more likely to have pelvic inflammatory disease than those who douched less than once per month. The doctors who conducted the study don't know for sure why douching may make you more susceptible to PID, but they have a couple of theories. One possible explanation is that douching may alter the vaginal environment to one less protective against germs that cause disease. They also suspect that douching could flush vaginal and cervical germs up into the uterine cavity, where they may cause inflammation and infection.

Also, germs that normally inhabit the vagina and organisms that enter the vagina through sloppy bathroom habits can invade the reproductive organs, says Dr. Hitchcock. Although doctors aren't sure how these germs enter these organs, they suspect that the normal defenses around the cervix break down and allow access to the uterus and fallopian tubes.

THE GIRL MOST LIKELY

Who's mostly likely to get PID? A sexually active young woman between 16 and 25 who has had multiple sexual partners, says Pamela Murray, M.D., director of adolescent medicine at Children's Hospital of Pittsburgh. This is partly because the reproductive organs of teenage girls are not completely mature, and once the cervix becomes infected, the infection is more likely to spread to the uterus and tubes. The more sex partners she has, the greater the risk of getting PID.

And she's most likely to get it again and again. One doctor told us that once a woman contracts PID, she is two to three times more likely to have a subsequent episode. Although the reasons for this are not clear, it could be that the initial infection destroys the cells lining the fallopian tubes, making them more susceptible to another infection.

But doctors do know that PID often causes permanent scarring in the fallopian tubes, a major cause of infertility and ectopic (tubal) pregnancy. In fact, says Dr. Murray, with each episode of PID, the chance of infertility increases. It's estimated that after one episode of PID, the risk of infertility is 11 percent. This increases to 20 percent after a second PID infection and climbs to about 50 percent after a third bout. A woman with PID also has a six- to tenfold risk of an ectopic pregnancy, a condition that can be life threatening to the mother and will result in the loss of the fetus.

BETTER SAFE THAN SORRY

As that old saw goes, "Forewarned is forearmed." And in the case of PID, it's about your best defense. In addition, consider these doctor-recommended precautions.

- Beware of the symptoms of sexually transmitted disease and PID, and go to your doctor if you suspect you have any. Don't delay. The longer you wait to get treated, the greater your chances of developing future complications, such as tubal scarring.
- Have as few sexual partners as possible, and use discretion in choosing them.
- Protect yourself against sexually transmitted disease by using a condom every time you have sex. Spermicidal foams and jellies, and diaphragms, probably offer some additional protection but are less reliable than condoms. They're best used along with condoms, not in place of them.
- Get treated for any sexually transmitted disease, and take all the medication prescribed, even if your symptoms disappear. Don't have sex until you are completely cured. Make sure all your sex partners get treated, too.
- If you use an IUD, get checkups regularly.
- If you're sexually active, have regular checkups.

See also Sexually Transmitted Diseases

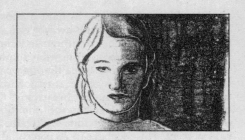

PHYSICAL ABUSE

FINDING A WAY OUT

*N*early ten years have passed, but she still relives the terror as if it were only yesterday. For three years, Elizabeth was married to a man who beat her, choked her senseless, forced her to take drugs and threatened to kill her. There were times she could hear their marriage vows ringing in her head—prophetically, she feared: 'til death do us part.

The violence was random. Rarely did she have any warning.

"I remember one Sunday before he went out he said, 'I love you more than anything else in the world.' The next time I saw him he pulled me off the sofa and throttled me until I passed out. When I came to, I was on the front lawn. I could have been dead."

At times he would throw her against the wall again and again until she couldn't get up any more. Once, he sat her on the couch and pointed his .357 magnum at her head, spun the chamber and fired, barely missing her. Another time, he dragged her to the cellar and forced her to watch him sharpen his ax.

But the worst part, she says, were the times when he "would make me get stoned and tear me apart verbally. I begged him, 'Please don't do this to me.' He took me apart verbally. He disassembled me and crushed everything there was."

She told no one what was happening. Her friends and family lived several states away. She was afraid they wouldn't believe her or would refuse to help her. She was afraid that they would confirm what she was beginning to believe, "that I am so horrible that anyone who is around me goes crazy and has to beat me." She didn't work, so she had no money to buy her way out. "When someone is holding a gun at you and says you're not getting a job, you don't get a job. I never had two cents in my wallet," she says.

So for three years Elizabeth was held captive by a terrorist who happened to be her husband. She was afraid to leave, afraid for her life. "I was frozen," she says, "like a deer caught in car headlights."

SCARED TO DEATH

In this country, a woman is beaten every 18 seconds. Every year, some three million women are smacked, hit, punched, kicked, stomped, scalded, burned, stabbed, shot, mutilated or sexually tortured by the men who say they love them. Four women a day are killed, many of them *after* they had left their abusers.

Experts agree that violence against women is a pervasive social problem. According to the Worldwatch Institute, a Washington-based research group, it is "the most pervasive yet least recognized human rights issue in the world." In 1989, Worldwatch found that in some Third World countries, up to 80 percent of women may be physically abused. In the United States, an estimated 16 percent of women are victims of violence by their mates.

The medical costs of abuse are astounding. Battered women are seen in emergency departments more frequently than patients with appendicitis. In one hospital, 70 percent of the victims of violence were battered women. In another, battering was the cause of half the injuries that brought women to the emergency room.

Many battered women suffer from a host of chronic psychological problems, including anxiety and depression.

In one study of 100 battered women, more than a third had tried to commit suicide.

Yet when battered women seek help from the usual sources—the police or medical personnel—they often meet with little sympathy. "She's the only crime victim in our society who is expected to disrupt her life and leave her home and abandon her possessions and perhaps her children in order to deal with the problem," says Cynthia Gillespie, a Seattle-based attorney and author of *Justifiable Homicide: Battered Women, Self-Defense and the Law*, a study of how the law treats women who kill their abusers.

"Many women come to the emergency room with bruises and fractures and lie about how they got their injuries," says Lila A. Wallis, M.D., clinical professor of medicine at Cornell University Medical College in New York City and past president of the American Medical Women's Association (AMWA). "The AMWA is now training women physicians to detect domestic violence despite a woman's denial or lack of history of abuse."

Very rarely are abused women even identified as victims of a crime. Although a number of studies have found a strong link between domestic disturbance calls to the police and homicide, sometimes the police won't even respond to a desperate call. One woman who called her local prosecutor's office for help was told by an assistant district attorney to "hire a hitman" to kill her abusive boyfriend. Instead, she killed him herself and, unlike most women who kill their abusers, was acquitted by a sympathetic jury.

A "PRIVATE PROBLEM"

Part of the problem, says Gillespie, is that in our society crime is defined as "something that happens to you at the hands of a stranger in a public place. What happens at home is something else. It's a problem, but it's a private problem. It's not the police's business, the public's business, the medical community's business—not anybody's business but your own."

In fact, Gillespie says, the law as well as the rest of

society does not view wife beating as a real crime. There is, unfortunately, a tacit belief that spouse abuse is justifiable.

"Traditionally, in our society it's been okay to hit your wife," says Deborah White, a social worker who has been involved for eight years in the domestic violence movement, first as a woman's advocate in a shelter and now as co-director of the National Coalition against Domestic Violence in Washington, D.C. "Some of our laws were founded on that notion. Combine that with the fact that when a woman did try to get some intervention she was basically told to go away and calm her nerves, and he was told to walk around the block and cool off. 'We know how these things happen with men.' These kinds of attitudes help support the whole idea that his behavior is somehow okay."

WHY DOESN'T SHE LEAVE?

There is also a wholesale lack of understanding of the dynamics of spouse abuse. Police and prosecutors complain that women, even when they do file charges, do not follow through. Judges and juries, friends and family struggle with the most perplexing question of all: Why doesn't she leave? Forensic psychologist Lenore E. Walker, Ed.D., author of *The Battered Woman Syndrome*, in her studies of hundreds of abused women, concluded that "doing anything other than leaving" will not end the violence. Yet she points out that many women find it difficult, often impossible, to extricate themselves from a relationship in which they may be physically, financially and psychologically prisoners.

Like Elizabeth, many battered women have been isolated by their spouses who, in an attempt to control them and make them more dependent, deprive them of family and friends or refuse to allow them to work. When they do work, they often must account for their time and mileage. In Dr. Walker's study, one woman, a doctor, was unavoidably delayed at work and was beaten so severely by her husband that she ended up losing a kidney.

When there are children involved, a financially dependent woman often must choose between staying and being beaten or escaping, leaving her children behind. In Dr. Walker's studies she found that more than half the batterers also physically abused their children. Few mothers will be willing to abandon their children to an uncertain fate at the hands of a violent father.

It's not uncommon for the abuser to threaten to take the children away. "He tells her, 'If you leave me, I'll go to court and prove you're a rotten mother,' and she believes him because he's been telling her she's a rotten mother all along," says Janice Rench, a national consultant on physical abuse and rape and former director of the Cleveland Rape Crisis Center in Ohio. "When you hear these tapes played in your head day after day, you begin to believe them. Your whole sense of self is twisted around."

Often, the law—and society—blames the battered woman for her own victimization, playing into the sense of responsibility women feel for keeping marriage and family together. "As women, we are conditioned to believe that we control our homes, our children, our husbands, and if we do everything right, then everybody around us will be happy," says Rench.

Her abuser often taps into that sense of responsibility that the woman may feel for her partner's well-being and the guilt she may experience because she feels she is to blame for the violence. She may try vainly to change herself, or him. Typically, an abuser is a man who holds traditional sex-role stereotypes and exhibits "macho" behaviors. He believes he is "the king of his castle" and his wife and children are subservient to him, says White. He may even quote Bible passages to prove he is justified in beating her. He will also try to justify his violent behavior by placing the blame on the woman.

LOOKING FOR DANGER SIGNALS

Even when they are being charming and loving in the early days of a relationship, many potential abusers give off clear signals what life could be like once the "honeymoon" wears off. If you're getting serious about a man, ask yourself these questions from the National Coalition against Domestic Violence.

- Did he grow up in an abusive family? Studies show that people who grow up in families where they have been abused or have witnessed abuse are more likely to grow up believing that violence is normal behavior.
- Does he use violence to solve problems? Does he get into fights, have a violent past or act tough? Does he overreact to little problems or punch walls when he's upset? Does he have a bad temper? Is he cruel to animals?
- Is he jealous or possessive of you? While it may seem flattering to have a man want to be with you all the time or know where you are, it may be a sign that he wants to control you.
- Does he hold traditional views of men and women? Does he believe a woman's place is in the home, serving her man? Does he think that women are second-rate?
- Does he have low self-esteem? Some men try to prove their masculinity by acting tough and macho to hide the fact that they are riddled with self-doubt.
- Is he moody, and do his moods rise and fall based on your behavior? For instance, does he get depressed if you have to go away and become affectionate and loving when you return? Can he be both extremely cruel and extremely kind?
- Does he abuse drugs or alcohol? There is a strong link between violence and substance abuse.
- Does he play with guns, knives or other weapons? Does he ever threaten to use them against people?
- Does he expect you to follow his orders or advice? Does he get angry when you don't, and are you afraid of him?
- Has he ever treated you roughly? Has he ever hit, pushed or kicked you? Has he ever used physical force to get you to do what he wants, even in play? If so, you are already being abused.
- Are you afraid of him? If you have already altered your life to avoid angering him, you are being abused and need to get help.

SUCH A NICE GUY

"He'll say, 'if you were a better person, if you were a better wife, if you were a better mother, I wouldn't have to do this to you,'" says Rench. "Often it's the psychological battering that puts her into a position of not being able to leave. Many women really come to believe that somehow they're just not being good enough, and if they were being good enough, he wouldn't have to do that."

Sometimes, the abusive spouse has a Jekyll and Hyde personality. He may be a pillar of the community and yet be uncontrollably violent at home, as in the case of John Fedders, former chief enforcement officer for the Securities and Exchange Commission who resigned his job when his wife of 17 years filed for divorce, citing years of physical and mental abuse. "The woman begins to think, well, maybe it is my fault, he doesn't act this way with anyone else," says White. "He's the head of our son's scout troop, goes to church every Sunday, and he's so well thought of at work, so it must be me."

Outsiders often overlook the fact that the battering partner wasn't always violent. Most of these relationships begin in "the tension-building phase," described by Dr. Walker in her cycle theory of violence. Although in most cases there are some clues to what is to come, the batterer is usually charming and attentive and often turns on the charm after a battering incident, apologizing, showing remorse, showering his partner with gifts and promises.

"That's the thing people find hard to understand, that batterers are often really nice guys," says Gillespie. "We have the tendency to think that they're slobbering beasts, ugly redneck caricatures, and they're not. They're often men who are charming. They're manipulators, controllers, who really need to have control over everything around them and the people in their lives. Often they're wonderful lovers and they're great dads, and when they're not angry and violent, they can be very loving. So women get jerked around in this up-and-down, on-and-off relationship."

IS IT MY FAULT?

Like many women, Elizabeth forgave her husband for his first violent episode. "He was more astonished and appalled than I was. He literally begged me to forgive him, out on the doorstep in tears in front of the neighbors." His remorse fed her hope that he would become his old self again or that she would be able to change him. What she did not do is get angry at him for his behavior. Although she was later able to associate his violence with drug use, during the brief respite in what was to become a cycle of abuse, Elizabeth found herself wondering, "What did I do to make him this way?"

"That is often the first reaction," says Gillespie. "Or they make excuses. This is a fluke. It happened because he lost his job, he had an argument with his boss. He's sorry. He says it won't happen again. The man loves me, I love him, we have children together, we have a happy marriage. Many battered women go through a long period of excusing violent behavior or accepting the guilt and blame, sometimes forever."

But what may be worse, when her repeated attempts to stop the abuse by being a "better" wife or mother, by arguing, pleading, even hiding or running away, all fail, as they usually do, she may begin to believe there *is* nothing she can do.

In fact, one study found that women who leave are at a 75 percent greater risk of being killed than those who stay. "Very often if a woman is faced with the choice of staying and being beaten and leaving and being killed, staying and being beaten is the more rational choice," says Gillespie.

For that same reason, battered women will not go to the police or tell the truth about their injuries in the doctor's office or emergency room. The woman who had been advised by the prosecutor to hire a hitman to kill her abusive boyfriend later told police she never filed charges against her boyfriend because she was afraid once he was free on bail he would come back and kill her. "It would have been like sticking a pin in an angry bee," she said.

THE GREAT ESCAPE

Despite the potential danger, the only effective way to break the cycle of abuse is to escape. "You're better off to leave, often the farther the better," says Gillespie.

Although there are not enough shelters for abused women, those that do exist can be very helpful in keeping a woman and her children safe. They're in undisclosed locations and some even have reciprocal agreements with other shelters to hide women and children in other states. Some shelters will help women develop job skills, find employment, a home and sometimes a new identity. Some provide day care. All provide understanding and sympathy.

Because leaving can put a woman and her children in peril, most experts advise planning in advance for a secret escape. "Start changing your life secretly," says Deborah White. "Save a few dollars out of your grocery fund, teach yourself a skill."

Elizabeth found a part-time job without telling her husband. "I saved every penny I made," she says, "and I moved out into a small apartment, got a full-time job and hired a lawyer. It was taking a chance and I was afraid, but I still had enough sanity left to know I couldn't stay."

Before you leave, you have to know where you are going. If friends, relatives or neighbors can't help you, or you are afraid of putting them in danger, check your phone book for the listing of your local shelter. Find out if they have room, and if necessary, have your name placed on a waiting list.

Meanwhile, to prepare for your escape and remain safe while you're still at home, here's what the experts suggest you should do.

- Rehearse your departure. Know exactly when and how you are going to leave—by cab, bus, train or car—and how you are going to get yourself and the children out of the house.
- Go to a class or support group while your husband is at work.
- Keep extra keys, copies of important papers, a list of phone numbers, some cash and a change of clothes

somewhere outside your house, ideally with a friend, family member or neighbor.

- If you have to leave in the middle of the night, find a safe place you can go: a motel, an all-night store or movie theater. Always back your car into the driveway or park in the street and keep the driver's door unlocked.
- Work out a signal system with a neighbor in case you need immediate help. "Tell them as soon as they hear a loud noise to call the police immediately," suggests White.
- Learn the signs of imminent violence. If you know he is more abusive when he is drinking, plan to be elsewhere when he comes in drunk. Don't tell him you are leaving. This may make him angrier. Slip away on an excuse ("I have to finish the laundry") or while he's still out.
- Avoid certain rooms in the house when he's violent, particularly the bathroom, which usually has only one door, and the kitchen, where he will have access to weapons.
- Hide household objects, such as knives and scissors, that can be used as weapons.
- If there are guns in the house, learn how to safely unload them. Store ammunition in another part of the house.

One of the most important things for your recovery is to get counseling. "You have taken tremendous blows, not only physically but to your sense of self-esteem, and you need to work with someone to discover why it is you were abused," says White. "Even when you get out of the relationship, you may leave thinking it was your fault. You need to learn that it's not."

CHAPTER 65

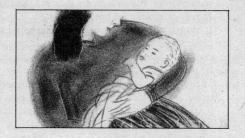

PREGNANCY

A NEW LIFE FOR EVERYONE

*T*here are few (if any) other times in a woman's life more intensely emotional than when she is pregnant. "An emotional roller coaster," it is frequently called in magazine articles and books on pregnancy, and in the sack of literature a woman receives at her first prenatal visit.

That barely does it justice.

Pregnancy, in psychological parlance, is a time of "crisis," an unfortunate word that suggests disaster but in meaning is closer to "upheaval." After all, pregnancy is a turning point in a woman's life, perhaps her only rite of passage in a society bereft of meaningful rituals for women.

The coming of a baby signals a new life for everyone. A woman who may have seen herself as daughter, wife, friend, coworker, boss, must now make room for a new identity: mother. And those around her are no longer who they were. Her partner becomes a father; her parents, grandparents; her siblings, aunts and uncles.

Her body changes, grows beautiful and ungainly, glowing and ponderous. These changes may damage or enhance her self-esteem, damage or enhance her sex life, but will almost certainly get her a seat on a crowded bus. As she becomes more and more preoccupied with her new role, ambition, drive, her career and even friendships are crowded out of her consciousness. Sad movies will make her sob. A so-so joke will make her laugh uproariously.

She struggles with conflicts over her abilities to mother and to rearrange her life to accommodate a child. She's troubled over mixed feelings toward a pregnancy that at first is nothing more than a missed period and perhaps a bout of what feels like a stomach flu but will end in a paroxysm of pain. Eventually, this gives way to overwhelming love for a child she can't see but who swells voluptuously and flutters gently under her heart.

There are times when her joys and fears seem to collide like atoms in a reactor. Her every fiber—physical and emotional—will be taxed by the nine months ahead. "This is an act of courage," writes Reva Rubin, one of the country's leading pregnancy researchers and theorists.

THE LOSS BEFORE THE REWARD

There's a tendency to blame this festival of emotions on the handy hormones that swell and surge during pregnancy. But most experts agree that hormones, while they can intensify feelings, can't produce them. A woman's pregnancy experience will be built on the foundation of her personal history. "We birth the way we live," says Christiane Northrup, M.D., a gynecologist at Women to Women in Yarmouth, Maine, who is also the co-president of the American Holistic Medical Association. "Check out how you are in a crisis and that's how you will be in your pregnancy."

Ask yourself how you've handled loss in the past. Although, as one expert points out, the root emotion of pregnancy is ecstasy, bearing a child triggers great ambivalence in many women because the joyous gains it represents are partnered with enormous losses.

"You're losing an identity, your freedom, and you're probably losing opportunities for career advancement at your prepregnancy pace," says Ellen McGrath, Ph.D., a mother of two who specializes in women's reproductive issues and is executive director of the Psychology Center in Laguna Beach, California. "You're making an active choice to go into role overload, especially if you work outside the home. You're definitely going to lose some of your female friendships in terms of quality and quantity because you don't have the time for them. There's also a lot of ambivalence about the physical vulnerability and jeopardy inherent in pregnancy and childbirth. How you've coped in the past with physical vulnerability, with being restricted in movement, is all going to come up again."

For some professional women who are having their first babies after a decade or more of career building, the time may be doubly difficult because they're so used to being in control. "Pregnancy is a primal experience and it's so physical; you're completely out of control in so many ways," says Dr. McGrath, herself a first-time mother at 40.

It's important to remember that all of these feelings, however troubling, are normal and human. Pregnancy is a time of enormous psychological growth—a shedding of one identity for another—and almost everyone experiences some anxiety around those periods in their lives. For most women, these feelings are productive. They are preparation for motherhood.

EMOTIONAL STAGES

For the most part, pregnancy is divided into three psychological stages that correspond to the medical trimesters. Almost every woman goes through one or many of the predictable emotional changes that will prepare her to be a mother.

If you are undergoing prenatal testing, your experiences may be slightly different. You may divide your pregnancy into three other distinct periods: before the test, waiting for the results and after the test. In the second trimester, while other women are falling in love with the child they feel moving within their womb, a woman waiting for the results of her amniocentesis may resist even thinking about her baby, to spare herself some grief if the test results are abnormal. If you develop a physical or emotional problem during pregnancy, you can usually expect your fears and anxieties to be intensified, and you may need professional help to ease your stress.

Although every pregnancy is different, researchers have cataloged some common emotions and physical sensations that you may feel during this special time in your life. Here's what they say you may experience during each stage of pregnancy.

FIRST TRIMESTER: A NEW AWARENESS

In its early stages, your pregnancy may be no more than a positive pregnancy test that may fill you simultaneously with delight and anxiety.

Gradually, you'll begin to notice some physical changes. You'll probably be unusually fatigued. "I was so tired in the early weeks of my pregnancy," says former publishing executive Lonnie Hagstrom-Benner, "I spent my lunch hours sacked out in the woman's restroom near my office. I fell sound asleep for half an hour, no matter how many times the door banged and the toilets flushed."

In the first trimester your breasts may swell and become tender. Although you haven't gained any weight, your waist may thicken and buttons may not meet buttonholes. You may become queasy or even vomit. Though it's called morning sickness, the nausea that sometimes accompanies pregnancy can hit anytime of the day or night. Your sense of taste and smell may change. You may find yourself craving foods you once disliked and spurning those you loved.

At this point, most researchers say, most women don't think of their unborn child as "real," which may be a psychological defense against miscarriage, which occurs more frequently in the first weeks of pregnancy. Studies of pregnancy stressors have found that one of the most intense fears a woman experiences in the first trimester is that her child will not be born normal and healthy, an anxiety that tends to resurface again nearer her due date. Some women may even wait until the first trimester is over before they announce their pregnancy because of this increased risk of

COPING TECHNIQUES THAT WORK

Experts say there are common fears and anxieties women go through during pregnancy. Here are the top six, along with the experts' advice on how to cope with them.

FEAR FOR YOUR CHILD'S WELL-BEING. Once your baby starts moving, you can keep a kick chart. Pick a time of the day you know your baby is awake and active and count the number of times it moves within a half-hour. If you haven't felt any fetal movement for 12 hours, contact your caregiver. But don't be alarmed. In one study, most of the women whose babies hadn't moved in 12 hours went on to have normal deliveries and healthy infants. If you are still worried, ask your caregiver to order an ultrasound—a harmless, non-invasive test that will allow you to see your baby in utero.

YOUR JOB. You may find you're less focused on your work during part of your pregnancy, especially if you're not feeling well. But studies have shown that most women can work throughout their pregnancies without their performance suffering. It will help if you use break times to eat nourishing food or to rest.

Certain jobs may make working until delivery difficult, however, especially those that call for a lot of standing, lifting or stair climbing. Discuss this with your caregiver. Also, find out from your employer if you may be exposed to toxic substances, such as lead, or to radiation. All hazardous substances must be labeled and employees are entitled to copies of Material Safety Data Sheets, which provide detailed information on exposure limits and special precautions. You may not be able to continue your job because of the increased risk to the fetus.

MORNING SICKNESS. Most women with morning sickness find it helps to eat small meals throughout the day, mainly carbohydrates. Some women eat several dry crackers upon waking since morning sickness seems to be worse on an empty stomach. Boston nurse-midwife Deborah Gowen says her patients get a great deal of relief by eating almonds.

STRESS. Get help. Depending on what is stressing you out, a cleaning service, an occasional babysitter, a psychologist or other pregnant women or mothers who offer a sympathetic shoulder can help. Studies have shown that the more support a woman has during pregnancy, the lower her anxiety levels. Look for help in unusual places. Your doctor's waiting room, your local breastfeeding support group, the prenatal exercise class at your local YMCA, YWCA or your PTA are all resources.

BEING A MOTHER. There are literally hundreds of books on the market that will help you develop your parenting skills. One recommendation: *A Good Enough Parent* by Bruno Bettleheim. The title alone should reassure you that there's no need for you to be the perfect mother. Good enough is good enough.

SEX. Some women find that their sex drive diminishes during pregnancy, although more women say theirs increases. If your lack of interest in sex is brought on by your fears of harming your unborn child, rest assured that there is no evidence that having sex is harmful to the fetus; and it may, in fact, increase your sense of well-being because you feel closer to your partner. Speak to your caregiver about alternate sexual positions and other forms of sexual expression. If you have a history of miscarriage or are having a problem pregnancy, ask your caregiver about your particular case.

miscarriage. This fear may also contribute to some women's preoccupation with death. Now keenly tuned-in to the entire cycle of life, you may find yourself feeling profoundly sad and weepy when you hear a story about a child being killed in an accident.

But in fact, in your first trimester you may be more preoccupied with yourself, your physical symptoms and what becoming a mother will mean to your life than you are with your baby. Some women get so sick in those early weeks that they find themselves wondering, "Is all this worth it?" Others find their physical symptoms comforting, even thrilling, since they serve as reassurance that the pregnancy is normal. And what if you don't have morning sickness? You may feel you're lucky, but don't be surprised if you feel anxious because you're deprived of this physical assurance that "everything is all right."

THE GREAT UNKNOWN

Faced with impending motherhood, some women even become panicky. They worry, "Can I do this?"

"When I found out I was pregnant, even though I desperately wanted a child, it scared the living daylights out of me," confesses Mimi Cohen, a medical technologist and mother of 2-year-old Amanda. "It was so irrevocable and I wasn't sure I had what it took to be a mom."

You may begin worrying about "the great unknown." How will a baby affect your life, your job, your marriage? How will it affect your sex life? And then there's childbirth. You may have already heard the horror stories, or, if you already have a child, have a horror story of your own you're not anxious to relive. Most experts believe that this early preoccupation with labor and delivery actually helps a woman prepare herself emotionally for the ordeal by letting her mentally rehearse it.

The most important date on your calendar will be your due date. You'll do all your scheduling around it. If it falls close to other anniversaries, you may see it as an omen, good or bad. Some women who have recently lost loved ones may think of the baby as a replacement. When high school art teacher Maria Bell found out she was pregnant, she realized she probably conceived a year to the day after her mother died. She doesn't believe it was a coincidence. "I think, somehow, I was trying to replace my mother," says Maria. "When we found out we were going to have a girl, my mother's family was beside themselves. They basically consider my daughter the reincarnation of my mother. I don't believe in reincarnation, but when I look at the baby, I think my mother's soul is in there, too."

As you face the future, you may find yourself becoming preoccupied with your past. Pregnancy tends to open a Pandora's box of memories, bad and good. You may find yourself reliving scenes from your childhood, reexperiencing both family conflicts and treasured moments. "Whatever unresolved issues you have are going to come up again," says Dr. McGrath. "Pregnancy brings you right back to past events. It's as though everything happened just yesterday. You can touch, feel and taste the whole thing just like you were there. You'll replay episodes of your childhood, paying special attention to how you related to your parents."

THOUGHTS OF MOM—
YOUR MOM

Facing parenthood yourself, you may turn to your first role models to help you develop your new mothering identity. Since you are literally following in your mother's footsteps, that relationship may be most important to you now. And depending on how it went, you may find yourself conflicted or comforted. Kathy Scott had barely emerged from a stormy adolescence, marked by raging battles with her mother, when she got pregnant. "I was so afraid I was going to be a mother like my mother was," says Kathy, the only child of older parents, who got pregnant at 20. "I remember writing in my baby diary, 'Am I going to turn into my mother? Please, God, don't let me turn into my mother.'"

Peggy Hathaway, on the other hand, had a storybook relationship with her mother. "She and I had this sort of mutual admiration society, and I identified very closely with her," she says. "When I got pregnant, I felt like I was fulfilling an unconscious need to be like her. It brought us even closer together."

SECOND TRIMESTER:
A NEW REALITY

If you had a bad relationship with your mother, you'll usually work through much of your anger and disappointment during the third to fifth months of pregnancy. You may find your other conflicts disappearing as you bring a new perspective to them. But if you find you aren't coping well, you may need short-term crisis counseling, says Deborah Gowen, a certified nurse-midwife with the Harvard Community Health Plan in Massachusetts and Boston's

Brigham and Women's Hospital. Studies have shown that stress in early pregnancy is one of the best predictors of pregnancy complications. Gowen and other childbirth experts also believe that stress, especially when it's brought on by unresolved issues in a woman's life, also can contribute to difficult or prolonged labors.

"Don't ignore these issues, because they're going to come up again," Gowen warns. "Pregnancy is the time when, if you face the unresolved conflicts from your past, you'll really be able to heal yourself."

THE CALM BEFORE THE STORM

For most women, the second trimester of pregnancy is a time of great joy and peace. Morning sickness is usually gone. Your body had adjusted to the flood of hormones. You can get back to life as you know it.

Two exciting events occur in the second trimester. You begin to show, which reveals your pregnancy to those around you. And you'll begin to feel the baby moving inside you. The experience is called quickening. Some women describe these first movements as a fluttering, like butterflies in the stomach. Others say it feels "like a muscle twitching." However it feels to you, this is the beginning of an intensely intimate relationship you will have with your baby, who is now very real to you. You'll be able to tell when he sleeps, when he hiccups, what foods he seems to like, even what side he likes to sleep on. In studies of couples' perceptions of their unborn babies, researchers found that parents, interpreting the child's movements in utero, gave it a personality: active, shy, happy, sweet.

A MEMBER OF THE CLUB

During the second trimester, you'll probably start wearing maternity clothes, again an outward sign of your condition that may affect the way others treat you. Studies have found that other people tend to want to help pregnant women. Friends and strangers will open doors for you, offer to carry your packages or give you their seats. You may also get

A WORD ABOUT STRETCH MARKS

Pregnancy, obesity and puberty are when they're most likely to appear, and until recently, you could be sure you'd have them for life. But now some doctors say that stretch marks—which settle in spots where the skin's collagen and elastic fibers have been pulled apart beyond their natural capacity—may fade with application of Retin-A, the same tretinoin cream used to treat wrinkles and acne.

Researchers say that Retin-A can help fade or completely eliminate stretch marks if used when the stretch marks are new. In other words, still pink and painful. Once they've turned white, the success rate plummets.

Retin-A works by boosting the movement of fibroblasts (cells that make collagen and elastic fibers) to the scar site. It can't be used during pregnancy, when stretch marks are most likely to appear, or during breastfeeding.

some unwanted advice and attention. "A complete stranger will go up to you when you're pregnant and pat you on the belly or tell you to wear a sweater," marvels Dr. Northrup. "You're seen as the divine baby carriage." You may want to rehearse a few polite ways to tell people you're not comfortable with their attention.

You'll find yourself treated especially well by other women. "What I see is that women in general want to be nice to other pregnant women," says Gowen.

At this stage, you may find yourself reaching out to other pregnant women and mothers, not only for their support but because you now feel like "a member of the club," an important sign that you're adjusting to the idea that you're about to become a mother, too.

FALLING IN LOVE

The pregnancy hormones that wreaked havoc with you in the first trimester may contribute to how good you look in the second trimester. Your skin may become clear and smooth. This is the time of the pregnancy "glow," which may draw you many compliments and make you feel that you're special. But, says Rubin in her book *Maternal Identity and the Maternal Experience*, that "glow" may be as much a result of your growing love for your baby as your hormones. "When a woman loves," writes Rubin, "her attractiveness is increased, there are social rewards and the love bond grows."

You may find yourself truly falling in love with your unborn child. You may have idyllic fantasies about your baby. Your love takes on a "romantic" quality that is fostered by your special relationship with this child whom only you can feel and with whom you alone can communicate. You may dream about your baby, look for clues to its sex ("It's so active it must be a boy"), talk to it, rest your hands on your growing abdomen and caress it.

FEARS AND DOUBTS

In your second trimester, you may very much want your husband to experience and accept the baby as well. You may draw his hand to your stomach to feel the baby kick. If he doesn't react the way you want him to, you may be upset.

"I was panicked because my husband wasn't 'into it' yet," recalls Maria Bell. "At this point, I was so excited about the baby and he was worried that his life was over. That would worry me and I remember getting very emotional sometimes and getting angry with him."

Although some studies have found that couples undergo more stress during pregnancy and that there may be more marital discord, many others reveal that a baby can draw a couple in a good marriage closer together. In one study, the researchers found that, although the couples they interviewed said they experienced more conflict during the pregnancy, they also felt more love for one another.

Some women worry about how their husbands will respond to their changing bodies. Most studies show that both women and men seem to adjust fairly well to the changes, although some women may have difficulty adjusting to their new shapes. Mimi Cohen was actually relieved when she began to look "really pregnant." "At four or five months people don't know you're pregnant to look at you," she says. "They think you're just pear-shaped, a particularly unattractive shape. I was less self-conscious when it became more obvious."

SEX IS FUN

There's more good news during the second trimester. Your sex life may return. Sex researchers Masters and Johnson found that 80 percent of women said there was a significant improvement in their sex lives over the first trimester and for some sex was even better than when they weren't pregnant. This may be due to the increased blood flow to the pelvic area and greater vaginal lubrication brought on by the pregnancy. But there may be psychological reasons as well.

"It was great," recalls Carol Tucker, a science writer and mother of two who says her pregnancy sex life was better than at any time in her marriage. "The best part was, you didn't have to worry about getting pregnant!"

THIRD TRIMESTER: SENSORY OVERLOAD

Suddenly the pregnant body that may have given you so much joy in the previous months becomes cumbersome. You'll describe yourself ruefully in terms of oversized things that bear life. You may think of yourself as "watermelon" or a "beached whale."

Your increasing size and the baby's position may make you very uncomfortable in the last months. The movements of the baby, once delightful, may be painful because of its size. You may have trouble catching your breath, getting up from an easy chair or picking your shoes up from the floor—if you can see them. You may suffer from heartburn and other assorted aches and pains. "Toward the end I had a pain in the pelvic area that felt exactly like I was wearing too-tight pants, although all I wore were dresses," recalls Becky Stern, a mother of two who writes fiction.

Emotionally, you may be on "sensory overload." Studies have shown that in the last months of pregnancy, some of the anxieties of the first trimester return with a vengeance. You may find yourself worrying about your health, your baby's health, the impending labor and delivery, your weight gain, your sagging breasts and stretch marks. You may begin to worry again about being a mother, something that was far off half a year before but now is imminent. You'll worry about how your other children are going to adjust to a new baby in the house. You'll also worry about how you are going to accomplish it all.

But at the same time, you have probably adjusted to the idea of motherhood and may go about gathering information that will help you allay some of your fears. Magazines, books, the other pregnant women in the doctor's waiting room are resources for you. You may keep yourself busy to avoid thinking about what's ahead.

But the last trimester isn't all worries and woe. You'll also be filled with great hope and anticipation. "All I could think about was getting my arms around this baby," remembers Lonnie Hagstrom-Benner. "In fact, there were many times that I was so anxious to get my hands on him, I forgot what it was going to take to get him out."

DREAMS OF CHILDBIRTH

As with motherhood, childbirth is never far from your mind. Studies have shown that the third trimester is a time when women have vivid dreams about being trapped or in great danger or of neglecting or forgetting a child. "With my second pregnancy, which coincided with the San Francisco earthquake, I would have these 'waking dreams' that came to me just before I would fall asleep," recalls Becky. "I would dream I was out shopping or at the bank with my 18-month-old and suddenly there would be an earthquake. A hole would open up and we would fall down into it. There I would be, with rubble on top of me, and I would suddenly go into labor. I had this dream many times, of falling into a hole and having my baby. I often wonder if it's the reason I named her Alice."

It's also possible to have pleasant "easy labor" dreams. One woman dreamed of going to the supermarket to get her baby and woke up thinking, "Wasn't that easy?"

Most experts believe the more negative dreams—nightmares, actually—may be a woman's way of preparing for the dangers and inevitability of childbirth and the responsibilities of motherhood. In fact, the entire uncomfortable experience of the last trimester may help you find it easier to face what's ahead. Jokes Lynda Rubin, an elementary school teacher with a 4-year-old daughter, "The way I look at it, the third trimester is just nature's way of making childbirth look good."

See also Prenatal Testing

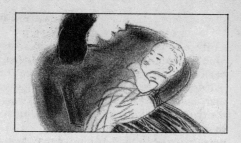

PREGNANCY AFTER 35

THE JOYS, THE RISKS, THE PITFALLS

When the nurse left the room, I sneaked a peek at my chart. There I found myself listed as an elderly primigravida. I was incensed. Since when is 36 elderly?
40-YEAR-OLD MOTHER OF A 4-YEAR-OLD

*L*onnie Hagstrom-Benner got married at 34 and got pregnant at 36. "This is the only time in my life I was ever really trendy," says the former publishing executive who had her son a month before her 37th birthday.

In fact, Lonnie is riding point on a trend that's expected to continue indefinitely: midlife childbearing. According to the National Center for Health Statistics, the number of first births to women between 30 and 39 has more than doubled during the last 15 years. During the same period, there has been a 50 percent increase in the number of women over 40 giving birth for the first time. Ten years ago, a woman's biological clock began chiming when she was 30. Today, it may first strike when she is in her midthirties or even early forties.

What's extended the baby deadline? For one thing, it's become safer to wait. Prenatal testing has made it possible for a woman of 40 to reduce her risk of bearing a child with a genetic abnormality to that of a woman in her twenties. Technology has also spawned a vast array of treatments for infertility, which tends to increase in women over 35. And the new field of maternal/fetal medicine has allowed women with chronic illnesses and those who develop health problems during their pregnancies to deliver normal, healthy babies and survive pregnancy themselves. Relatively safe forms of contraception and public role models such as Bette Midler and Glenn Close—both first-time mothers in their forties—have also contributed to this pervasive it's-never-too-late attitude. Today, many women believe that they can safely postpone childbearing until the "right" time, which for most has meant after they've finished their educations, established their careers and their bank accounts and entered into stable relationships.

The truth is that many women have not deliberately delayed childbearing. Midlife pregnancy may simply be the side effect of infertility, marrying later or marrying for a second time.

"I didn't consciously set out to put off having a baby," says Lonnie. "It just so happens that I didn't meet my husband until I was 33, after many years of unwed serial monogamy. I didn't want to get pregnant on my honeymoon. Bruce and I wanted a *little* time to ourselves before we had children. In retrospect, however, I can see it was the 'right' time for me. My career was in place, we were financially secure and I was emotionally stable, something I couldn't have said about myself as a 24-year-old. But it really wasn't a conscious decision of mine to wait to have children. It was the circumstances."

PRIME-TIME CHILDBEARING

Although, medically speaking, the best time for a woman to have a baby is between the ages of 20 and 24, many feel that is not their emotional "prime time." For some women (and men) who grew up in the 1950s and 1960s, their twenties were more part of a prolonged adolescence than the anteroom of adulthood. In terms of childbearing, this shifting of adulthood has meant that women are peaking emotionally a decade, sometimes longer, after they peak physically. But the fact is, the "elderly primigravida" ain't what she used to be. Even the term, used in the medical textbooks, is becoming passé. Today a woman of 35 who

CALCULATING THE RISKS

Pregnancy over 35 is certainly not without its risks, but they may not be as dramatic as you think, and in many cases they can be minimized. Here's what an older woman may be up against when trying for a first baby.

First, you may have trouble getting pregnant. It has been well-documented that fertility diminishes gradually after a woman reaches 35. "But the important factor here is that it diminishes *gradually*," says New York obstetrician/gynecologist Sally Faith Dorfman, M.D. "Barring a major adverse event such as premature menopause, it's not that you can conceive one day and can't conceive the next. So it may take you 6 to 12 months to conceive instead of 4."

But an even greater risk an older first-time mother faces is delivering a child with genetic abnormalities, particularly Down syndrome. Statistics show that a 40-year-old woman's chances of having a Down syndrome baby are nine times greater than that of a 30-year-old. "But," says Dr. Dorfman, "you've got to look at the numbers as well as the rate." A 40-year-old woman has *less than a 1 percent* chance of having a child with Down syndrome. Although the risks increase with age, a woman of 45 has only a 3 percent chance of having a Down syndrome child—or, to look at it another way, a 97 percent chance of having a healthy baby. "Of course, playing with those numbers has its limits," cautions Dr. Dorfman. "If it happens to you, it's 100 percent."

Women over 35 are more likely than younger women to have some health complications of pregnancy, particularly diabetes and high blood pressure, both problems that are more prevalent at older ages. About 6 percent of all women over 35 develop these complications, compared to 1.3 percent of younger women. Statistically, older women also have an increased risk of pregnancy complications, including placental failures and fetal distress, all of which can lead to more medical interventions and serious health consequences for both mother and child. There is also an increased risk of miscarriage. The evidence shows that older women may have more difficult or prolonged labors, a leading factor in the current epidemic of cesarean sections. However, Dr. Dorfman found in reviewing some studies of older women's labor that the average increase was only 45 minutes.

There's also a greater chance—simply because of "time

PREGNANCY AFTER 35   461

spent on this planet," as Dr. Dorfman puts it—that an older woman has been exposed to potentially harmful environmental toxins. A woman over 35 also runs a higher risk of problems associated with endometriosis and fibroid tumors, which can affect fertility and pregnancy.

But all of these risks can be minimized if an older woman, who is likely to have a very planned pregnancy, prepares herself physically to become pregnant. Prepregnancy care allows a woman to take care of herself in an *optimal* way before she is even pregnant. Fetal organs form in the first 12 weeks of pregnancy and are at their most vulnerable, say doctors, so if you're eating a healthful diet, avoiding cigarettes, alcohol, caffeine and drugs, taking vitamins and exercising *before* you become pregnant, you have an improved chance of having a healthy pregnancy and a healthy baby. But pregnancy is no time to *start* an exercise program, doctors warn. It's better to be physically fit before you become pregnant to help you handle the rigors ahead.

becomes pregnant is not automatically "high risk." That's one less anxiety to face.

In fact, if a woman over 35 is physically healthy and has not had a history of infertility, miscarriage or stillbirth, her chances of having a normal, healthy baby are not significantly different from that of a 20-year-old, according to a study of 3,917 women who had babies at Mount Sinai Hospital in New York City. The study, headed by Gertrud Berkowitz, Ph.D., contradicted previous studies that found older women were more likely to have premature or smaller babies and babies who were more likely to die or have health problems.

Having a clear understanding of the real risks you face as an older, first-time mother is the first step to reducing stress during pregnancy, which can lead to labor and delivery complications, says Christiane Northrup, M.D., a gynecologist at Women to Women in Yarmouth, Maine, and co-president of the American Holistic Medical Association. "The worst thing for you, if you are healthy, is to be called high-risk, because the language alone may affect you psychologically. Every emotion is accompanied by changes in the body's biochemistry. If you think of yourself as sick, you can make yourself sick."

Leslie Steele, a 38-year-old marketing executive who developed mild pregnancy-related high blood pressure in her second trimester, thinks that may have happened to her. "My obstetrician was one of those nervous nellies who basically treated my pregnancy as an illness," she says. "I was stressed out from the get-go. When my blood pressure began to inch up, he sent me to a maternal/fetal medicine specialist in the city near where I live. Every week I drove 30 miles to have my blood pressure checked, ultrasounds done, blood taken and urine tested, with the occasional really high-tech test thrown in. Now I know I had the best care available. I knew it was all in the best interest of my baby. But I swear that my blood pressure literally leaped every time I saw a white coat. I went from being nervous to being downright scared. I mean, why would they put me through all that if there weren't something drastically wrong with me?"

DOCTOR ANXIETY

If such meticulous care seems overzealous, if not alarming to the soon-to-be older mom, it's not perhaps to the obstetrician who, in his or her training, has come to consider the older first-time mother as a high-risk patient.

A number of studies have suggested that what one doctor calls the obstetrical "nerve" factor may be at least partly responsible for the significantly higher cesarean rate for women over 35. In some cases, C-section rates are three times higher for older women than for younger women.

"Generations of obstetricians have been taught that maternal age is a risk factor," explains obstetrician/gynecologist Sally Faith Dorfman, M.D., commissioner of health in Orange County, New York. "If a woman is in her forties and having her first child, at the first sign of any problem the obstetrician isn't just going to sit there. She's going to want to intervene. Unfortunately, the studies of older pregnant women have been pretty biased and skewed. Years ago, older women who were delivering generally had one of two situations: Either they had already had many kids so their bodies might have been worn out, or they had tried for the last 15 years to conceive and had had a series of miscarriages."

More recent research, such as the Mount Sinai study, has focused on the more demographically current older mother who is likely to be middle-class and well-educated, having a first, not a tenth, baby. When fertility factors are removed from the picture, the older woman and her younger sister aren't all that different.

And new obstetricians are being trained and medical textbooks are being rewritten, notes Dr. Dorfman. "I don't have the same kinds of prejudices as many other doctors," she explains. "I was born when my parents were 43."

GOOD TIMING

It's becoming abundantly clear that older motherhood has some distinct advantages. In fact, when Wellesley College researchers Pamela Daniels and Kathy Weingarten asked a group of parents who had had children in their twenties if they would make the same decision again, more than half said that, given a second chance, they would wait. When the same question was posed to a group of parents who had waited until their thirties or forties to start a family, almost all said they thought their timing had been just right.

Women who wait are, truly, as ready as they'll ever be to take on the challenging task of bearing and raising children. Research has shown that older mothers are less likely to be ambivalent and have fewer conflicts about their pregnancies. In fact, they're likely to regard pregnancy as a blessing, and not simply because they've beaten the fertility odds. With age and experience comes knowledge—of who you are and what you want.

"You're more in control, more at ease with yourself," says Corinne Nye, a professional photographer who married for the second time when her only child, a daughter, was 16 years old. "You have some idea what you're giving up and what's coming. When I got pregnant at 41, I not only considered myself lucky, but I knew unimaginable joy was about to hit. I knew having a child was a great responsibility. While it is sometimes difficult, it has brought more joy than I could have ever expected or hoped."

Pregnancy at midlife is usually the culmination of years of thoughtful consideration, the decision of two people of maturity and experience. Depending on the couple's age, it may be looked upon as a "last chance" and, therefore, as a precious gift.

"Research has shown that a child born to an older mother has a very special meaning for the mother, and older women are often less stressed and more open to and appreciative of the experience than younger mothers," says Ellen McGrath, Ph.D., executive director of the Psychology Center in Laguna Beach, California, who had the first of her two children when she was 40, the second at 43. "The child of the older mother comes into the world highly valued by a woman who is very clear on her values."

In a study done at Toronto General Hospital, comparing the feelings of older and younger first-time mothers, researchers found that the older women experienced less distress during their pregnancies than the younger women, despite the greater danger of having a child with genetic abnormalities and the perhaps more significant change a baby would mean in their lives. The researchers speculated that the older women, most of whom had married later in life, had, by virtue of their years, more opportunities to increase their feelings of self-esteem, confidence and independence, which contributed to their sense of well-being during pregnancy. Even though the women grew more depressed as labor approached, they were still less distressed than the younger women.

Also, the older woman, who has spent most of her adult life building her career, may see the pregnancy as a way to explore what is, for her, uncharted territory: her femininity. "I see a lot of women, particularly women in their thirties who have had successful careers, who want to affirm the parts of themselves that have been dormant, that weren't brought out by simply being a wife or being in business," says Dr. McGrath. "For these women, having a baby represents the epitome of femininity. They feel they've had to

THE SANDWICH GENERATION

Bonnie Kin's father is 72, terminally ill and living on the East Coast. But her daughter is 3, barely a preschooler and living on the West Coast.

Where is Bonnie? "I'm somewhere in the middle," replies the 45-year-old California State University psychologist. And she's only partly joking.

That's because, like a lot of women today, Bonnie Kin, Ph.D., is caught both geographically and emotionally between the needs of the generation ahead and the needs of the generation behind. It's a position that makes her a charter member of what demographers have dubbed the sandwich generation, the generation of women "sandwiched" between parent and child.

It's also a sociological phenomenon that is turning legions of women into wilted watercress, adds Dr. Kin. Created by the collision of three different cultural trends—parents living longer with chronic illnesses, women delaying marriage and women having children in their late thirties and early forties—the "sandwiching" of American women is rapidly turning what should be the most exhilarating and productive years of a woman's life into a time of exhausted servitude.

Women have traditionally nurtured family members who are either leaving the cradle or approaching the grave, explains Dr. Kin. But in our culture they generally haven't been expected to work from 9 to 5 and care for both ends of the generational spectrum at the same time. Especially not when both ends of that spectrum frequently live in two entirely different places.

Unfortunately, the demands on women in this position are frequently so ferocious that women are forced to put their own development—as professionals, as women, as creatures on this planet—on ice.

Some women think their lives are over when this happens, says Dr. Kin. But it simply means putting your personal growth on hold for a certain period of time. And it is intense. Most women come out of their holding pattern either completely crazy or so bursting with creative growth that they take off like a rocket.

How can you make sure the sandwich you're in becomes a launch pad and not a one-way ticket to the Far Side?

(continued on page 466)

Get clear. Clarify your priorities, emphasizes Dr. Kin. Know who you are and what you want. Know what you want for your kids, yourself and your parent.

Look at the long-range implications. If you decide to take Grandpa in, for example, that will take resources—both in terms of time and money—away from your children. How will that affect your children's emotional health? Or your ability to pay for college?

Recognize your own limitations. Despite advertisements that insist we can do anything as long as we've been energized by the right pair of pantyhose, we can't. Some of us lack patience, others lack time. Recognize your own limitations, says Dr. Kin. If you regularly exceed your limits, they'll eventually pop up later and drown you in guilt.

Talk about expectations. What do you expect of yourself as a daughter? What does your parent expect of you? What's a "good" daughter, anyway? Is a good daughter someone who invites an aging mother to come live with her? Is she someone who arranges for a neighbor to stop in and give her mother lunch? Is she someone who puts her mother in a nursing home? We all have different expectations of ourselves and one another, says Dr. Kin. The only way to really know what is best for everybody is to sit down and have an honest and open discussion.

Talk about money. It's probably easier to talk with your parent about death or sex than money, says Dr. Kin. But do it before you assume any responsibility for a parent's care. Your relationship is much more likely to remain intact if everyone knows where they stand.

Set limits. Decide what it is you can and cannot do for your family. Then stick to those limits—no matter what anybody else says.

Schedule family meetings. It's easy for siblings to forget that the parent who needs care belongs to them, too. Call a meeting, itemize all the caretaking tasks your parent requires— grocery shopping, rides to the doctor, laundry—and then calmly ask each sibling which task he or she would like to do.

Swap tips with other caring children. Groups such as Caring Children of Aging Parents are popping up all over the country, says Dr. Kin. They're a great way to meet others wrestling with some of the same problems, swap parent-care tips, discover new resources and vent the steam that "sandwiches" seem to absorb.

keep the masculine sides of themselves dominant for so long in order to survive, they hunger for that kind of balance."

Unlike a younger woman who, perhaps, has still not made her mark on the world, the older mother is less likely to look to her child to fulfill her. She is also less likely to feel "held back" by a child while she tries to go about her unfinished business. Most older first-time mothers have already taken care of business. "I remember my mother saying there were certain things she wanted to achieve in her life to prove she was as good as any man in her field, and she did, so she never had any resentment of children holding her back," says Dr. Dorfman.

THE DOWN SIDE

Older parenthood has its down side, of course. Older mothers may not "bounce back" from childbirth as quickly as younger women. "After Danny was born, I kept a list of at least a dozen things that were wrong with my body," laughs Corinne Nye, who discovered during her pregnancy that she had early degenerative arthritis in her spine. She did water exercises during her pregnancy and continues exercising, keeping her weight in check and getting chiropractic treatments regularly to keep her condition under control.

Like many older mothers, she finds she has less energy than she did as a young woman. She relies on exercise classes and biofeedback, which uses electronic sensors to detect changes in body temperature and muscle tension, to help her keep up with an active 3-year-old. "But I'm basically no good with Danny the three days a week that I work," she says. "I'm not up for anything physical with him. On those days, the most I can manage is reading to him. Fortunately, my husband is great with Danny and they throw each other around, so the balance is there."

Some older women may also find it difficult to adjust to a demanding infant after decades of only looking after their own wants and needs. The woman who is highly organized may be caught short when everything from pregnancy to childbirth to mothering doesn't go according to plan, as often happens.

There are some other sobering realities to midlife pregnancy. Although it has been stretched, there *is* a childbearing deadline. Older parents may be forced to limit their families to one, or to space their children more closely than they may want to. Some critics of older parenthood have pointed out there is often a tendency among late-in-life parents to indulge their children—the too-precious child syndrome—particularly if the child is an "only." But that is by no means a tendency restricted to any one age group.

And there's some arithmetic to consider. At 35 or 40, a woman may find herself in a dual role: new mother and caretaker of her own aged parents. Karen Hutchinson, who had her daughter, Jamie, when she was 39, was forced to quit her well-paying managerial job to take part-time work after her father was diagnosed with Alzheimer's disease. "I thought juggling a baby and work was hard," she says. "The stress grows exponentially when an ill parent is added to the equation."

And it's something for which Hutchinson's own daughter may need to prepare. When she is 35, her parents will be in their midseventies. She may be part of a generation—called the sandwich generation—burdened with the responsibility of caring for aging parents *before* they've had a chance to establish their own lives.

GRAY-HAIRED MAMAS

And what kind of role models will gray-haired parents make to teenagers? Because of the wide age gap between parent and child, the potential for a virtual generation chasm is there, something Corinne worried about "for a few minutes" before dismissing it.

"I may not be young in years but I'm young in spirit," says Corinne. "When I was a young mother, I remember thinking that all the other parents around me were old fuddy-duddies. When I look around me now, no matter how old they are, I think we're the same age."

In fact, while a younger mother may joke that "kids make you old," late-in-life mothers may find parenthood rejuvenating. Dr. Dorfman doesn't recall thinking of her mother as old. In fact, she says, she suspects many older parents find they're too busy to feel old.

"I remember asking my mother about menopause," says Dr. Dorfman. "She said, 'Hardly noticed it. I was too busy chasing young thoughts and challenges from a 9-year-old, getting her to ballet lessons and Girl Scouts.' Late parenthood keeps you young. It keeps you vibrant and tuned-in. I saw it myself. When my parents' contemporaries were talking about retirement and moving to Florida, my mother was still active in the PTA!"

See also Prenatal Testing

CHAPTER 67

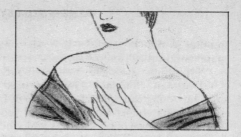

PREMENSTRUAL SYNDROME

A MYSTERY WITH TOO MANY CLUES

*A*t some point in her life, just about every woman has some unpleasant symptom associated with menstruation, from breast pain to the blues, from irritability to acne. Contrary to popular notions, very few women—10 percent or less—suffer from debilitating symptoms that cause them to lose work, alienate loved ones, or as one expert wryly put it, "try to stick their cats in the dryer."

Despite its near universality, little is known about premenstrual syndrome (PMS), the mysterious condition that strikes millions of women once a month, to varying degrees of misery, with one or more of the 150-plus reported symptoms. Although PMS has been suffered with, studied, diagnosed and occasionally used as a legal defense, doctors can't agree on the nature—or even the name—of the beast.

BAFFLING DOCTORS

Is PMS hormonal or psychosocial? There's very persuasive circumstantial evidence that PMS is hormonal, since it accompanies the swing of the female hormones, estrogen and progesterone, in the week preceding menstruation, and its monthly symptoms disappear at menopause. Researchers who have hospitalized women with severe PMS and measured their hormonal levels around the clock, however, have never found any significant alteration of normal circulating hormone levels. Early work by British physician Katharina Dalton pointed to progesterone as the antidote to PMS. Although some women suffering from PMS have reported relief from taking progesterone—even swear by it—so far, most studies have not found the hormone to be any better than a placebo in relieving PMS symptoms. In at least one small study, women suffering from severe PMS reported some relief using a common treatment for the symptoms of menopause—estrogen administered topically through skin patches.

Some of the latest evidence casts little light on the hormone controversy. In a study published in the *New England Journal of Medicine*, government researchers gave PMS sufferers a drug that would eliminate the hormonal changes that occur during the premenstrual (or luteal) phase. The PMS sufferers suffered anyway, leading the researchers to speculate the problem may be triggered by hormonal changes in *another* part of the cycle—or it may be an entirely different mood disorder that is synchronized with but not caused by the menstrual cycle.

Some researchers have investigated possible connections between PMS and a dysfunctional thyroid gland and between seasonal affective disorder, a disturbance of circadian rhythms that is treated with doses of bright, full-spectrum light. But so far, PMS is almost as mysterious as it was in 1931, when obstetrician/gynecologist Robert Frank, M.D., first coined the term to describe the cyclical psychological condition suffered by a number of his patients.

THE MIND CONNECTION

The theories on the psychological roots of PMS have come a long way since the prevailing thought was—and may still be, among some clinicians—that PMS sufferers were neurotic, mentally unstable, hysterical "typical females."

There is some evidence that PMS can be exacerbated by stress, which leads some researchers to speculate that the reason PMS seems to peak when a woman is in her thirties is because this time of life can be quite stressful, especially if a woman is juggling marriage, career and children. It also appears that existing emotional problems can be exacerbated by PMS, something one physician calls premenstrual magnification. A number of researchers have found that those suffering from the binge/purge eating disorder known as bulimia may increase their bingeing premenstrually and drug and alcohol abusers may also increase their intake right before their periods.

Psychiatrist Leslie Hartley Gise, M.D., director of the Premenstrual Syndromes Program at Mount Sinai Medical Center in New York City, says that evidence suggests that having a past or family history of mental disorder, mood instability, significant adjustment problems or substance abuse seems to predispose women to PMS. There are some researchers who even think PMS may be manic-depressive disorder.

As for its name, scientists also disagree. Should it be called premenstrual syndrome, premenstrual tension or premenstrual disorder? Since each woman may suffer from her own unique clutch of symptoms, which may change in severity each month and may have different origins, some researchers believe it is more technically correct to refer to it in the plural. The most cumbersome of its names is late luteal phase dysphoric disorder, which is how it is listed in the American Psychiatric Association's manual of psychiatric disorders, much to the dismay of feminists and others who fear that its ranking as a psychiatric illness may work against women.

FEELING GOOD AGAIN

With little scientific data behind them, those who treat PMS use an arsenal of largely unproven treatments, from diet and exercise to antidepressant drugs to hormones, based apparently on the philosophy that if it helps, do it. Unscientific though it may be, rarely does it do any harm, and often, it works. According to PMS expert Jean Endicott, Ph.D., of Columbia-Presbyterian Medical Center in New York City, "some people say you can't try to treat a disease without knowing its etiology. My response is that if all medical treatments had waited until people understood the etiology, there would be a lot more sick people out there."

In fact, although there are some women for whom only drug or hormone therapy brings relief, many PMS treatment programs focus on healthful changes in diet and exercise and stress reduction—modest, harmless alterations that most doctors can prescribe with confidence. "You can't get sick from going on a healthy diet," says Michelle Harrison, M.D., author of *Self-Help for Premenstrual Syndrome* and assistant professor of psychiatry at the University of Pittsburgh School of Medicine. When she began treating PMS patients several years ago, Dr. Harrison says, she brought to the practice a certain dubiousness about diet as therapy.

She changed her thinking when, on a hunch—based on the strong resemblance between PMS symptoms and those of low blood sugar (hypoglycemia)—she developed a modified hypoglycemic diet for her patients. The high-carbohydrate diet—full of whole grains, fruits and vegetables, potatoes and pasta—was low in fat and eliminated sugar, caffeine, alcohol and artificial sweeteners. She encouraged her patients to eat frequent small meals during the day.

"And it worked," she marvels. "I was astonished. I have a lot of high-tech education behind me and if anyone had ever told me that one day I would be telling women to cut out sugar and caffeine and eat complex carbohydrates to feel better I would have thought they were nuts. There are a lot of treatments for PMS that seem to work for a month or two, after which they don't work anymore. The diet doesn't always work, but when it does, it has lasting effects."

Other clinicians who use similar programs report similar results—never a complete cure, but a significant reduction in symptoms. Dr. Gise says lifestyle changes "make the difference between women having symptoms that interfere with their lives and women whose symptoms are short-lived and mild enough that they feel they can manage without medication."

THE MOOD-ALTERING DIET

Though there's no evidence that women with PMS are truly hypoglycemic, there is growing evidence that food may be

THE PMS DIET

If you suffer from premenstrual syndrome (PMS), following the high-carbohydrate, low-protein diet designed by Susan Lark, M.D., director of PMS Self-Help Center in Los Angeles, may help relieve the symptoms. In order to work, she says, you should follow the diet—which she calls The Women's Diet—all the time.

WHAT TO EAT: Complex carbohydrates—whole grains, breads, cereals, rice, potatoes, pasta, seasonal fruits and vegetables.

WHAT TO LIMIT: Protein.

WHAT TO AVOID: Sugar—candy, cookies, cakes, soft drinks and cereals; caffeine—coffee, tea and colas; fatty foods—chips, fried foods, chocolate; alcohol; salt (only if you are prone to fluid retention).

a large part of the answer to the PMS mystery. Strong links have been found between caffeine and PMS. And ironically, the typical premenstrual bingeing many women experience—and despise—provided one of the most important clues.

Massachusetts Institute of Technology researcher Judith Wurtman, Ph.D., who has done research on the appetite- and mood-altering effects of carbohydrates, wanted to find out if the foods PMS sufferers craved might be a form of self-medication, an attempt to readjust internal mood regulators. She invited 19 carefully selected PMS sufferers to live at her research lab for two days before their periods and two days postmenstrually so she could measure and monitor their food intake and compare it to nonPMS women. What she found was that PMS sufferers reached more often for carbohydrates premenstrually than they did when they were postmenstrual.

But do carbohydrates improve mood? To find out, Dr. Wurtman gave another group of premenstrual women—who had all taken psychological tests—a bowl of cornflakes in nondairy creamer. "It worked like Valium," says Dr. Wurtman. The women, who were glum and sluggish, suddenly became more alert and happier and less angry, irritable and depressed. When she gave them the same meal after their periods, their moods didn't change.

What makes complex carbohydrates an upper to PMS women? Research done by Dr. Wurtman and her husband, Richard Wurtman, M.D., has shown that carbohydrates raise the levels of a brain chemical called serotonin, which elevates mood and regulates sleep. It may be the only brain chemical so directly influenced by food. To be effective, however, the carbohydrate meal must be taken without protein, which is why Dr. Wurtman gave her study subjects cornflakes in nondairy creamer instead of the usual milk. "Protein interferes with serotonin synthesis," she says.

One antidepressant drug that affects serotonin—fluoxetine, marketed under the name Prozac—has also been shown to be effective in treating PMS in some women, though, unlike carbohydrates, it is expensive and has side effects. Be sure to use the smallest dose to minimize side effects.

KEEP MOVING

No one is sure why exercise helps PMS symptoms, but it does. "Women get angry when I tell them to exercise. They say they could have read *that* in a woman's magazine," says Dr. Gise. "But when they really make a commitment to a regular exercise program, they report feeling a lot better."

Why? Many experts suggest it's the increase in endorphins that accompanies vigorous exercise. "We know there is a release of endorphins, which are the body's natural opiates, so there's a sense of well-being that comes from exercise," says Stephanie DeGraff Bender, clinical psychology director of The PMS Clinic in Boulder, and author of *PMS: Questions & Answers.*

In one study, in fact, the researchers found that women's endorphin levels dropped during the premenstrual phase. Another study has hinted at a link between endorphin levels and fluid retention and breast tenderness.

BACK IN CONTROL

"A lot of taking care of PMS is taking care of ourselves, which a lot of us don't do," says Bender, who herself has suffered from PMS. "A 15-minute walk gives you a break and time to yourself in the fresh air. Your energy isn't being tapped in an emotional way. You're being revitalized. I don't know what I'd do without my morning run. I feel so good taking care of myself."

In fact, says Bender, doing just about anything to take care of PMS can have some positive effect because it gives a woman the sense that she can control what often seems like an unpredictable, uncontrollable condition.

"Women who have PMS frequently look at their bodies as having betrayed them. They've been told that it's part of being female, it's all in their heads, they have to learn how to live with it. Control is *the* issue with PMS. We've been told it's something we can expect and there's nothing we can do. But when you take that first step to gain control of it, you've turned the corner. If I had not gotten my PMS under control, I would not have been able to start a clinic. I would not have been able to write two books, I would not be able to do public speaking appearances."

HELP FOR SEVERE CASES

If your PMS interferes significantly with your life, your work and your relationships, you should get help. Ask your doctor to recommend a book or clinic that offers a variety of sensible treatments for PMS, since no one diet, drug or program works for everyone. Be wary of claims that your PMS can be "cured." The best programs can help relieve but not eliminate all your symptoms.

Good programs will start you off keeping a daily diary of your symptoms so you and the professional treating you can determine if you suffer from true PMS—which requires that your mood drop premenstrually and swing back up at or around the onset of menses—or if you have an underlying emotional or physical problem that worsens premenstrually. Treating an underlying problem through psychological therapy or with medication may by itself eliminate most of your PMS symptoms. Sometimes just keeping a diary can help a woman feel she's in control of her condition.

Says one woman who charts her periods religiously: "When I start to feel irritable, I just check the calendar. Once I know it's just my period coming, I tend to downplay whatever is bothering me. I avoid situations where I think I might lose control. I know it's not the time to have a serious discussion with my husband or the kids. I don't exactly hibernate, but I lay low for the duration."

FAMILIES SUFFER, TOO

If your PMS is severe, chances are you've noticed that it's affected your relationships with the important people in

---

THE TERRIBLE 20

Ninety percent of all women experience one or more of the 150-plus reported symptoms of PMS. Here are the top 20 on the list of monthly miseries and the percentage of women who get them.

70 to 90 Percent
- Anxiety
- Irritability
- Mood swings
- Tension

60 Percent
- Bloating
- Breast tenderness
- Fluid retention
- Weight gain

30 to 40 Percent
- Cravings for sweets
- Dizziness
- Fatigue
- Headache
- Increased appetite
- Palpitations

1 to 20 Percent
- Confusion
- Crying
- Depression
- Forgetfulness
- Insomnia
- Withdrawal

your life. "The number one problem that motivates women to seek help is that they're afraid of the emotional scars they're leaving on their children," says Bender.

Bender, who has two teenage sons, says she was always grateful that she was never a physical disciplinarian when she flew into one of her PMS rages. "But my tongue could do a lot of damage, too." She sought help when her children were young and involved them and her husband in the process. "My family really came together. It was my project, but it became a group project."

She recommends that you explain to your children that you are suffering from a physical problem that sometimes makes you upset, but that you are working on taking care of it. "Ask for their help," says Bender. "Who wouldn't want to help Mommy with her problem? You need to take them off the hook, assure them that they are not responsible."

Your husband needs to understand the same thing you do—that you are suffering from a medical problem that can be treated and controlled, not a peculiar mental aberration or a self-indulgent case of the blues.

It's also not a good idea to use PMS as an excuse for bad moods or to control those around you. "It's not okay every month to turn into a person who needs to be taken care of," says Bender. "If PMS is that significant, then it behooves the woman to do something about it."

See also Menstrual Problems

CHAPTER 68

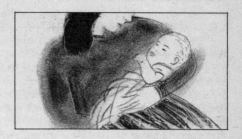

PRENATAL TESTING

PUTTING EMOTIONS ON HOLD

*H*er doctor suspected that the baby Gloria Higgs was carrying wasn't growing normally. "I was petrified," says Gloria, who was 36 at the time. "The diagnosis, fetal growth retardation, sounds so ominous."

Gloria's doctor sent her to a nearby university hospital, which had a maternal/fetal medicine department. There specialists performed an ultrasound. Using high-frequency sound waves, fetal ultrasonography produces an image of the fetus moving within the womb. In obstetrical care, it's used for everything from determining the age of the fetus to detecting structural abnormalities to guiding the needle during diagnostic uterine testing. "I was almost afraid to look at the screen," Gloria admits. "But when I did, I felt an indescribable joy wash over me. I could see my baby. He was moving his arms and legs the way I've seen babies do, trying to shake off their blankets. Up until that point, he had just been an idea to me. Now, he was a real baby."

For Gloria, the experience was glorious. Although the test revealed her baby was smaller than average, it was not considered alarmingly so. Doctors advised her to have repeat ultrasounds periodically during her pregnancy and she happily agreed. She started referring to her upcoming hospital appointments as "visiting the baby."

HEALTHFUL BENEFITS

Prenatal testing—usually accompanied by genetic counseling—has dramatically changed the experience of pregnancy for the thousands of women who undergo it every year. For some it relieves the anxious months of worrying, "Is my baby all right?" For others, like Gloria, it turns the idea of a baby into a real baby, sometimes hastening motherly feelings. For a few, it offers the grim choice: to terminate the pregnancy or prepare for a child with birth defects.

Today, doctors have a vast armament of genetic tests that can diagnose up to 250 diseases, most of which can't be treated or cured. Today, parents can learn if their child will be born with a cleft palate, be mentally retarded or be doomed to succumb to brain deterioration and death in middle age from Huntington's disease. For many parents, this opportunity to learn their child's fate—and their own—is both reassuring and anxiety provoking.

"It all sounds so simple," says Lonnie Hagstrom-Benner,

WHO SHOULD SEEK GENETIC COUNSELING?

Anyone who is concerned about the possibility of a birth defect, a genetic syndrome or a structural abnormality is a candidate for genetic counseling, says Ann Garber, Dr. P.H., genetic counselor at Cedars-Sinai Hospital in Los Angeles.

The majority of those seeking genetic counseling are women over 35 who are at a slightly higher risk of having a child with Down syndrome. But 35 isn't a magic number. It's simply the age at which the risks of bearing a defective child outweigh the risks of the tests, Dr. Garber points out. Anyone who is concerned about birth defects should see a genetic counselor. "If you're 32 and are anxious, if you have a friend who had a baby with Down syndrome at 26 and you're feeling concerned, then it's time to sit down with somebody who is going to be objective about it and go over with you exactly what the risks are and what the risks and limitations of the prenatal diagnostic tests are."

And there are statistics you need to know before you make what will be a very personal decision, based on your own circumstances. A woman who is finally pregnant after seven years of trying may decide that the small risk of miscarriage in amniocentesis is still too great a risk for her to take. Another woman, without a history of infertility, may perceive that same small risk of miscarriage quite acceptable when weighed against her chance of bearing a child with a birth defect.

Counseling is also recommended if either partner has or suspects a genetic disorder in the family. Certain ethnic groups—blacks, hispanics, Italians, Greeks, Asians and Eastern European Jews—are offered screening for genetic disorders that are more prevalent in their groups, such as sickle-cell anemia in blacks, Tay-Sachs disease in Jews and beta thalassemia in those of Mediterranean ancestry. Women who have had an infant death or one or more miscarriages as well as those who believe they may have been exposed to any substance known to cause birth defects should also be counseled.

Ideally, says Dr. Garber, those women who may be more likely to have a child with a genetic disorder for any reason should see a genetic counselor before becoming pregnant. "For certain disorders special family studies need to be done in order to complete a prenatal diagnosis. Sometimes these can take months to complete," she says.

A visit to a genetic counselor will not always be followed by a battery of tests. A counselor will go over a couple's family and obstetrical history and help them evaluate their chances of bearing a baby with a birth defect. In fact, studies have shown that encouraging genetic counseling prior to amniocentesis actually reduces the use of prenatal tests, specifically amniocentesis.

When she became pregnant, Louise Petrillo and her husband sought genetic counseling because Louise had an aunt with Down syndrome.

"The genetic counselor told us that our risks, based on a simple blood test and a family history, were only slightly higher than normal, so we stopped worrying about it at that point," says Louise, whose daughter was born healthy and normal. "We didn't feel the need to 'confirm' anything with further tests. When we walked out of her office, we already felt as though a great weight had been lifted from our shoulders."

who underwent genetic counseling and amniocentesis because of her age—36—when her son was born. "But you realize that this test is going to determine whether you're going to become a mother or not. I think I tried not to think about the baby too much until after the test results came back. I didn't want to give my heart away if it was just going to bring me grief."

Lonnie's experience isn't unique. Nor is Gloria's. A number of studies have shown that viewing the living, moving child on a monitor can hasten a woman's acceptance of her pregnancy as something real long before quickening, the second-trimester event when she feels the fluttery movements of the baby in her womb. Up until that point, as Gloria noted, the baby is just an idea, the cause of fatigue and nausea but not a physical presence. In this way, a woman gets a head start on her relationship with her child.

The sight of her baby—thrashing its arms and legs, sucking its thumb, somersaulting—can be so moving that, studies show, a woman who has an ultrasound is more likely to stick to a healthful diet and give up harmful habits such as smoking and drinking. In studies of women undergoing ultrasound for a high-risk pregnancy, the sight of their unborn child, moving and apparently normal, brought them enormous relief, even when they had to undergo other, more accurate, diagnostic tests such as amniocentesis. Some caregivers will order ultrasounds for women who may be overly anxious about a pregnancy with no sign of a problem, simply to reduce their stress. Ultrasound also provides fathers with a tangible baby to relate to since they're deprived of other physical sensations of pregnancy.

TOO WORRIED TO CARE

Amniocentesis and chorionic villus sampling (CVS) are the two diagnostic tests most women will have because they are used to diagnose chromosome abnormalities, such as Down syndrome, which are the most common birth defects. While such testing is usually reassuring to many women, this reassurance is undercut by the fear that the test results may reveal a serious genetic disorder. Studies have shown that women who are to undergo amniocentesis tend to pull back from bonding with their unborn babies and many don't even consider the pregnancy "real" until after the test results are in. Some may not even announce they are pregnant until after they learn of their prenatal test results, which, in the case of amniocentesis, may not be until 20 or more weeks into the pregnancy, after the woman may have already felt fetal movement.

The advantage of CVS, though it may be a slightly riskier procedure, is that it is done earlier in pregnancy, long before quickening. "Although genetic termination is never something anybody looks forward to, the longer a pregnancy progresses, the more difficult it seems to be for most couples," says Ann Garber, Dr.P.H., a reproductive geneticist at Cedars-Sinai Medical Center in Los Angeles. "To be able to get that information prior to feeling the fetus move, prior to having your body change dramatically, is really important for the would-be mother and father."

Researchers at Simon Fraser University in British Columbia found that women who underwent CVS testing had a briefer period of anxiety than women who had amniocentesis, presumably because they got their test results earlier. Significantly, the reason the researchers were interested in the stress levels of these women was because anxiety early in pregnancy is associated statistically with pregnancy complications. The CVS women's anxiety declined by the third month, but the women undergoing amniocentesis did not have their stress relieved until the fifth month, "precisely the period of highest risk," the researchers pointed out.

Even the most well-adjusted woman with finely honed coping skills may find the waiting period unbearable. Corinne Nye, who was 40 when she became pregnant with her second child, doesn't recall feeling anxious before she underwent amniocentesis. "But I know that I was," she says. "I know because after we got the test results, which were good, I got a three-day migraine."

The extent to which a woman can put her emotions on hold before prenatal tests may be limited. In a Swedish study, researchers found that, although women said they tried to distance themselves from their babies to spare themselves if they got bad news, it was clear that they could not.

One woman who claimed to have stopped thinking about her fetus confided to the researchers she had bought clothes for the baby but had hidden them. Another confessed that as much as she tried to fight her feelings for her child, she realized the baby "is in the back of my head all the time." In fact, the researchers said, "all the women displayed emotional engagement with the child-to-be through smiles, changes of voice and gestures, no matter how they reported withdrawing and dreaming."

The truth was, the women may have been even more focused on their unborn babies simply because the testing itself made the child "more alive" for them, the researchers said.

WHAT IF . . . ?

"Although I tried not to think of my baby, I knew in the end it was futile," says Lonnie Hagstrom-Benner, who had seen her child on ultrasound before undergoing early amniocentesis. "Once you find out you're pregnant, you begin thinking of yourself as somebody's mother, a somebody you can't see, feel, hear or touch but who is still vaguely real to you. Your life begins revolving around your due date, the time you expect to finally meet this little stranger. I know if I would have lost my baby, I would have been devastated. You can't steel yourself against loss. If you love someone, even if it's just the 'idea' of someone, you're going to grieve."

Most genetic counselors, while they don't provide therapy, can recommend support groups and therapists skilled in dealing either with pregnancy loss or birth defects. "For some who have already had an experience with a diagnosis of an abnormality, returning in a subsequent pregnancy to the same physical surroundings brings that difficult time right back home," says Dr. Garber. If you are unduly distressed, she says, it would be best to seek professional help, even if it's limited to helping you get through the few weeks you have to wait for test results.

PRENATAL TESTS: REASONS AND RISKS

Test	Detects	Timetable	Procedure	Accuracy	Risks
Traditional amniocentesis	Chromosome abnormalities, such as Down's syndrome, sex-chromosome abnormalities, neural tube defects, a large and growing number of single gene defects, such as spina bifida, baby's sex	16–18 weeks; results within 2–3 weeks	With ultrasound guidance, a needle is inserted abdominally into the womb to draw out amniotic fluid, which is tested for fetal cells, proteins and enzymes. Local anesthesia used.	Nearly 100% for chromosome defects; slightly less for other conditions	0.3%–0.5% for miscarriage. Because test results may follow quickening, waiting period, and decisions may be more emotionally charged. Termination procedure more complicated in second trimester.
Early amniocentesis	Same as traditional amniocentesis, except for neural tube defects, such as spina bifida	12–13 weeks; results within 2–3 weeks	Same as traditional amniocentesis	Same as traditional amniocentesis	About 0.5% for miscarriage

(continued on page 486)

PRENATAL TESTS (continued)

Test	Detects	Timetable	Procedure	Accuracy	Risks
Chorionic villus sampling (CVS)	Same as traditional amniocentesis, except for neural tube defects, such as spina bifida	8–12 weeks	Under ultrasound guidance, a small-volume catheter is inserted vaginally through the cervix or abdominally to the chorionic villi (preplacenta), which will become the placenta and is of the same genetic makeup as fetus	99%	0.5%–1% for miscarriage; some researchers claim 8%
Ultrasonography	Neural tube defects, such as spina bifida, structural abnormalities, heart defects, multiple pregnancies, fetal age and size, sometimes baby's sex	Anytime	Using high-frequency sound waves, fetus is viewed on monitor from within uterus	Varied; should be followed by other, more sensitive tests if abnormality is detected	None known

Maternal serum alpha-fetoprotein screening test (AFP)	Risk of neural tube defects, such as spina bifida, and risk of Down's syndrome	15–20 weeks	Simple blood test measures protein produced in fetal kidneys, which circulates in maternal blood	AFP is a screening, not a diagnostic test like amniocentesis. Over 40% of women with elevated AFP will have a normal child.	None for blood test; more emotional turmoil for parents because of false-positive results
Percutaneous umbilical blood sampling (PUBS)	Same as traditional amniocentesis, except for neural tube defects, such as spina bifida	Late pregnancy	With ultrasound guidance, a thin needle is inserted abdominally into the umbilical vein to draw out fetal blood. Local anesthesia used.	Nearly 100%; test is used for rapid confirmation of other ambiguous test results	2% for miscarriage; emotionally charged because test is done late in pregnancy to confirm earlier abnormal findings; test is still somewhat experimental

It's also important not to overestimate prenatal testing. "Even in the best circumstances, there is still a 3 to 4 percent chance of some kind of congenital problem, usually correctable," says Dr. Garber. "Sometimes testing can give parents a *false* sense of reassurance."

By accepting the notion that prenatal testing will "guarantee" her a perfect baby, a woman may also inadvertently invite more medical intervention, which itself can be anxiety provoking. All the poking and prodding, all the searching for something gone wrong, tends to equate pregnancy with illness. "It can lead to what I call medical terrorism," says Christiane Northrup, M.D., a gynecologist at Women to Women in Yarmouth, Maine, and the co-president of the American Holistic Medical Association. "A woman submits to all these tests and the testing itself leads her to fear that something is going to go wrong. We've come to think that with every test in the book and the best prenatal care possible, we can prevent every possibility of a poor outcome and we can't. We all need to understand that."

See also Pregnancy after 35

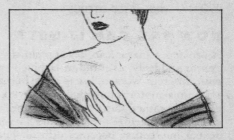

PROLAPSED UTERUS

HEALTH TURNED INSIDE OUT

*D*ebbie Barrone knew something was wrong as soon as she got out of bed and stood up. "It felt like something from inside me was hanging down in my vagina," says the 38-year-old housewife. "At first I thought it was a tumor that sprang up overnight. But on second thought I knew that was unlikely. Lifting anything—including my 4-year-old son—made it feel worse, like my insides were going to fall out and come crashing to the floor."

Debbie went to her gynecologist, who explained that the bulge in her vagina wasn't a tumor at all. It was her bladder being pushed down by her uterus, a condition known as a prolapsed uterus. "No wonder I had to urinate all the time," says Debbie.

"A prolapse is caused by a weakening of the supporting muscles and ligaments around the uterus, which makes it sag or slip down into the vagina, sometimes even reaching the vaginal opening," says Yvonne S. Thornton, M.D., associate professor of obstetrics and gynecology at Cornell University Medical College in New York City. "In some cases, bladder or bowel function can be affected, too.

"Having children through vaginal delivery is the most common cause of a prolapsed uterus. But the strain of simply carrying a child in the womb can cause it, too. Obesity and the chronic coughing common to cigarette smokers can also contribute to the problem."

HOW BAD CAN IT GET?

A prolapsed uterus can develop slowly over the years or appear suddenly, as it did in Debbie's case. "It's different with different women," says Dr. Thornton. "You can go from no symptoms to seeing your cervix through your vagina in a rather short period of time. At that point it's called a third-degree prolapse, and it's very uncomfortable. Sexual intercourse becomes difficult because the penis is constantly bumping up against the cervix."

On the other hand, you may be unaware of your prolapsed uterus even during intercourse or when inserting a tampon. Some women have lived with the condition for 30 years or more before requiring attention for their symptoms. It just depends on how much discomfort you care to live with, says Dr. Thornton.

Debbie says that her prolapsed uterus bothered her mostly at the time of menstruation or when she tried to lift anything heavier than a 5-pound sack of sugar. But there were occasions—especially when urinating—that she half expected to see something plop into the toilet. "It was *that* bad," she says.

EMBARRASSING MOMENTS

Some women endure the discomfort until the last possible moment because it's so difficult to go to the doctor to complain about "this 'thing' between their legs," says Dr. Thornton. She says a woman is more inclined to come forward if her doctor is a woman. "At first, women are reluctant to talk about it because they find it embarrassing," she says. "Of course I reassure them. After all, they're not responsible for their prolapse," she points out.

Depending on the severity of the prolapse, some women can't even walk freely or do any of the sports activities that they did before the prolapse. And sex can be a real problem. One woman admitted to Dr. Thornton that she has to push her uterus back up with her finger before she and her husband can make love. No wonder it causes a lot of emotional stress.

WHAT YOU CAN DO

"The first thing my doctor suggested to me was a hysterectomy," says Debbie. "But to her credit, she also suggested that I try doing Kegel exercises before making a final decision about surgery."

The fact is, about 16 percent of all hysterectomies (and 33 percent for women over age 55) are done for uterine prolapse. But unless you have a third-degree prolapse, there are other, less drastic options to consider—Kegels being tops on the list. (See "Training for Labor" on page 102 for directions on how to do Kegel exercises.)

"Kegel exercises help strengthen your pelvic floor muscles, but you must do about 200 of them a day to notice an improvement if you have a prolapse," stresses Dr. Thornton. Debbie says that she started doing the exercises as soon as her doctor recommended them. "I was motivated to keep my uterus," she admits. "I knew that a hysterectomy could mean weeks of recovery and besides, what if I wanted to have another child someday?"

After two months of doing 200 Kegels a day, Debbie says it made a tremendous difference. "I no longer could feel my uterus or bladder bulging out. In fact, they helped so much that I don't do them as conscientiously as I first did. When I realized I could cure my symptoms, I felt on top of the world," adds Debbie. "I felt powerful, in control of my body. And it validated my decision not to have a hysterectomy."

OTHER OPTIONS

Another nonsurgical option is a pessary—a ring-shaped device that fits around the cervix and props up the uterus. It's even effective for third-degree prolapses, says Dr. Thornton. But it's not without drawbacks. The pessary most commonly used today needs to be initially inserted by a doctor. It's deflated when you put it in, and then you inflate it to the point of comfort. It must be cleaned frequently and removed for intercourse. But if you're not sexually active or a good candidate for surgery, this could be right for you.

There's also a surgical alternative that's not a hysterectomy. It involves resuspending the uterus in the abdomen. This is major surgery usually requiring general anesthesia, but if you want to save your uterus for any reason, you may want to consider it.

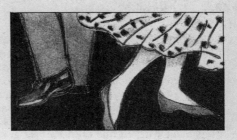

PSLQ

COMMITMENT WITHOUT MARRIAGE

*M*arriage is an institution, so the old joke goes, and who wants to be committed to an institution? Well, according to the U.S. Census, about 2.9 million of us don't. That's the number of couples the 1990 Census says are living together without officially tying the knot—PSLQs, as they're sometimes called, an acronym for Persons Sharing Living Quarters. And their numbers are on the rise. Back in 1980, there were only about 1.6 million unmarried couples cohabitating. By 1985, that number had risen to 2.0 million. Clearly, it's a relationship whose time has come.

Why? For one thing, living together is more socially acceptable. We have successful role models, most of them celebrities like the long and happily unmarried actors Kurt Russell and Goldie Hawn.

And, in many cases, it's a relationship that works. For some, living with a lover is a rehearsal for marriage, a temporary thing, a test. For others, it's an end in itself. Some women, particularly those who have been through an unhappy marriage (or two) or for whom procreation isn't an issue, do find unwedded bliss. Other women like the psychological independence of not being "tied" legally to another. For others, living together is simply a marriage without documentation, as strong and committed as any good marriage in which both partners feel responsible for one another.

But, like any relationship, it has its pitfalls, as Pamela Armstrong discovered. Pamela, who is a producer in Washington, D.C., and is herself the child of unmarried parents, once lived with a man who was divorced and had joint custody of his two young children. Because she was out of work at the time, she stayed home and cared for her lover's children and took care of the household chores. The arrangement worked fine until Pamela got sick.

"He was making $40,000 and I was staying home with his children. But when I got sick, I was expected to take care of my own medical bills because I wasn't covered on his medical insurance," Pamela says. "Not long afterward, I left. I realized I was giving a lot more than I was receiving. I had nothing legal on my side. I could not be on his insurance plan although I was performing the duties of wife and mother. I realized there's a reason marriage is an institution. It's an institution to protect women."

HIDDEN AGENDAS

There are other reasons why live-in relationships may not be right for you. For one thing, by their very nature live-in relationships imply lack of full commitment, says Iris Sanguiliano, Ph.D., a psychologist in private practice in New York City. There's a measure of uncertainty and insecurity about them that can sometimes be exciting and other times frightening. There's also the risk that a relationship that's not held together firmly can come apart.

"In working with couples I have found what I term a roommate syndrome, where the man and woman are leading almost parallel lives but are not truly intercoursing socially. They don't really feel responsible for each other. There is a lack of commitment in many areas," she says.

For those who are afraid to commit or to be close to another person, a live-in relationship can look like a good alternative to marriage—but it simply is a way to avoid dealing with those issues that stand in the way of real intimacy, she says.

Although there are certainly many people who live long, happy lives together unmarried, most experts see the ones for whom it all goes sour. Clinical psychologist Diana Kirschner, Ph.D., sees many women in her private practice in Gwynedd Valley, Pennsylvania, who are in live-in relationships. She says the great majority of them go into the relationship with a hidden agenda—hidden even from themselves. "No matter what they tell you, they often harbor a secret desire to be married," says Dr. Kirschner. "It's a fairly well-developed inner fantasy. Sometimes they barely know they're feeling it. They will actually repress it. I've seen women who thought of themselves as tough career women, vehemently denying these feelings. My clients say things like, 'I don't really care that we're just living together. I don't know why I cried at the wedding scene in the movie. It had nothing to do with me wanting to get married.' But, of course, it does."

Sometimes, she says, these women become involved with men who have been burned by a past marriage and aren't in the market for another one. "Often, he doesn't want to go through bringing up another family as he's still paying for the first one," she says.

If you harbor a secret desire for marriage and are involved with a man vehemently opposed to tying the knot, you're in the same position as the woman who goes into a relationship figuring she'll "change him." It rarely happens, warns Dr. Kirschner. Instead, you set yourself up for unhappiness.

"Over time it has a debilitating effect. You're hoping for a feast and you're starving to death," she says. "Not only that, but it can lower your self-esteem so much you feel like you don't even deserve to be fed."

MARRIAGE PHOBIA

Women who fall into half-a-loaf relationships out of fear—fear that this is "the best I can do" or fears of being intimate with another person—are also setting themselves up for failure.

Dr. Kirschner says she sees many women who fall in love with a man who is "not the marrying kind" and stick with him, unhappily, because their sense of self-worth is so damaged they think it's all they can hope for. "She may think to herself, 'I'm getting older living with him. I'm wasting time in this thing, I don't have any security.' And she begins to feel she's losing currency.

"Unfortunately, women are discriminated against in the marriage 'market.' We need to have youth and physical attractiveness to get a man, and the fact is that as you age, there are fewer and fewer men available. These women become unhappy but don't leave. They'd rather have something than be alone."

Some women enter into live-in relationships because *they're* afraid of marriage, says Dr. Sanguiliano. "All of us will equate marriage with the only marriage we've known intimately, our parents', which may have been bad. There's an inclination to feel, 'Well, I'm never going to do anything like that.' It's a social thing, too. When we look around us, we see that half the population is divorced or comes from a broken home. So it's not only our personal history. In society as a whole there's a sense of instability."

Some women are afraid that they'll be "swallowed up" by marriage, just as their mothers were, says Dr. Sanguiliano. Others may fear commitment or intimacy or simply want to circumvent the heartache of a marriage gone sour. Some women—and men—have what amounts to marriage phobia. "We live with many illusions and myths—one being that if you're not married, somehow you're free," says Dr. Sanguiliano. "That may be the reason some couples who marry after years of living together break up."

THE ULTIMATE TEST

How do you know if a live-in relationship is right for you? Dr. Kirschner gives her clients a revealing test. "I tell them to envision their ideal life five years from now," she explains. "When you do this, describe exactly what is happening, who you're living with, what his relationship is to you, what your house looks like, what it feels like, what it sounds like. Using those three sensory modalities, you can create a vision real to the mind. When you envision your ideal life, you will know if you want to be married to this man, whether you love him or even like him."

If you realize that your problem is lack of self-esteem, says Dr. Kirschner, do a little reality testing. "Get out, get active, flirt," she recommends. "What do you have to lose?"

If you're involved in a live-in relationship that seems more like a dead end to you yet you're too afraid to leave, it's important to keep up your activities outside the relationship. "Some women will give up everything for the relationship," says Dr. Kirschner. "Staying involved with life, your hobbies, your friends all tend to raise your self-esteem."

Take a look at your personal history. Do you tend to be impulsive? Are you afraid of getting too close to another person because you fear being hurt? Do you tend to pick partners who allow you to replay scenarios from your past in the hope that it will turn out differently? Do you think you can change this man if you live with him?

You need to be aware of your motives, say the experts. A successful live-in relationship, like marriage, requires love, honesty and commitment. Anything less really is just roommates.

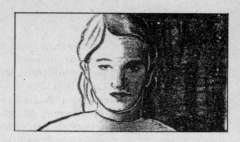

RAPE

LOOKING FOR SENSE IN A SENSELESS CRIME

Now women must worry about crowded offices, local restaurants and comfortable homes. For women, there is no longer any place that they can call secure.
UNITED STATES SENATE MAJORITY STAFF REPORT

Robin Warshaw was 20 years old when she learned that painful truth. While she was a college student in Philadelphia, Warshaw was held at knifepoint for hours and raped, not by a masked stranger in a darkened street, but by her ex-boyfriend in the apartment of a friend. But because he had been her boyfriend, because they had had sex before, it took her three years to call what happened rape.

"I was handicapped by the same kinds of things that young women are handicapped by today," says Warshaw, now 41, married and author of the Ms. Foundation's landmark book on date and acquaintance rape *I Never Called It Rape*. "At the time it happened to me, nobody was talking about acquaintance rape. I knew something cataclysmic had happened because of the threat, the fear I felt, but I focused more on fearing for my life."

THE SHOCKING STATISTICS

One in five women will be raped at some point in her life, according to one of the country's leading rape experts, Mary Koss, Ph.D., professor of psychiatry at the University of Arizona. Nearly 300 women are raped every day. In fact, rape in this country is epidemic. In 1990, according to a report by the U.S. Senate Judiciary Committee, more women were raped than in any year in United States history. The rape rate has increased four times faster than the overall crime rate in the last decade. "Today, as never before, women in the United States are forced to live in fear," the Senate report concluded. Knowing that one in five women will be raped at some point in her life, each woman must ask herself—every day of her life—"Will it be me?" and if so, "Will it happen today?"

In order to collect accurate figures, the committee, chaired by Senator Joseph Biden of Delaware, was forced to go beyond the usual police and FBI reports and contact rape crisis centers in over half the states in the country. The reason? Rape is one of the few crimes in which the victim risks being blamed for her own victimization. Many women, fearful of being held responsible for the rape or of having every aspect of their sex lives exposed and judged in open court, do not report the crime. Some do not even tell family or friends what has happened. Not surprisingly, rape is also the crime least often reported to the authorities. Only about 7 percent of all rapes are reported to the police.

Another reason rape is so underreported is that in most cases, the victim, like Robin Warshaw, knows her attacker. Because of that, she may not realize that what has happened to her is rape. Part of society's rape mythology is that the rapist is always a stranger and that what goes on between two people who know each other, even if force is involved, is seduction and sex. But, the experts point out, the truth is that *any* form of forced sex is rape, whether it is committed by a masked stranger who jumps out of the bushes or by your best friend's brother, accompanied by wine, flowers and music.

In fact, you are four times more likely to be raped by someone you know than by someone you don't know. "According to the myth, the rapist is an 'other,' " says Warshaw. "He's poor, black, Latino, anything other than what you are. But you are more likely to be raped by someone who is most like you are. This is not something people readily accept. You're cautious about parking lots and darkened streets. You don't expect to be attacked in your own living room or in a car by a guy you're out with for the first time."

PROTECT YOURSELF FROM RAPE

You avoid dark subway stations and alleys and cross the street when you see a suspicious stranger. But that's not enough. There are other high-risk settings and people you should avoid, warn experts who examine rape and its causes.

Many men give off danger signals that they are potentially date rapists. Be wary of men who don't view you as an equal or emotionally belittle you or women in general, men who are jealous or intimidating. "One of the things we know about the guys who do this is they see themselves as being more important than the woman they target, which is why so much acquaintance rape goes on in closed cultural systems like a college campus with its pecking order of status," says Robin Warshaw, rape victim and author of *I Never Called It Rape*.

When you are at a party or with a man you don't know well, stay sober. Stick with close friends or double-date. Pay your own way and, on a first date, take your own car.

Trust your feelings. If a man makes you feel uneasy, don't be so quick to dismiss your thoughts. Many of the rape victims Warshaw interviewed had put aside their misgivings. "We want to be nice—that's the watch-word of being a girl," she says. "We don't want to embarrass him or seem foolish ourselves. You're out with the guy because you initially found him attractive or nice. You think, he's cute, he went out with Rochelle or he's Brian's roommate. Many women are talked into irrevocable situations by not trusting their own reactions."

Read about rape. There are a number of things you should know to help you avoid becoming a victim. For example, many studies have shown that men and women have widely different interpretations of social interactions. What is rape to a woman may seem like a normal sexual encounter to a man who sees more sexual overtones in social situations than a woman does. Men are also socialized with a sense of entitlement that makes them believe—often unconsciously—that they are more important than women and do not have to listen to what a woman says, especially when what she's saying is no.

A particularly telling statistic: In a study of reported rape on 32 college campuses across the United States, by leading rape expert Mary Koss, Ph.D., of the University of Arizona, 84 percent of the men who committed what was by legal definition rape said what they did was *definitely* not rape.

RAMPANT SELF-BLAME

Many rape victims struggle for years with feelings of guilt and self-blame, which, psychologists say, can lengthen and increase the severity of their symptoms. Rape is a serious trauma with far-reaching consequences. According to one study, rape is second only to military combat in its impact on a person's life. Being raped is a risk factor for every serious mental illness except schizophrenia.

"After a rape a woman just rakes herself over the coals. What signals did she give? What did she communicate? Why did she decide to go to this bar or that place with that person? What did she do wrong?" says Dr. Koss.

Society at large—and often, the people around her—support her in the view that somehow she is the architect of her own suffering. "If only you hadn't worn that mini-skirt." "If only you hadn't gone to that party." "If only you hadn't gotten drunk." "If only you had fought back." These thinly veiled accusations mirror her own regrets and may keep her from seeking help.

She may bury her feelings—what psychologists call denial—but they rarely stay buried. Many go on to suffer from post-traumatic stress disorder, a diagnosis originally designed to describe the delayed psychological symptoms of Vietnam veterans. In fact, the largest group of sufferers are rape victims, says Dr. Koss. In one study, 94 percent suffered some of the symptoms of post-traumatic stress disorder within 12 days of the rape. Three months later, 47 percent were experiencing *all* of the symptoms.

FLASHBACKS AND NIGHTMARES

Like combat veterans, rape victims often reexperience their trauma through flashbacks, intrusive thoughts, nightmares and other images that may erupt years, even decades after the original event.

"If they're exposed to anything that reminds them of the trauma, they can become very anxious," says Constance V. Dancu, Ph.D., director of the Crime Victims Program at the Medical College of Pennsylvania in Philadelphia and co-investigator of a long-term government-funded study on the efficacy of treatment for women victims of crime.

"Walking in the mall and seeing someone who looks like their assailant can make them physically shaky and cause them to have flashbacks of the event. Some women try to avoid thoughts, activities or situations that remind them of the assault. To avoid feelings of anxiety and fear, they avoid going out. When they do venture out, they may become very upset by people walking behind them. They become hypervigilant, always scanning the environment, fearful, the thoughts going through their heads, 'He's going to hurt me,' 'I'm in danger,' 'I'm not safe.' "

Some women's current relationships may suffer. "They may suffer from sexual dysfunctions," says Dr. Dancu. "They may find it very difficult to have loving feelings. Just being hugged or touched by a male is upsetting, even a father or an uncle or significant other who they know is not going to hurt them."

WHAT IF IT HAPPENS TO YOU?

There's no guarantee that any of these techniques will work in all situations, and how you respond to a sexual attack is going to depend on a number of things, including how you appraise the potential threat of the situation. Remember, your first responsibility to yourself is to stay alive, even if it means being raped.

Stay calm and appraise your situation. If you yell, will

someone hear you? Is there a means of escape? Does your attacker have a weapon? How likely is he to hurt you if you act? You need to think and act quickly if you want to get away.

Run away. "This is the most effective defense," says Robin Warshaw, rape victim and author of *I Never Called It Rape.* Often, fleeing will take your attacker off guard, and if you are able to run to a public place where people are around, it may discourage him from following you. Yell, scream, wave your arms—don't be afraid of appearing ridiculous. You need to get attention.

Get angry. Studies have found that women who escape from threatening situations have a higher sense of anger, says Warshaw. "They're so angry they don't become debilitated by the fear of being killed."

Fight back. Although common wisdom has it that women who fight back will only be hurt worse or killed, recent studies cast doubt on this. Psychologist Sarah Ullman, Ph.D., then at Brandeis University in Massachusetts, analyzed a number of violent stranger rapes and found that "fighting back was related to fewer completed rapes and unrelated to physical injury that could result from the offender's physical violence." There is no guarantee that fighting back will always work.

"Every situation is different," says Dr. Ullman, a psychologist at the University of California, Los Angeles. "But my research shows that the more women don't resist, the more there will be completed rapes." Since it's unlikely that a woman will be able to overpower a man because of the difference in size and physical strength, Warshaw advises, "Fight dirty, but decisively. Your goal is to incapacitate him long enough for you to get away. Do not worry about hurting him."

Act crazy or vulgar. One woman Warshaw interviewed foiled a rape by feigning hysterics, which destroyed her attacker's fantasy of a seduction scene. In her book, which concerns acquaintance rather than stranger rapists, Warshaw recommends telling your attacker you have a sexually transmitted disease, have your period or are pregnant. "You might do physical things to turn him off: Urinate on the floor, pick your nose, belch, pass gas, even vomit," she suggests. Warshaw cautions that these methods should be used as a last resort.

Diane was assaulted by a teenage friend of her brother when she was 12. "He sneaked into my bedroom when I was sleeping and ripped off my panties," recalls Diane, now in her midthirties and the mother of two. "I was afraid to tell anyone because I was afraid they would ask me what I had done to encourage him." Her "crime," as she saw it, was that she was "more well-endowed than most 12-year-olds."

As a result of her rape, Diane has never felt comfortable around men. For many years, when she walked into a public place, she was sure everyone was staring at her. Once very slim, she has struggled with a chronic weight problem and with depression. But, for 15 years, she never associated her problems with her rape. Then, something—she's not sure what—triggered the memory. She began having nightmares and panic attacks. Unable to eat, she began losing weight and suffered from a host of physical symptoms, including colitis. She ended up in therapy, where she discussed her assault for the first time. But her greatest relief came when she learned that the boy who assaulted her had been killed.

NEVER THE SAME AGAIN

Ironically, self-blame is often a woman's attempt to regain her equilibrium after a rape, which can irrevocably change her view of herself as a good person and of the world as a safe place. "It's a form of pseudo-recovery," says Dr. Koss. "If you blame yourself, then you've at least got an explanation for why it happened. That gives you some sense of control. 'If I know why it happened, then there's something about my life that I can change so it won't happen again.' But it's all an illusion."

It's an illusion many people share, however, which is why rape victims may have difficulty getting the support they need from those around them, from the police to their loved ones. Many people prefer to believe that bad things only happen to bad people.

One reason rape is so traumatic, says Dr. Koss, is that "rape involves the violation of your most intimate private spaces. It's not only penetration of the personal space around your body, but it's penetration of the actual boundaries of your body. It's a loss of control over a part of your body that girls are raised from a very early age to feel they have a responsibility to protect. It is an experience that immediately makes women realize that something has happened to them that potentially affects their value in the eyes of other people."

Acquaintance rape adds another dimension to the psychological damage. "When it's someone we know, there is that terrible sense of violation of personal trust," says Dr. Koss.

GETTING HELP, GETTING BETTER

Rarely are women able to recover from so profound a trauma alone. Most experts agree that the best place to go for help is a rape crisis center.

"Adding to the trauma is the idea that what has been done to them has now made them mental patients," says Dr. Koss. "For that reason, a rape crisis center is a good place to go because it's not part of the formal mental health system."

Trained crisis workers, through their sympathy and understanding, can help a rape victim through the roller coaster of emotions that follows sexual assault. They can provide counseling and advocacy work for the victims. If the rape just happened, a volunteer often will accompany a woman to the hospital and stay with her through the examination, which for some women can be very difficult.

Many women need counseling after a sexual assault, says Dr. Koss, but not all counselors will be equally helpful. Because of the nature of psychological counseling, some professionals may unwittingly focus on the victim's perceived role in her own assault.

PLACING THE BLAME WHERE IT BELONGS

If you have been the victim of a sexual assault, one of the best things you can do for yourself, aside from seeking help, is to believe in yourself, say rape experts. "A terrible thing happened to you and *it was not your fault*," says Dr. Koss. "That seems like such a simple thought, but many women go for years and years not being able to believe that."

Even if you knew your assailant, even if you were dressed and acting provocatively, even if you were drunk or locked together in passion, even if you did not fight back, if at any moment you decided you did not want to have sex and said no and the man proceeded, what happened to you was rape. As a rape counselor told Robin Warshaw, "Bad judgment is not a rapable offense."

One of the rape myths that even women hold is that men, once sexually aroused, lose control of themselves, the thought behind the wry greeting card punch line, "When you unzip a man's pants his brains fall out."

For a study, Dr. Koss asked a group of men and women whether they believed there is a point after which men cannot control themselves sexually. "A number of women did believe that, whereas the men realized that, of course, that is not the case at all," she says. "If it *were* true that men are out of control, it seems to me we would have to establish procedures for the vice-president to take over for the president when he was sexually aroused."

Women are not, as Warshaw points out, "the gatekeepers of the furies of sex. It's not true that if a woman's guard slips, she deserves it. Men have to accept some responsibility. It was *his* decision to do what he did, clearly not yours."

LET YOURSELF OFF THE HOOK

Recognize blame—your own and others'—for what it is: unwarranted. As Warshaw points out, "As a society we don't blame the victims of most crimes. A mugging victim is not believed to 'deserve it' for wearing a watch or carrying a pocketbook on the street. Likewise, a company is not 'asking for it' when its profits are embezzled; a store owner is not to blame for handing over a cash drawer when threatened. These crimes occur because the perpetrator decides to commit them." Why, then, do we blame the victims of rape?

Talk about your experience to a trained counselor or to a close, supportive friend, or find a support group. Although it may seem painful at first, you will find it will help you come to grips with your experience and salvage your self-esteem. "A group of women who have had the same experiences as you can validate you and reinforce your worth as a person," says Dr. Koss.

Recognize that you are not the only woman this has happened to. "It's really, really helpful to understand how common this is," says Warshaw. "If it's happened to you, it's happened to thousands of other women like you."

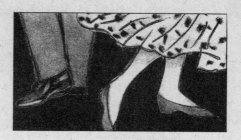

REMARRIAGE

WHEN HIS KIDS STEP INTO THE PICTURE

*G*etting married for the second time was so different than getting married the first time," says Jean Saunders, a 46-year-old teacher who remarried two years after her divorce. "I expected our married life to be smooth sailing, because we are so compatible. The fact is, we're still compatible, but it hasn't always been a piece of cake. That's because we had to contend with my two children, his two children, his ex-wife, my ex-husband. You get the picture.

"All in all, we've fared beautifully, probably because we love and support each other so much, no matter what problems are swirling around us. But I can certainly understand how second marriages, especially those with stepchildren, can fall apart."

And fall apart they do—in vast numbers. According to statistics, 50 percent of first marriages fail, approximately 80 percent of divorced people remarry, and about 60 percent of *those* marriages end in divorce.

"Most alarming, perhaps, is the fact that remarried couples give up on their marriages much sooner than first-time married couples," according to researchers Deena Mandell and Esther Birenzweig, who counsel families in Toronto. Indeed, divorce is 50 percent higher in the first five years of a second marriage than it is in a first marriage, suggesting that those first five years may be the critical phase of adjustment.

So if you're contemplating remarriage or have already taken the plunge, what can you do to make sure that your new relationship doesn't become a grim statistic?

A SECOND CHANCE

To begin with, you can be aware that if children are involved, you face a greater challenge, says Emily Visher, Ph.D., a clinical psychologist and family therapist from Lafayette, California.

Not that there aren't some concerns anyway. "If you've been through a messy divorce, for example, you may have a harder time trusting your new relationship," says Dr. Visher, who is cofounder, with her husband, John Visher, M.D., of the Stepfamily Association of America, located in Lincoln, Nebraska.

"You may wonder, 'If I failed in my first marriage, will I be able to make this one work?' I suggest that you view that first experience as a failure of the *marriage*," Dr. Visher points out, "rather than as an individual failure. After all, marriage is a relationship that two people build together. So it is the relationship that has failed. It helps, though, to try to figure out what didn't work in your first marriage so you don't repeat the same mistakes in your second one."

Your adjustment to a second marriage also depends very much on whether your first marriage ended in divorce or widowhood.

"If divorce ended it, you usually want the second marriage to be quite different," says Dr. Visher. "But if the marriage ended because of the death of a spouse, and it was a good relationship, then you usually want it to be the same. It should be noted, however, that nothing can ever be the same. It can certainly still be wonderful, but it will be different." Expecting it to be different and *allowing* it to be different can be helpful.

The social stigma often attached to second marriages varies along the same lines. One woman confided to Dr. Visher that she couldn't get over how different the reaction was following her second marriage (which took place following a divorce) and her third marriage (which took place after her second husband died).

"When she married her second husband, everyone was very chilly, wondering who is this person coming in here? No one seemed that thrilled for her," said Dr. Visher. "But now, since her second husband died, everyone is so happy that she's found husband number three. They've opened their arms to him and think he's so wonderful."

MULTIPLE MARRIAGES

Normally, however, if you marry and divorce more than twice, the social stigma increases. "People start to wonder what's wrong with you," says Dr. Visher. "In fact, multiple marriages may indicate that intimate relationships are difficult for you. Understanding why this is so can make intimacy more rewarding."

Studies on multiple marriage are scant, but one done at the Medical College of Georgia in Augusta may shed some light on the subject. Even though it was conducted using mostly men, it's interesting to note the researchers' conclusions. They suspect that people who divorce and remarry over and over again are more likely to be socially nonconforming and impulsive and need lots of stimulation.

People who are impulsive, for example, may have a shorter courtship, leading to a poor choice of spouse, with incompatibility and conflict more likely, they say. And those who need lots of stimulation may bore easily, leading in turn to less tolerance of routine. A certain amount of routine is helpful for maintaining a stable marriage.

FAMILY FUSION

Sixty percent of those who remarry are parents. And that means there are more than two people involved in establishing a new relationship. It's more complicated, and consequently, more can go wrong. The variations and permutations can seem endless, likewise the potential problems they elicit.

There are households in which the husband *or* the wife has children, ones in which both have children and a whole variety of possible custody arrangements, says Dr. Visher. In a sense, it's as though the kids have dual citizenship.

"Think about it. With two countries the money is different, the food is different, the customs are different and the language is different," she explains. "But what happens when the two countries are at war with one another? Then the person with dual citizenship has tremendous loyalty conflicts. That's what stepchildren must often confront and master."

In fact, Dr. Visher says that she herself had to learn all of this when she remarried many years ago. She and her husband each had four children from previous relationships. Since he's a psychiatrist and she's a psychologist, they thought that combining their two families would be a breeze. "But were we ever wrong," she says.

THE STAGES OF STEPPARENTING

Getting used to a whole new family is a transition that takes time, sometimes lots of time, and is often hampered by false expectations. The greatest myth of all is that everybody will love each other right away.

"That's just setting everyone up for a major disappointment," says Dr. Visher. "Adapting to a new family arrangement is a slow process, and there are emotional stages stepfamilies go through before adjustment and cooperation within the new family unit finally set in."

The typical period of adjustment, she says, goes something like this:

FANTASY STAGE. You think you're going to be the Brady Bunch, that everything is going to be so wonderful and easy. You're so happy, for instance, that your kids will have a new father figure and new siblings.

PSEUDO-ASSIMILATION STAGE. You try to make it the way you fantasized, but it isn't working out quite as you expected. Here's where fantasy hits reality.

AWARENESS STAGE. You know that something is wrong here and that some changes have to be made. You suddenly get tired of your stepdaughter sitting up front in the car next to her daddy, for example, instead of you sitting next to him. The tensions are mounting and someone usually explodes during this stage.

MOBILIZATION STAGE. At this middle stage, the family starts to unfreeze and talk about what they don't like. Expect a lot of arguments.

ACTION STAGE. The parents begin to form an executive team in the household, working together to figure out how to settle the complex needs of their new family.

CONTACT STAGE. You are finally getting a deepening of the stepparent/stepchild relationship.

RESOLUTION STAGE. Now you know each other well; new rules have been set and are being followed. You've become a solidified family.

Some families make it through the entire adjustment cycle within four years, says Dr. Visher. For others it takes five to seven years. And some never make it through, finding that divorce is their only option.

Jean Saunders made it, although it was hard at first for her to accept her husband's children. "My kids were teenagers and his were under 10 when we married," she remembers. "I hated the idea of having to deal with little children again, and his were so rambunctious. At first, I just tried to grin and bear their bad behavior, but eventually I was able to reprimand them myself, just like I would my own children. That was a milestone.

"It took five or six years to get really comfortable with his kids, to feel that special kinship. On the other hand, my children accepted their new stepfather with relative ease, and vice versa. There was a short period of time in the beginning when my kids worried that loving my new husband meant that they were being disloyal to their father. But we talked about it extensively, and eventually they understood that it was okay to love both."

MAKING IT WORK

There are a few things you can do to make sure that you and your new family successfully make it through that challenging adjustment cycle.

"Good relationships grow from positive shared memories, and feelings of belonging develop from familiar ways of doing things," says Dr. Visher. "The establishment of rituals and traditions is an important characteristic of successful stepfamilies."

Jean says that she used to moan to her new husband that they had no shared history. "I felt like I had amnesia," she recalls. "All my memories were current. There was no past to recall. But after a while we developed our own rituals. Each Christmas, for example, my husband and his children go to the same place to cut a tree. We've accumulated our own set of ornaments that have special meaning just for us. We can also all look back now and recall events that pleased or frightened us. I think that's part of what makes us feel like a family."

All the differences that each of you brings into a stepfamily situation have a positive side to them, says Dr. Visher. "Even the changes and the losses can offer an up side," she says. "I've had children tell me that learning to live and get along with the whole stepfamily scene has given them a sense of mastery. They feel that they can handle anything that life dishes out. They've learned to live with adversity, and thrive in spite of it."

One child told Dr. Visher that she considered herself lucky to be part of two households. "Now I have four adults who love me," she said.

MAKE TIME FOR THE TWO OF YOU

There's also the likelihood that you will not have to parent 24 hours a day, seven days a week—if the children spend time with their other parent. New couples are often left trying to have a honeymoon in the midst of a crowd, says Dr. Visher. It's important for them to plan for time alone to nourish their relationship. "In well-functioning stepfamilies, remarried parents realize that, while their children continue to need them, the children also need the sense of security that comes from a stable couple and the assurance that the stepfamily unit will continue. It also gives the children a model of a couple that can work together—lessons they'll appreciate later on in their lives."

You and your new husband need that special time for yourselves, too, she says. Don't feel guilty about making it; your brand-new marriage may depend on it.

CHAPTER 73

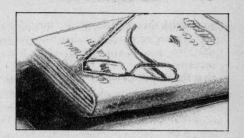

RETIREMENT PLANNING

THE BEST WAY TO BEAT THE BAG-LADY BLUES

Will you retire to a cabana on Sanibel Island or a tenement in New Jersey? Or, as some women fear, will you become a bag lady in Anywhere, U.S.A.?

"Most of the women who come to my seminars are afraid of exactly that," admits financial planner Judith Martindale, who hosts a radio talk show and a weekly TV segment on money issues in San Luis Obispo, California. "I hear it over and over again. Women come in and say, 'Oh, Judi, I don't want to end up a bag lady.' I even have one woman who puts extra clothes, blankets and bedding into a trunk, just in case. And this is a woman who owns her own business and does very well in this town."

DOES OLD EQUAL POOR?

Like Martindale, some psychologists also have detected a new anxiety among our aging population. Although not confined to one sex, it seems to plague many single, widowed or divorced women who, peering into their futures, see themselves alone, huddled next to the pile of their belongings on a steam grate.

"I'm a single woman and I'm self-employed and I know

when there is nobody else, it is really scary," says Martindale, who is divorced and has no children. "There was a time when I was panic-stricken that I would be a bag lady, too."

Her solution to calming her fears was to plan. She realized that the quality of her life after retirement was dependent on her health and how much money she had. So she takes care of herself and her finances, good advice for all women who face a number of grim financial realities particular to their sex.

Consider these facts.

- Most married women will face old age as widows.
- The median income of women over 60 is $6,300.
- Most women earn less than men, so they have less available for retirement funding. Retired women also receive substantially less from Social Security than men.
- Women who take time out to care for their families, work part-time or not at all or start careers after their children have grown have less income to put aside for their old age. Plus, at retirement they also find themselves hit with the "motherhood penalty": a lower Social Security payment because of less time spent and less money made in the work force.
- Wives who don't work receive at age 65 only 50 percent of what their husbands earn in Social Security.
- Although the average age at which a woman is widowed in the United States is 56, women aren't eligible for Social Security widow's benefits until they are 60.
- Women tend to live longer and suffer from chronic illness more than men, so unless a woman plans well for her later years, she may well outlive her retirement nest egg.

PLANNING AHEAD

Like Martindale, Lynn Scherzer is planning for her retirement. She and her husband, Jack, have a very clear vision of what it will be like. Lynn, who is self-employed, and Jack, a tenured university professor, who are both nearing

50, are able to take Thursdays off to spend time together, shopping, cooking, walking and taking horseback riding lessons. "When we think about retirement, we think we'll be living the way we do on Thursday every day of the year," says Lynn. "I'm looking forward to doing the things I enjoy in my old age. And I don't want to spend the next few years worrying about what's going to happen to us. So we're planning for it not only financially but healthwise, too."

Both Lynn and Jack are vested in pension programs. One of their priorities is to put the maximum allowable amount in Individual Retirement Accounts every year, even when there are other bills clamoring to be paid. They take good advantage of Jack's medical benefits, which cover yearly physicals for both of them, and bought a home gym, where they both work out three times a week.

"This is very important to us," says Lynn. "We don't want to be destitute and we want to spend our retirement years traveling to interesting places, not doctor's offices."

In fact, financial planners and psychologists agree the time to lay the foundation for your retirement is now, no matter what your age.

If, like Lynn, you know how you want to spend your golden years, you'll be best able to plan for them psychologically and financially. If, for example, your plan is to use your leisure time to see America from a mobile home, Martindale points out, you'll need to set up a savings plan to finance your travel—which might get pretty pricey. If, on the other hand, you see yourself spending your later years doing volunteer work, your financial needs—and thus your savings plan—might be more modest.

Decide how long you want to work—or, in the case of many women, *have* to work. A woman who enjoys her work, the financial independence it gives her and the camaraderie of the workplace may want to stay a "working girl" past traditional retirement age. Others, who got a late start in the job market or who have little savings, may *need* to work longer to support themselves.

And, if you're married, you and your spouse should talk

WHAT IF . . . ? COUNT ON IT!

Married women need to consider the very real possibility that they will spend their retirement years alone. "You need to get comfortable with the idea that you might be living single," says California financial planner Judith Martindale. "About 41 percent of all women who retire are not married."

But it doesn't have to be a scary thought, says Martindale. In fact, she says, you can plan now by developing in yourself the skills you need to survive alone. Among her suggestions:

- Identify three situations in your life where you faced adversity and survived.
- Imagine yourself in a negative situation and then see yourself resolving the problem.
- Learn to be flexible. Perhaps the simplest way to do that, she says, is to identify one of your daily routines and vary it. "Get out of your bed on a different side in the morning," she says.
- Learn to be assertive and independent. If you don't know how to go about it, says Martindale, ask someone you know whose independence you admire how he or she does it.
- Make friends. Your best hedge against loneliness is to have people in your life you care about and who care about you. Because old age is a time when we often lose the friends of a lifetime, you need to be skilled at making new friends, says Martindale. "I think this is where our cultural bias toward being nurturers is really good for us," she says. "We know how to relate to other people. But we often get busy and lose track of our friendships, so we have to remember to nurture them."

about your vision of the future. If you're planning to spend it together, you need to agree on your itinerary.

"You need to know what you want and you have to know what the other person wants," Martindale says. "I've come to the conclusion that more people live by default than by choice. Only about 3 percent of our population sets goals. If you're not setting goals, you're living by default."

HAVE A PLAN B

In looking for a retirement plan, take into consideration the fact that we do not always live happily ever after. There's a very good chance that at some time during your golden years, you may become disabled, says Dorothy Litwin, Ph.D., a psychologist in private practice in New York City and suburban Larchmont who works with older women in psychotherapy.

"When you reach your fifties, that's the transition period. Things start changing. Fatigue sets in. You can't do what you once were able to do. Good things happen, too. You're more secure financially during that decade. That's when people should really start thinking about what they are going to do when they get older and possibly more disabled."

Check your health coverage—private plans and Medicare—to make sure you'll have enough to cover the medical bills that mount when you have a chronic illness. Statistically speaking, women have more chronic illnesses than men, so their health care needs will be different. Chronic illnesses can require long-term nursing care that may not be covered by Medicare or private plans.

If you got a later start in the workplace, make sure you find out from the Social Security Administration if you qualify for Social Security when you retire. Nearly twice as many women receive payments as wives of workers than as workers themselves. Remember that a dependent wife is entitled to only half of what her husband earns in Social Security. "If this is her only source of income, she will face severe financial constraint," warns Martindale. You may be better off claiming retirement benefits under your own account—but you have to have one first.

KNOW YOURSELF

Retirement can put a great deal of psychological strain on a woman and, if she is married, her marital relationship. Some introspection now can ward off problems, says Dr. Litwin.

For example, ask yourself how you're going to cope when you have—as one wag put it—"half as much money and twice as much husband." A staple of newspaper advice columns are letters from wives whose retired husbands are annoyingly underfoot—offering cost-saving suggestions at the supermarket and work-saving suggestions at home. "When he retires, a husband loses his social contacts and may become more dependent on his wife," says Dr. Litwin. "He loses his power base, so his wife can become his audience."

And ask yourself if you're going to be ready to retire when your husband does. Some women, who've gotten a late start at a career, aren't ready to put their feet up when he's 65 and she's only 60. "In some cases when the husband is ready to retire, the woman is still going gung-ho at her job," says Dr. Litwin. "Women's life expectancy is longer, so she might not be ready to retire even at 65."

GET A LIFE

Unless you have interests beyond your job, your spouse and your family, your retirement years can loom before you like a vacuum rather than as time you fill with joy and fun.

"The more interests you have, the better off you are," says Dr. Litwin. "The people who look forward to their retirement see it as the leisure time they've always wanted so they can indulge their hobbies."

Consider this part of your plan B when, for some reason, plan A doesn't work out. Dr. Litwin says she has seen the difference outside interests can make in an older woman's life. "I had a patient who was divorced in her seventies. Her husband was her job. She planned her whole day around him. He was the organizing principle of her life. But she eventually did okay because she had a skill she could fall back on, and her loss then was not so devastating. In contrast, I saw a woman who was in her seventies when her husband died. She was a very dependent person her entire life, in growing up as well as in her two marriages. Without an occupation, she's terribly depressed because of her loss. She doesn't seem to have the resources the other woman has."

HEALTH—FIRST AND FOREMOST

Taking care of your health is one of the best investments you can make in your future. Like a nest egg, good health will keep you independent longer.

Although she's a financial planner, not a gerontologist, Judith Martindale heartily seconds doctors' recommendations for preventive health care. She tells her clients to start and keep up with an exercise program, which will improve their health and mobility, to take an interest in and improve their diets and to have yearly checkups. She warns women in particular to pay attention to their calcium intake, to avoid osteoporosis and to do regular breast self-exams and have mammograms for early detection of breast cancer.

LEARN TO SAVE

Martindale tells her clients to calculate their net worth to give them a clearer idea of their current financial picture. Many women quake at the thought, she says, in part because they think what they're going to find out will be a blow to their self-esteem, not to mention their sense of financial security. "Many joke that they don't own enough to even bother. But they often find that they have more than they think they do," says Martindale.

Also, she says, women—especially married women—tend to be a little intimidated by finances, which they feel they lack the expertise to understand. "Even if a wife does the day-to-day bills and really feels she's involved in the family finances, her husband still traditionally makes the decisions on the investments they make," Martindale says. "She has the illusion that she is managing the money, when the real money management comes from long-term planning."

Martindale also asks women to examine their attitudes toward money in part to determine if they have any psychological stumbling blocks to starting a savings plan. To explore their feelings and thoughts about money, she asks them to complete sentences that begin, "Money to me means . . ." or "At the thought of being responsible for my own financial future, I . . ."

She also requires them to examine their spending habits and keep track of where their money goes for two or three months to help them determine whether they spend for today and never plan for tomorrow, or save everything for tomorrow and never enjoy today.

She recommends beginning a retirement savings plan as soon as possible. A financial planner can help tremendously, she says, but shop around until you find one you can work with. "You need to learn the language first so you can participate in your investment strategies. You don't just want to turn over everything to someone else."

And don't think you don't have enough money to get started. Even saving $10 a month can help. In 25 years in an investment vehicle paying only 5.25 percent interest a month, that monthly $10 will be $6,193. In an investment that pays 10 percent, it will be $11,295.

Make sure you appear in your budget, following the old admonition to "pay yourself first," says Martindale. If saving is tough for you, take advantage of "painless" methods of saving, including 401(k) pension plans offered by many employers or direct-deposit programs.

CHAPTER 74

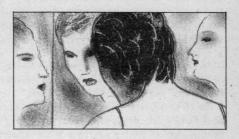

ROLE MODELS

MENTORS ARE CHARACTER BUILDERS

Who's your role model? Your mother? Your dad? Margaret Mead, Meryl Streep, your French professor, the woman next door? It may be a celebrity or someone you know, but chances are there's someone you admire and in whose footsteps you're following.

And that's good, because having someone to emulate can have a strong and positive impact on your life, says Michele Paludi, Ph.D., coordinator of the Women's Studies Program at Hunter College in New York City who has studied women's mentoring relationships.

And they can also have a lasting effect on your life, even when they're no longer in your life. "When I was in my twenties and insecure, I met an older woman at work who was the single mother of three and a newspaper reporter like me," says Mary Cameron, 39. "She not only knew lots about the business—things I didn't know—she had self-confidence to the max. I was always impressed by how she handled everything with such a sense of humor. Things just rolled off her back. Nothing was so terrible she couldn't crack a joke. I learned a lot from her about being a good journalist—and a together person. Over the years, I know I've adopted some of her traits. I can sometimes even hear myself saying things I've heard her say."

SOMEONE TO ADMIRE

In Mary's case, her role model became her friend and mentor, a term usually used to refer to an influential individual who takes a special interest in you and who helps you achieve academic or career success.

And everyone can benefit from having one.

"For many women, mentors perform a psychosocial function," says Dr. Paludi. Your "mentor" may be a woman you know who is successful at combining her career and family life or someone who's experienced in the field you'd like to enter, whether it's management or motherhood. She may be someone whose personal style you admire or who struggled successfully with the same problem you have. Her life may serve as a guide for yours.

THE NEW AGE OF MENTORING

Role models are important to have, says Dr. Paludi. The problem for women today is they have fewer role models for the many roles they've taken on.

But a role model can be anyone. It can even be each other, says Dr. Paludi. "A mentor doesn't have to be someone older. It can be and frequently is someone from your same age group. It's a more reciprocal relationship. We call it networking mentoring."

You may have many role models throughout your life. In one of Dr. Paludi's studies, she found that men's role models generally didn't change from the time they were children, but women changed role models each time they took on a new role. "They had different people at different stages of their lives," she says.

Where do you find these "hands-on" role models? They may be in your office or in your neighborhood, or you may have to join a professional or support group to meet other women who share your interests. In a study of people who identified themselves as mentors, researchers asked how their mentoring relationships got started, says Dr. Paludi. "Many of them just said, 'chemistry.'"

CHAPTER 75

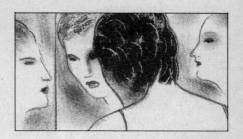

SELF-ESTEEM

GETTING FROM LOW TO HIGH

*W*hen psychotherapist Linda Tschirhart Sanford and her partner, Mary Ellen Donovan, were writing their landmark book *Women and Self-Esteem*, their friends gave it another, more accurate working title.

"They called it The Blind Leading the Blind," admits Sanford, who has conducted self-esteem enhancement workshops for women across the country. "I grew up with low self-esteem, and perhaps the most important thing we learned by writing this book was that there is really nothing innate or God-given about self-esteem. It has to be learned along the way."

And, oh, what we learn. "When I was a teenager, I was tall and wasn't part of the in-group, so I got this idea that I was big and gawky," says Robin Tucker, a slim, stunning woman who, in her late forties, looks a decade younger. "At 16, I felt unattractive and undesirable, even though I had lots of dates. I did very well in school, but I didn't think I was smart. I thought I was lucky."

SMART WOMEN, FOOLISH CHOICES

Like many women with low self-esteem, Robin made choices based on her skewed self-image. She thought she was lucky when, at 17, she met Michael, a handsome blond with a lifeguard's physique with whom, she says, "I fell in lust." They were married right out of high school and Robin became a mother a year later. "But I knew almost from the first day of the marriage that I'd made a big mistake," says Robin. "I married because I thought no other man would ever want me, and I gave up the idea of college because I thought I wasn't smart enough. I was wrong on both counts, but it took me 15 unhappy years to figure that out."

Robin's story isn't unusual. Some experts believe that low self-esteem is epidemic among women whose lives and happiness, say Sanford and Donovan, "have been constricted" because of their fundamental feelings of inadequacy. Self-esteem, they believe, is at the bottom of many other problems women have, from overeating to alcoholism. Neither liking nor respecting ourselves, we marry men unworthy of us, choose jobs for which we're overskilled and make other unfortunate choices—from substance abuse to tolerating abuse—"based," says Sanford, "on what we *think* we deserve."

She even suggests that, in some ways, gender is a risk factor for poor self-image because we live in a society that values male, not female, traits. Presidents aren't elected because they're warm and compassionate. It's the rare CEO who gets high marks in sensitivity. It's men, not women, who dominate most of our society's venerable institutions, from the Congress to the Church. "The fact is we live in a patriarchy in which women are in a subordinate position," says Sanford. "It's hard to have self-esteem when you are constantly being told by society that by definition you're not good enough."

GETTING THE WRONG MESSAGE

Many women have internalized that message, spending their lives pursuing, as one self-esteem expert puts it, "the Holy Grail of enoughness." In her book *Perfect Women: Hidden Fears of Inadequacy and the Drive to Perform*, Colette Dowling suggests that for many woman "enoughness" is nothing short of perfection, a standard that, once reached, will finally put to rest nagging feelings of worthlessness. Plagued by the "if only" syndrome—if only I were smarter, prettier, thinner . . . fill in your own inadequacy—women embark on a perpetual course of self-improvement aimed at winning approval. We spend years struggling to "fix" ourselves to earn the final nod that assures us that yes, we are good enough. We are literally driven to excel in the workplace, to stay model-thin, to be Super Somebody whose place at the top will make us invulnerable, complete—even if it means we have driven ourselves into exhaustion, drug abuse or eating disorders.

In her work, Sanford has found that many women who seem to be aware of their good points nevertheless give more weight to all the things they're not. "Almost all women have aspects of themselves they're satisfied with, particular skills and competences, but those aren't the most important things in their lives. Those aren't what they measure their worth by."

No, it's their flaws by which they gauge themselves. Many women write off their own good points because they assume, says Sanford, "that if I'm good at it, it must not matter." It's also not unusual, says Sanford, for a woman to acknowledge that she's bright, attractive, a good mother, a good secretary, but to add with a certain wistfulness, "but I could certainly stand to lose 10 pounds," making it clear that all those positives notwithstanding, she thinks of herself first and foremost as overweight.

Studies have shown that self-defeating behaviors, such as focusing on flaws or making too much of failure, are hallmarks of depression. In fact, according to the American Psychological Association's Task Force on Women, low self-esteem is clearly an important factor in depression. Low self-esteem was identified as leading to the higher incidence of depression among women, who suffer from the blues twice as often as men.

CHANGING THE MESSAGE

What can you do about your self-esteem? After all, you weren't born with those "worthless me" messages. They came from somewhere outside of you—from the parents who told you that you were bad, the classmates who made fun of your red hair, your nose or your slowness at math. "None of us got into low self-esteem in isolation," says Sanford. "None of us is going to get out of it alone."

Counseling and support groups can help you become aware of the false messages you've been receiving about yourself and offer you some affirmation about who you truly are. But there's plenty you can do on your own, too.

Sanford suggests that you start with a physical reflection of your self-image: a self-concept collage. Take a piece of paper and arrange on it symbols that represent how you view yourself—positive, negative and neutral—using words, drawings or photographs and illustrations from magazines. Place the one most crucial to your identity in the center. For many women, this simple artistic act is an awakening, says Sanford. "When I've done this in workshops with women who say they have low self-esteem and we count what's positive, negative and neutral, there are really very few negatives there. This is a very good way to get to know yourself."

The self-concept collage can also help you come to see yourself as the sum of your parts, so those extra 10 pounds, the heavy thighs and the crooked nose that are so important to your identity become simply part of it, along with your sense of humor, warmth, skill at illustrating or managing people or caring for your children. Instead of focusing on your flaws, you literally can see the "big picture."

Often negative images become such an integral part of our identities, even reality can't convince us to give them up. Sanford suggests doing a little reality testing. Ask someone close to you, someone you trust, to describe you, "Ask them for three adjectives," she says. "Asking for feedback from other people is really important. After all, it was other people who told you who you were in the first place."

This requires some risk, but you have to take some risks if you're going to change how you see yourself. As Rebecca Curtis, Ph.D., professor of psychology at Adelphi University in Garden City, New York, and author of *Self-Defeating Behaviors*, points out, "It's not possible to sit there by yourself and change your self-image. You have to get confirmation from other people and the environment that you're different. We need to have a view of ourselves that other people validate."

It also means doing the kinds of things the "real" you would do. For Robin Tucker, reality testing took great courage. To see herself as smart and attractive, it meant applying to college—and filing for divorce. It paid off. "I walked into the college classroom with my head down, and by the end of the first year I felt like a queen. The teachers all loved me. I got straight A's. And then I married someone who believed in me. I felt like a different person. But all that really happened was that I discovered who I was all along."

RELABEL YOURSELF

Another way to help shed those outdated labels is to re-frame them. One of Sanford's techniques involves making two lists, one starting with "You are," followed by all the adjectives your parents might have used to describe you, and the second starting with "I am," which is followed by those same qualities reframed in a positive light. For example, if your parents drummed it into your head that you were stubborn or slow, come up with positive attributes of those traits. A stubborn person could also be seen as independent or persistent. Someone who is slow may be thoughtful or purposeful.

"Improving self-esteem doesn't mean a major overhaul," says Sanford. "It means shifting a little bit, putting some of the things you do well into the core of your self-concept and putting less emphasis on the aspects of yourself that are less than perfect. It's really clear that men are conditioned to take the things they do best and build their identity around them. The aspects of themselves that are less than perfect they tend to dismiss."

NO OVERNIGHT SUCCESS

But don't expect a metamorphosis overnight. This is not necessarily going to be easy. Unfortunately, says Sanford, "it's considered very feminine to be self-denigrating. There's a false nobility about not liking yourself."

The truth is, you need to toot your own horn once in a while. Some sincere and subtle bragging isn't going to hurt every now and then. If you find the thought terrifying—after all, you don't want to be seen as vain or self-centered—you can start slowly by learning to accept compliments. Many women find it very difficult to accept praise, let alone heap it on themselves, says Linda Dunlap, Ph.D., assistant professor of psychology at Marist College in Poughkeepsie, New York. The proper response to a compliment is not an embarrassed denial that you are or did anything remarkable, she says. "It's 'Thank you.'"

Declare a moratorium on negative put-downs. Consider mistakes and failures as learning experiences, rather than conclusive proof you're as incapable as you think you are. Rather than being harsh and accusing with yourself, suggests Dr. Dunlap, "turn it around and say, I learned something from that. I'm going to try my very best next time and accept whatever happens, so at least I can say to myself, 'I tried my best.'"

And you need to recognize that your "best," no matter how good it is, will never be perfect. No one is perfect. So lower your expectations to something within the realm of possible. It's more important, say the experts, to be the best you can be than to be the best. Above all, says Sanford, don't become one of those people "who end up with low self-esteem about having low self-esteem."

See also Body Image

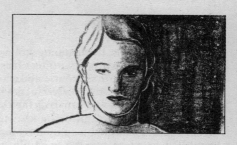

SEXUAL ABUSE

HOW THERAPY CAN HELP

*U*ntil she was 36, Jessie kept her memories buried in an alcoholic fog. The only child of an auto executive and his wife, she began getting drunk regularly when she was only 13. "I didn't know at the time, but I was really covering up a lot of pain," says Jessie, now 43. At 36, she went into alcoholism recovery—and the memories of being sexually abused by her father began to surface.

In therapy, Jessie found that she had been using booze to distance herself from the pain. Even now, her fear of men lingers, as does her fear of intimacy. She managed to earn a master's degree in social work but has had trouble holding down a job. "I went through six jobs in 11 years because I was so angry and volatile, and I couldn't trust authority. I rebelled against anyone who had power over me," she remembers. Like a lot of women who have been abused, Jessie became a loner, haunted by an amorphous anxiety that alcohol could not erase.

THE SECRET CRIME

Jessie is the victim of what has been until recently a hidden epidemic. Current research indicates that an astonishing one in four women—maybe more—was sexually abused as a child. Many, like Jessie, are victims of "the last taboo"— incest. Others were molested by older relatives, authority figures, or in smaller numbers, by strangers. For many, the struggle to keep their secret, oftentimes even from themselves, has led to serious mental and physical illness.

Researchers in fields as diverse as childbirth and substance abuse are finding alarmingly high numbers of women whose lives have been tainted and twisted by childhood sexual abuse. For example, one study found that anywhere from 30 percent to two-thirds of all women with eating disorders were abused at some point in their past. And a startling 70 percent of female substance abusers—alcoholics and drug users—were sexually or physically abused. In one 1990 study of women seeking outpatient psychiatric help for a variety of reasons, 63 percent had been victims of childhood physical or sexual abuse.

In recent years two celebrities—former Miss America Marilyn Van Derbur and comedian Roseanne Arnold—came forward with their own shocking stories of childhood sexual abuse. Many experts believe those revelations may have ended once and for all the secrecy that has cloaked this devastating trauma.

For too long, it has been a crime that was easy to hide. "Years ago, you simply did not talk about it," says Virginia Revere, Ph.D., a psychologist in private practice in Alexandria, Virginia, who works with sexual abuse victims. "If you got run over by a car and survived, you could tell everybody, 'Hey, I got run over by a car,' and it was all acceptable. But you couldn't talk about abuse."

In some cases, no one would listen. "People who were abused may have been told that they seduced their abuser and are terrible people," says Dr. Revere. "It's very common for the parent to blame the child for what happened."

Often the child believes she is at fault, says Linda Tschirhart Sanford of Quincy, Massachusetts, a therapist and author of *Strong at the Broken Places: Overcoming the Trauma of Childhood Abuse*. Trying to make sense out of the abuse, she may come to believe it happened because she deserved it or provoked it.

HEALING THE PAIN

But in many cases, the abuse remains a secret because the child represses the painful memories. Even when her memories do intrude on conscious thought, they may be dismissed as imagination. In other cases, victims have excruciatingly clear memories but remain emotionally numb in order to distance themselves from the pain. One of Sanford's clients described herself at the age of 5 as "having calluses on the heart."

Sometimes these repressed memories gradually begin to emerge. In the short run, the victim doesn't have to face them, but she may suffer many physical and psychological symptoms that seem to have no cause. "What the mind forgets, the body remembers," says Christine Courtois, Ph.D., a psychologist who works with sexually abused women in the Washington, D.C., area and author of *Healing the Incest Wound*.

In fact, many victims live their lives in the thrall of compulsive and destructive urges whose source is maddeningly elusive. As Roseanne Arnold, who struggled her whole life with drug, food and alcohol abuse, told a reporter from *Time* magazine, "It's the secret that's been killing me my whole life."

Usually abuse victims regain their memories when they begin to feel safe enough to recall them, such as when they become involved in an intimate relationship with someone they trust or when they enter therapy, often for another problem. Jessie believes it was no coincidence that her memories began to return when she entered an alcoholism treatment program that helped her rebuild her self-esteem.

Therapy, which is usually necessary, can be "extremely difficult and extremely painful," says Dr. Courtois. Because a woman who was sexually abused as a child may have trouble trusting other people, it's very important to seek out a therapist who is trustworthy and who is experienced in dealing with such abuse, she says.

"I went through a couple of therapists who just didn't believe me," says Jessie. "They told me they thought my memories were linked to my having had polio at the age of 7. I knew there was more to it than that."

Many victims, says Dr. Courtois, "alternate between facing it and blocking it off, tuning in and taking time out. However, once it's faced head-on, healing can begin."

THE SURVIVORS

But the victim of childhood sexual abuse is by no means doomed to a lifetime of psychological trauma. In a study of two groups of incest survivors by sexual abuse experts Judith Herman, M.D., Diana Russell, Ph.D., and Karen Trocki, Ph.D., the majority said they had been deeply disturbed by their experiences but about half the women said they felt they had recovered well.

In fact, some women cope with their experience in a positive way. "A lot of survivors become very high achievers and do well in life," says Dr. Revere. "They feel a lot of shame, and one way to overcome shame is to achieve."

Healing, although it eventually comes, is often slow. Along with a sensitive therapist, many victims may benefit from a self-help group, such as Incest Survivors Anonymous, to which Jessie belongs. "I go to Incest Survivors Anonymous and Alcoholics Anonymous," she says. "The groups are one way I stay out of isolation. One big benefit I've realized is coming to know the men in these groups who were also abused. It's been healing for me to see that they go through the same pain and are as vulnerable as I am. Being with other people like myself helps to remind me that, although it happened, I *survived* it."

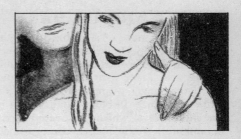

SEXUAL DYSFUNCTION

A PROBLEM TOO EASY TO HIDE

o read about it you'd think it's a problem that only happens to men. Yet nearly every woman—or at the very least most women—will experience a sexual problem at some time in their lives. It's not that they don't want to have sex. They can't. Or they can but it's just not satisfying. Sort of the female version of impotence.

For men, it's pretty hard to hide an erection problem or premature ejaculation, two of their more common sexual dysfunctions. But when women have a sex problem it's often invisible—they feel inhibited, they have trouble reaching an orgasm or they can't have one at all. It's the type of stuff women tend not to discuss, so it's a problem that often gets ignored. They can go through the act of making love, usually, but remain unfulfilled. And the sexual frustration, just like for a man, can threaten happiness, contentment and self-esteem. It can even threaten your marriage.

By far the most common sex problem for women is inhibition, which often stems from that sense of exploring "the forbidden" that dates back to the times when even a turn of the ankle was viewed with a raised brow. "There's a lifetime of history behind inhibited sexuality," says Judith H. Seifer, R.N., Ph.D., associate clinical professor in the departments of psychiatry and obstetrics and gynecology at the Wright State University School of Medicine in Dayton, Ohio.

INHIBITION DIES HARD

"Inhibition is more of a problem in younger women *and* in older women," Dr. Seifer says. "The ones in the middle— the 30- to 45-year-olds—have fewer inhibitions, probably because they made their way through the Sexual Revolution. For younger women inhibition has more to do with sexual ignorance. In older women it's a throwback to the time in society in which they were raised."

Inhibition is the main reason women have difficulty reaching orgasm, says Dr. Seifer. All the angst and anxiety they go through to make love the first time or first few times leaves them with the letdown: "Is that all there is?"

Yet once a woman learns to reach orgasm, she rarely loses the ability, adds Lonnie Barbach, Ph.D., psychologist and sex therapist and author of *For Yourself: The Fulfillment of Female Sexuality* and *For Each Other: Sharing Sexual Intimacy.* But to achieve orgasm in the first place often requires self-exploration, something many women still find embarrassing or guilt producing. Younger women have also discovered self-help books to help them get to orgasm, says Dr. Seifer.

Dr. Seifer admits, though, that all this talk of sexual fulfillment may be lost on older women, who came from a generation in which a healthy female sexual appetite was seen as more wrong than right. "My sister-in-law and I often sit around and joke and laugh about sex with our teenage daughters," Dr. Seifer says. "But my dear mother-in-law, who is sitting there with us, can't understand why everybody is so excited about sex. To her it's no big deal. She's managed to maintain her sense of self-worth because she believes that she is a 'good' woman. She's had a successful, loving marriage, and she's proud that she never said no to her husband. But she'll also live out the balance of her life never knowing sexual fulfillment."

LET LOOSE A LITTLE

But let's forget lost causes. How do you go about discovering sexual bliss?

"Orgasm depends on your ability to 'let go,' " say Maurice Yaffe and Elizabeth Fenwick, authors of *Sexual Happiness for Women: A Practical Approach*. If you're the kind of person who likes to be in control of yourself, to remain unemotional no matter what happens, then the idea of being carried away by an orgasm might seem quite scary. Or it might be that the loss of control involved during orgasm might make you look unattractive, undignified, even ridiculous to your partner, they suggest.

"Sometimes women are trying so hard to have an orgasm that they concentrate on the act instead of the feeling," says Dr. Seifer. "They start doing what's known as 'spectatoring.' They can see themselves responding, and they're saying to themselves, 'this is it, it's going to happen, I can feel it this time.' And then they lose it. It just dries up because they've climbed out of that experience. I tell them," she says, " 'you can't be in two places at the same time. You can't be in your crotch experiencing all the good feelings that go along with lovemaking and in your head thinking about it at the same time.' "

Dr. Seifer explains to couples during therapy that the orgasm in and of itself is not where it's at. "We're all very productively oriented in our society. We want outcomes and we want them now. The outcome of a successful sexual encounter in our culture is that the man ejaculates and the woman has an orgasm. But that's not what sex is really all about. *Getting there* is what sex is all about."

SEXUAL SHUTDOWN

Lack of orgasm, however, isn't all there is when it comes to sexual dysfunction in women. Some women live very happy, very satisfying sex lives until one day something else takes the place of pleasure—like pain.

It's called vaginismus and it's the third most common cause of sexual dysfunction in women. What happens? There's an involuntary tightening of the muscles surrounding the opening of the vagina and the outer one-third of the vagina that prevents the penis from penetrating. It means that sex is impossible at worst, or sporadic and painful at best. The strange thing is that you may be capable of becoming aroused, and even have orgasms, in spite of it all.

This, too, has a psychological basis. "It's the body reacting to taboos and fears," says New York sex therapist Shirley Zussman, Ed.D. Having negative sexual attitudes pounded in by parents since childhood, or too rigidly following the dictates of a strict, disapproving religion, for example, are common themes. Or it could be that the woman has intimacy problems. She can't open up to others and is emotionally guarded and not sexually responsive, Dr. Zussman continues.

"When I see a woman with vaginismus," adds Dr. Seifer, "she is often extraordinarily competent. In other words, she's compensated eloquently for her sexual inadequacies. She's often a high-powered, upwardly mobile career woman who has in many cases had a history of sexual misuse," she explains. "It's as if she says to herself, 'Well, sex isn't going to be important to me. I'm going to make my mark in the business world.' "

Meanwhile her sex life or her marriage is falling apart. Even though she knows something is wrong, she'll often ignore the problem, especially if she can tolerate intercourse at least some of the time, according to Jo Marie Kessler, a nurse practitioner at the Crenshaw Clinic in San Diego, California. What's worse is that a doctor may dismiss her symptoms when he can find "nothing wrong" on examination. And, in fact, there is nothing to see if her condition is sporadic. Only when a woman comes in because of an unconsummated marriage will a doctor be alerted to this condition, says Kessler. Not surprisingly, women with vaginismus feel guilt, shame, fear and distrust. Eventually, those feelings give way to frustration, anger, resentment and hostility as well as feelings of helplessness, hoplessness and powerlessness, notes Kessler.

SEXUAL REAWAKENING

As devastating as vaginismus sounds—some therapists have even called it a sexual emergency—there are positive outcomes for most seeking treatment. Therapists have developed a program using plastic, rubber or glass dilators in graduated sizes. You begin with the smallest-size dilator and, after a warm bath to relax tissues, gently insert the smallest one to stretch the vagina. This is done several times a day, until the largest dilator can be comfortably inserted. Once you can then accept someone else doing this with you, you may soon be tolerant of penile insertion. Fingers can also be used instead of dilators.

Doctors have also found that Kegel exercises—voluntary tightening and releasing of the pelvic muscles—can give you a sense of control over your vaginal muscles. And others have found success with relaxation techniques and hypnotically guided imagery.

"Both men and women usually do very well and gain a satisfying sex life after therapy," says Dr. Zussman. "Just talking about the sexual problem is therapeutic; for many, it's the first time they've ever talked about it at all. Everyone feels better once they realize a sex problem is not as scary or embarrassing as they had thought."

See also Inhibited Sexual Desire

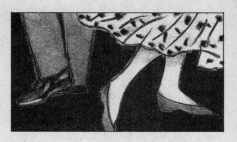

SEXUAL HARASSMENT

GETTING CAUGHT IN A POWER PLAY

*J*ennifer Leidy, a 30-year-old single mother with two young sons, was hired as a clerk at a small firm 10 minutes from her house. Before the first week was up, her boss, a 36-year-old single man who ran the family business with his mother, asked her out. She refused.

"I told him I never date anyone I work with," says Jennifer. "But he kept bugging me. He would hang around my desk during the day, ask me if I needed anything, make small talk. He asked me out a few more times and I refused each time. But it was making me nervous. He never said I would be fired if I didn't go out with him, but I always thought it was a possibility. After all, he owned the company. Then one day, I saw him driving slowly past my house and it really gave me the creeps."

Jennifer wasted little time finding another job, but she never told anyone the real reason she wanted to quit. "I didn't like the job that much anyway, which was the excuse I used. But I wonder what I would have done if I had to stay there," she says.

ON-THE-JOB AGGRAVATION

In the now-classic 1981 Merit Systems Protection Board random survey of government employees, 42 percent of the more than 10,000 women who responded said they had been sexually harassed on the job. Sixty-two percent said they had been touched in a sexual manner and 20 percent reported actual or attempted rape or assault on the job.

Other surveys have found that about 50 percent of women have been sexually harassed on the job. And at least one expert says it's even worse. Midge Wilson, Ph.D., associate professor of psychology and women's studies at De Paul University in Chicago, says she tells her students, "I've never met a woman who hasn't been harassed at some point in her work life."

While the Merit survey shed some light on what is obviously a pervasive social problem, it focused on the number of women sexually harassed on the job and not what happened to them because of it. The consequences of sexual harassment can be profound.

In the same year the Merit survey was conducted, researchers at the Working Women's Institute in New York City found that 42 percent of the women they surveyed, like Jennifer, had left jobs where they were harassed, and 24 percent had been fired, either as retaliation for complaining about the harassment or because their work had suffered as a consequence.

In fact, the researchers discovered, 75 percent of the women reported that their work performance deteriorated because they were unable to concentrate, had lost confidence in their skills and accomplishments or lost their motivation to perform because they were victims of retaliation. Almost all the women reported one or more psychological stress symptoms, such as tension, nervousness, anger, fear or helplessness. Some suffered serious psychological distress, similar to that experienced by rape and incest victims. Many also had physical symptoms, including nausea, headache and chronic fatigue. Some even turned to alcohol and drugs to ease their stress.

NO ESSAY OPTIONS

Jennifer exercised one of the few options available to women who are sexually harassed on the job. But what about women who can't leave their jobs for one reason or another? They can either stay and suffer or file charges against their harasser. Many employers have guidelines and grievance procedures to handle sexual harassment cases. In 1980, the Equal Employment Opportunity Commission (EEOC), the federal agency that handles sexual harassment cases, allowed women to literally make a federal case out of harassment. Sexual harassment is considered a violation of a woman's civil rights, under Title VII of the 1964 Civil Rights Act, and harassment cases are heard in federal court.

"Yet a very tiny percentage of women are ever actually going to file a complaint, get a lawyer and follow it through," says Dr. Wilson.

Why? The reasons are myriad. A recent study of female college students—frequent victims of what one expert refers to wryly as the lecherous professors—found that many women are hesitant about bringing charges against a harasser for fear that they will ruin his life. "A lot of sexual harassment policies are very punishment-oriented and a lot of women really are not interested in seeing a professor lose a job or a supervisor get fired," says Dr. Wilson. "They don't want to carry that guilt around—and women are just guilt magnets."

FEARS OF RETRIBUTION

There's also the fear of retaliation. Although the law prohibits companies from retaliating against a woman who files charges against her harasser, she can become persona non grata in her office, shunned even by coworkers who, fearing for their own jobs, refuse to support her even when they may be victims themselves or have been aware of the problem.

Kathleen Neville, an account executive with a New York TV station who charged that she was harassed by her supervisor, received death threats even before she filed her complaint with the EEOC. She was fired from her job and took another job at $28,000 a year less than she had been making. In her book *Corporate Attractions* she writes that her new employer, upset that she was bringing suit against her old boss, told her he was sorry he had hired her and put pressure on her by forcing her to account for every minute of her time, including time spent in the ladies' room.

Women also fear repeated victimization in court. Unfortunately, the courts, in hearing sexual harassment cases, have also permitted testimony on the victim's conduct in much the same way a rape victim's life becomes an open book. In doing so, writes law professor Susan Estrich in *The Stanford Law Review*, the court has reinforced "some of the most demeaning sexual sterotypes of women." A woman's conduct—even the way she speaks or dresses—is considered a relevant issue. In reality both she and her harasser are on trial. Her conduct is scrutinized so that the court can determine if she made it clear his advances were unwelcome, which reinforces the idea that women have a gatekeeper role in sexual matters. In effect, writes Estrich, professor of law and political science at the University of Southern California in Los Angeles, the court has ruled that "men are legally entitled to treat women whose clothes fit snugly with less respect than women whose clothes fit loosely."

"I have tremendous admiration for the courage of women who have brought these charges and followed them through," says Dr. Wilson. "It takes courage just to risk being considered a troublemaker in a society that expects women to not complain when things happen to them."

WHAT IS HARASSMENT?

The courts have also wrestled with the definition of sexual harassment. In some cases, it's easy to recognize. The so-called quid pro quo harassment—you do something for me, I'll do something for you—usually involves a promise of employment benefits in exchange for sexual favors. That's when the boss asks you to sleep with him in exchange for a job or a promotion. Not as easy to recognize is the type of harassment that creates what the law calls a hostile work environment. Suggestive remarks, teasing, jokes or gestures, even sexually explicit drawings or photographs posted in the workplace, also constitute sexual harassment, but many companies and the courts—even some women—have found it difficult to distinguish between what's harmless and what's not.

Part of the problem has been that, as studies have shown, men may view a situation quite differently than women do. Many men are flattered by sexual advances and think women are, too. Until 1991 the courts tended to look upon sexual harassment cases more as a "reasonable man" might view them than a "reasonable woman." But in January 1991 the 9th U.S. Circuit Court of Appeals reversed an earlier ruling that found that an IRS agent who deluged a female coworker with love letters had not been guilty of sexual harassment. Any "reasonable woman," the court concluded, would have been frightened and disturbed by the letters.

ABUSING POWER

"It's a power difference that creates harassment," says Dr. Wilson. Usually, a victim of sexual harassment is in a position subordinate to that of her harasser, as in Jennifer Leidy's case. Although her boss made no overt threats about her job, the fact that he owned the company made her feel intimidated. If you are a working woman, chances are your boss is a man. According to one study, 75 percent of women are employed in sex-segregated jobs supervised by men, making the workplace a fertile ground for harassment.

But it's not only bosses who are to blame. What happens to secretaries can also happen to neurosurgeons. Even if a man is not in a more powerful position at work, our society regards men, by virtue of their gender, as more powerful than women. "In work settings, men are viewed as more competent, responsible, committed and valuable than women," write sexual harassment experts Donna M. Stringer, Ph.D., Helen Remick, Ph.D., Jan Salisbury and Angela B. Ginorio, Ph.D., in *Public Personnel Management*. A woman—even if she has achieved power in an organization—is less likely to be believed than a man and may even be seen as less powerful because she was harassed and unable to stop it.

Since a man at any level of achievement may regard himself as more powerful than any woman, no woman is immune. In 1991 a female brain surgeon at Stanford University School of Medicine resigned her tenured professorship after years of harassment during which her colleagues called her Honey in the operating room and fondled her legs under the operating table.

"One of the deans at this school was harassed by a member of a site visiting team for accreditation," says Dr. Wilson. "She was hosting a party for the team and he refused to leave her hotel room when everyone else had left. She was shocked. She said, 'I didn't think it would ever happen to me. I have so much power at the university and I felt that if I didn't sleep with him he wasn't going to accredit us.' So it happens at every level."

Especially at risk are women in traditionally male occupations, such as construction workers, police officers and firefighters. Jacquelyn L. Morris was a machinist in the Pevely, Missouri, bottle-making plant operated by American National Can Corporation. In 1987, she had achieved top seniority in a unit with 12 men and was consistently rated good or excellent in her work performance. She left her job, however, because her bosses and coworkers made her life there untenable. Several made crude comments about her anatomy and one morning she arrived at work to find a photo of an erect penis on her toolbox. She filed suit and won $16,000 in back pay, with interest.

SAYING NO IS NOT ENOUGH

If you are the victim of sexual harassment, "the most effective thing you can do is confront your harasser," says Dr. Wilson.

"The moment you see it, say, 'I don't like what you just said and I prefer that you not talk to me this way,' " she advises. "Try to say it in front of other people. Get an audience so that other people can document that you recognized what it was and responded to it the first time it occurred. And don't smile when you say it. That sends a lot of mixed messages. It's very difficult for women to be assertive and to talk to someone directly without smiling and sort of disclaiming, 'I'm sorry to say this'—smile, smile—'but I really don't like that'—smile, smile.''

According to Susan Estrich, the court will be looking at your conduct as well as your words. "Just say no" may be a good slogan for the war on drugs, but it won't hold up in court. If your no is delivered with a smile, the court could view your attitude to the harassment as ambivalent and rule against you. You may be embarrassed, but get angry instead, says Dr. Wilson.

If the harassment persists or escalates, report it to your supervisor or your harasser's supervisor or the personnel manager, says Dr. Wilson.

Be aware of your company's own grievance procedures. If there aren't any, suggest that they be instituted. It's in your employer's best interest to attend to the law. A company may be held liable for sexual harassment that occurs in the workplace and, in addition to damages assessed by the court, may have to pay its own and your attorneys' fees, back pay and unemployment. They may have to pay in other ways, too—in the loss of customers or prospective employees put off by the attendant bad publicity.

INVITING TROUBLE

Dating in the workplace has its risks. One well-known trigger for sexual harassment is an office love affair gone sour. Unless you know with complete confidence that you are "among friends" in your office, avoid becoming overly friendly with the men you work with.

What can get you into trouble? According to Estrich, acting in stereotypical ways—complimenting men, straightening their ties or remaining on good terms with a man who makes advances—can hurt your chances if you wind up in court. Conversely, women who act like men—using lewd language, going out "with the boys"—can be adversely affected.

If, after using the grievance procedures at your workplace, the harassment continues or your supervisors retaliate against you, contact the EEOC office nearest you (they're not in every city) and ask about filing charges. Even if the EEOC does not take legal action, you can still file a private suit.

CHAPTER
79

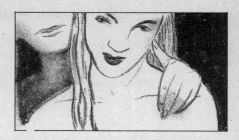

SEXUALLY TRANSMITTED DISEASES

NO SUCH THING AS TOO CAREFUL

he mid-twentieth-century sexual revolution that was ushered in by the Pill is quickly being ushered out by an epidemic of sexually transmitted diseases (STDs).

Besides the gonorrhea and syphilis that we were warned about a generation ago, today's microscopes have revealed that there are now other diseases that can be transmitted during what is supposed to be one of the most sublime moments of human existence.

Maybe that's why many of us resist protecting ourselves from sexually transmitted diseases. To actually think that genital herpes, chlamydia, genital warts, trichomoniasis or AIDS might be passed on to us during an exquisite burst of human-to-human communication is to somehow tarnish the feelings and the humans involved. But anyone who's ever been saddled with an STD will tell you that it's no fair exchange for a few moments of ecstasy.

Approximately 50 percent of the population has or will have an experience with a sexually transmitted disease sometime in their lives, says Dr. Penny Hitchcock, acting chief of the Sexually Transmitted Diseases Branch of the National Institute of Allergy and Infectious Diseases in Bethesda, Maryland. Yet, it always has been and still is one of those subjects no one dares talk about it in polite company. Or in *any* company, for that matter.

"It's quite amazing when you think about it," she says.

THE FACTS AND FIGURES ON STDs

Disease	Number Infected in U.S.	Cause	How Transmitted	Symptoms	Diagnostic Tests	Treatments	Complications
AIDS	1 million (150,000 women)	Human immuno-deficiency virus (HIV)	Exchange of body fluids through genital contact	May be no symptoms for years. ARC (AIDS-related complex) eventually develops with such symptoms as persistent swollen glands and chronic infections that don't respond to medication. Malignancies or severe infections develop when the immune system is compromised.	Blood test determines presence of HIV anti-bodies	Experimental drugs such as AZT. No cure.	May be passed from mother to baby in the womb or at birth and is often fatal to the child as well as the mother

(continued on page 550)

THE FACTS AND FIGURES ON STDs (continued)

Disease	Number Infected in U.S.	Cause	How Transmitted	Symptoms	Diagnostic Tests	Treatments	Complications
Chlamydia	4 million each year (1.3 men to every woman)	*Chlamydia trachomatis* bacteria	Direct contact with infected mucous membranes and secretions in genitals, mouth and throat	75% of women have no symptoms. For those who do, usually appear 1–3 weeks after exposure; include burning urination, unusual vaginal discharge, abdominal pain, painful intercourse and bleeding between periods.	Sample of vaginal secretions can give results in 30 minutes	Antibiotics	Major cause of pelvic inflammatory disease. Infants exposed during birth may develop eye infections or pneumonia.
Genital herpes	30 million affected; about 500,000 each year (2 women to every man)	Herpes simplex virus	Direct contact with an active sore or virus-containing genital secretions. Can lie dormant for	Generally develop 2–20 days after contact with virus. Blisters or bumps appear, which	Sample from a sore	Prescription Acyclovir is effective in reducing frequency and duration of	Self-infection of eyes, fingers and other body parts possible if infected area is touched. Ba-

Disease	Incidence	Cause	Transmission	Symptoms	Diagnosis	Treatment	Complications
			months or years. Can be transmitted even when there are no symptoms.	may itch, burn or tingle. May cause flulike symptoms with first outbreak. May cause painful urination. Recurrences likely.		outbreaks. During outbreaks, keep area clean and dry. No cure.	bies can be infected during birth.
Genital warts	1 million each year (men and women equally affected)	Human papilloma virus	Direct skin-to-skin contact with an infected person during sex, whether warts are visible or not	Warts appear in or near vagina several weeks to 9 months after exposure. May appear raised or flat, singly or in multiples. Often no symptoms and usually painless, but can cause itching and burning.	Direct visual examination, Pap smear	Doctor may apply a liquid to gradually remove the warts. Warts may be removed by freezing or burning. Surgery is occasionally needed to remove large warts.	Strongly associated with cervical cancer

(continued on page 552)

THE FACTS AND FIGURES ON STDs (continued)

Disease	Number Infected in U.S.	Cause	How Transmitted	Symptoms	Diagnostic Tests	Treatments	Complications
Gonorrhea	1.4 million each year (1.3 men to every woman)	*Neisseria gonorrhoeae* bacteria	Direct contact with infected mucous membranes and secretions in genitals, mouth and throat	Often mild or nonexistent, especially in women. If they develop, it is usually within 2–10 days of sexual contact with infected person. Symptoms include painful urination and yellowish vaginal discharge.	Sample of discharge	Antibiotics; newer drugs may be needed for strains resistant to standard antibiotics	Common cause of PID. If untreated, may cause arthritis, skin sores and heart or brain infection. Infection of infants during birth may lead to blindness.
Syphilis	130,000 each year (1.3 men to every woman)	*Treponema pallidum* bacteria	Direct contact with ulcers of someone with active infection. The germs can also pass	Painless open sore, called a chancre, appears in or near vagina within 10 days to 3	Blood tests and microscopic identification of bacteria using a sample	Antibiotics	Bacteria can damage heart, eyes, brain, spinal cord, bones and joints. Can cause miscar-

Disease	Number of cases	Cause	How spread	Symptoms	Diagnosis	Treatment	Effects on babies
			through broken skin on other parts of the body. Untreated infected people (even with mild or no symptoms) can infect others during first two stages of the disease—up to 2 years.	months after exposure. Later symptoms include skin rash over body or on palms of hands and soles of feet and flulike symptoms. All may vanish, but the infection may not, unless treated.	from the chancre		riage or birth defects. Babies acquire the infection in the womb and may develop symptoms later in childhood.
Tricho-moniasis	3 million each year (male/female ratio unavailable)	Trichomonas vaginalis protozoan	Through intercourse	Heavy, yellow-green or gray vaginal discharge, abdominal pain, discomfort during intercourse and painful urination occur within 4–20 days after exposure.	Microscopic examination of vaginal fluid	The drug metronidazole eliminates the parasite	Bladder or urethra inflammation

"We're perfectly comfortable with the idea that we catch the flu or a cold from one another. Yet we squirm at the idea that we might catch a disease when we are being physically intimate with someone. And this discomfort cuts across all levels of society—rich, poor, black, white, highly educated or not."

To prove her point, Dr. Hitchcock often does a little exercise with the many audiences she speaks to about STDs. "These audiences are made up of professionals who deal with STDs and whose job it is to prevent and control the spread of these infections," she points out. "You would expect these people to be the most open about their personal experiences with STDs.

"So first I ask everyone to please raise their hands if they are sexually active. People are comfortable acknowledging this, so almost everyone's hands go up. Then I ask all those who have had a sexually transmitted disease to please keep their hands up. And of course, everyone's hands come down. Only once did a few brave souls keep their hands up. Yet, considering how widespread STDs are in our society, you might expect a significant number of those hands to remain in the air," she says.

PLAYING IT SAFE

This hush-hush attitude is, in large part, responsible for all the confusion and lack of communication concerning these diseases. People know they are out there, but they're too timid to ask how to protect themselves.

But if you had the nerve to ask (and you *should*), this is what you'd be told: Be *very* careful.

Take it for granted that when you're in bed with someone you're not alone, advises Dr. Hitchcock. His partners before you and *their* partners before them all increase your risk of contracting an STD. There's no denying it, the fewer partners you have, the less chance of acquiring an STD, says Dr. Hitchcock.

Careful also means using a condom. In fact, using a condom should be considered an act of caring rather than an act of suspicion, says Dr. Hitchcock. The only people who shouldn't be using condoms are those who have been in a mutually monogamous relationship with an uninfected partner for years. You may want to protect yourself even further by using a diaphragm and spermicide along with a condom. There is some evidence indicating that spermicides that contain nonoxynol-9 may reduce the risk of transmitting some STDs. Keep in mind, though, that having intercourse with an unsafe person is never safe.

BE ON THE LOOKOUT

You should enter any new sexual relationship with your eyes open—literally. Know the signs and symptoms of sexually transmitted diseases, says Dr. Hitchcock. Take note of unusual warts, rashes or sores in the genital area.

Inspect your own body as well. Warts and sores in the genital area, unusual discharge, including bloody discharge, tingling and burning in the vagina and painful intercourse are some of the more obvious symptoms. (See "The Facts and Figures on STDs" on page 000 for more details.) And seek medical help immediately if you suspect that you may have been exposed or infected, even if the symptoms are mild.

You should also have an annual pelvic exam and a Pap smear, even if you have no symptoms, says Dr. Hitchcock. Some sexually transmitted diseases are so subtle that they can be missed, but tests can reveal their presence.

If you discover you have an STD, you should consider it your obligation to notify all your recent sex partners and urge them to get checkups, says Dr. Hitchcock. You should refrain from having sex during treatment.

HERPES AND AIDS: TODAY'S BUG-OFF WORDS

Sexually transmitted diseases caused by bacteria—gonorrhea, chlamydia, syphilis—are completely curable. Those caused by a virus—AIDS, genital herpes and genital warts—are not.

If you contract herpes, you may have five to eight recurrences a year. You will have to abstain from sex during those outbreaks, which run 10 to 14 days. Condoms offer some but not full protection, doctors report, since the virus is transmitted by secretions not only from the genital tract but also from ulcers outside the genital area. What's more, even when signs and symptoms of herpes aren't present, an infected person can be shedding the virus, making disease transmission possible.

Fortunately, the drug acyclovir can eliminate 90 percent of all outbreaks when taken as prescribed, says Dr. Hitchcock. Partly because of acyclovir, herpes is no longer quite the focus of women's anxiety that it once was. Today AIDS stands at that unenviable pinnacle, and the numbers of women infected with the AIDS virus is increasing at a rate greater than for any other group.

The primary mode of transmission to women is sexual intercourse. So unless women are in a long-term, mutually monogamous relationship, experts agree, women simply cannot remain "safe" unless they use condoms. Fear of AIDS is the reason condoms are becoming as common as a comb when it comes to essential carry-along items. Today, women are just as likely to carry them as men.

Unfortunately, not enough men or women are taking this threat seriously. At least that's what the statistics bear out. In one study, 58 percent of college women surveyed said their partners seldom or never used a condom. In another study, only 24.8 percent of the men and 15.6 percent of the women always used a condom during sexual intercourse.

What's worse is that among the 21.3 percent of men and 8.6 percent of women with ten or more partners, regular condom use was reported in only 21 percent and 7.5 percent, respectively.

See also Contraception

CHAPTER 80

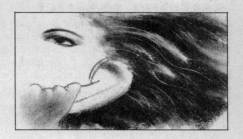

SIBLINGS

THE MAKING OF A
LOVE/HATE RELATIONSHIP

*Y*ou've shared parents, genes, history, sometimes a bedroom and clothes. You've been friends and rivals, co-conspirators and mortal enemies. There are times when you feel as close as Siamese twins, as distant as strangers. You can provoke in one another the most profound love and the most virulent hate.

If you're a sibling—someone's sister—you are in one of the most complex relationships known to human beings.

"It's 'I can't stand you. I hate your guts . . . I love you. You're a part of me,' " says Adele Faber, coauthor with Elaine Mazlish of *Siblings without Rivalry* and *Between Brothers and Sisters*. "It can be a volatile, ambivalent relationship."

In her studies of sibling relationships among adults, University of Indianapolis researcher Victoria Hilkevitch Bedford, Ph.D., found that for most people, the sibling relationship is fraught with expectation, obligation and conflict. Siblings at all ages and with all sorts of relationships believe that they can always rely on one another, although they rarely tap one another for help. Sisters, especially, view breaches and breaks in the relationship as temporary. "When they separate," she says, "they expect to reconnect later, and they do."

BREEDING CONFLICT

Yet Dr. Bedford, who studies same-sex siblings, also found that sisters are more likely to have conflict than brothers, possibly because throughout their lives they are more emotionally involved with one another. "Intimacy breeds conflict," she says.

With few exceptions, siblinghood, not just sisterhood, seems to breed conflict. "People carry scars from their sibling relationships," says Faber, who conducts sibling rivalry workshops for parents across the country. "There are deep hurts that siblings are able to inflict. 'I was the ugly sister; she was the beauty. I was stupid, she was the smart one.' It hurts so deeply. Often we define ourselves in terms of our sibling."

And these first impressions tend to be lasting; we hold onto them and the rivalries of our childhood well into adulthood. "In the workshops I do around the country," says Faber, "I tell everyone in the audience to close their eyes, then I ask, 'How many of you still have some vestiges of sibling rivalry that persist?' The hands slowly, cautiously go up. Then I tell them to open their eyes and look around. They gasp. There are so many hands up, so many people admitting to this secret they hesitated to share even with their eyes closed."

TIME CREATES NEW WOUNDS

Sibs who as children fought over who would sit in the front seat and who Mom liked best, in adulthood wrangle over who makes more money, whose kids are smarter and who's going to take care of Mom. In Dr. Bedford's studies, she found that sisters tended to become embroiled in conflict over inheritances.

Sibs also cross boundaries no one else dares to cross. You will resurrect the most embarrassing moments of each other's lives at the most inopportune times. You will remind each other of who you used to be ("a jerk," "a pig," "a selfish brat") while you fail to see who you have become. You regard no aspect of each other's life as beyond your right to scrutinize and criticize.

"My sister is incredibly tactless," says Karen Spaulding,

48, of her 54-year-old big sister. "I've learned over the years not to take it personally. One time I showed up at her beach house wearing walking sandals. She said, 'What are those orthopedic old-lady sandals you're wearing?' I burst out laughing. I think she wears old-lady clothes, but I wouldn't dream of saying anything. But when we were younger, that kind of thing would make me cry."

Although there's some research evidence that sibling relationships get better as we get older, sometimes even time and reality can't change long-held impressions. Dr. Bedford recalls rushing to the home of a woman in her research study to finally meet the woman's sister, whom she had described vividly as the family beauty. "This was *no* beauty, except in her sister's eyes," says Dr. Bedford. "To me, the sister in my study was the beautiful one. She had a sparkle in her eyes, she was interesting, she had untold talents and approached life with fantastic joy. Her sister was a dull, uninteresting, formerly pretty person."

THE ROOTS OF RIVALRY

It's not hard to track down the roots of sibling rivalry. "It all goes back to the beginning, having to share Mom and Dad's love with each other," says Faber. "On the last plane ride I took, I observed a mother with a baby about 6 or 7 months old and a 3-year-old boy, who was obviously still needful of his mother's attention. The mother was completely absorbed in her baby, singing to him, making him laugh. It was so sweet to watch the quality of loving between them. But the look on the face of this 3-year-old! It was, 'How can you do this? You're *my* mother!' "

Even if your parents were sensitive to your feelings and took judicious efforts to treat everyone in the family equally, siblings may still regard one another as rivals. To a child, writes Faber, a sibling is "a robber of time . . . a stealer of songs, stories and smiles for you alone."

"You don't need parents to foster it," says Faber. "In fact, it's my personal theory that people get married because the vow 'to forsake all others' means 'you're mine. It's what I wanted all my life, a human being that's mine alone!' "

But it's not just the initial rivalry and the scars we bear from childhood that stand between us and friendship with a sibling. Despite the fact that sibs share roughly half of the same genes, we may be no more alike than two strangers on the street, say researchers Judy Dunn and Robert Plomin in their book, *Separate Lives: Why Siblings Are So Different*. Although we may be genetically related, we may be dramatically different people who experience what seems to be a common life in dramatically different ways, screening it through our diverse personalities. Asked to relate the same story from your childhood, you and your siblings would probably sound like characters from the Japanese play *Rashomon*, in which eyewitnesses to a crime give wildly differing accounts.

Faber tells a story about herself as a young girl of 10 waiting eagerly for her much-adored big brother to come home from his job in the city. When he arrived, he asked her to take a walk with him after supper. "It was what I was waiting for—he wanted to talk to me," recalls Faber. But when they had gotten 50 yards from the house, her brother handed her a dime and asked her to cover for him. He was going to meet a girl. "I was devastated. It was my first male rejection," she says. But when, as adults, she brought up the incident, her brother had only a sketchy recollection of it. "It's so typical of siblings," she says. "The single most devastating memory to one isn't remembered at all by the other."

GRAVITATIONAL PULL

Yet no matter how far apart we are, geographically, experientially or psychologically, the sibling bond can be a strong one. We may be drawn together by some kind of emotional gravity.

"I'm so different from my brother and sister," says Faber. "My sister is a pragmatic person, good with numbers. My brother is a businessman. I'm more emotional. It wouldn't appear that there's a close connection between us. Yet one Sunday we decided to visit my father at his nursing home. My brother and sister came to pick me up.

I was about to get into the back of the car when they said, 'No, sit up front with us.' When I slipped into the front seat, I felt so snug, so overwhelmed with how good it felt, how primitively *family* it felt sitting in the car between my brother and sister. There was something physical about it. It was as if my genetic cells were saying, 'Oh happiness, happiness, the family is together again.' "

In her research, Dr. Bedford discovered a few events that seem to help patch up some sibling relationships gone awry. Aging, she says, is "a leveler. As we get older we value family more and feel more obliged to maintain contact." Making a geographical move also seems to remind us of how much we need our sibs. "You lose your neighbors so you begin to rely on your sister. You're on the phone yakking with her."

Although it can have the opposite effect, the death of a parent can bring siblings closer together, particularly if it brings them into closer contact, says Dr. Bedford. "People like each other the more they see each other. Circumstances such as a parent's death that give you more reason for contact helped some of the people in my research group. The emotional aspects of their relationship improved. Often what's not so great about the relationship in the past fades away, as interacting helps you make more contact with the present."

Of course, she says, close contact can also resurrect old hurts. "That former child may be hiding, all the time waiting to sabotage you," she says.

If time hasn't healed those old wounds, says Faber, you have two choices. You can bury them, for the sake of your relationship, or talk out your problems with your sibs.

"Some sibs have to have that long, heartfelt talk," says Faber. " 'I never hated you, I felt jealous.' 'I thought you hated me, that's why I did what I did.' You laugh, cry and then suddenly you're on a new footing."

CHAPTER 81

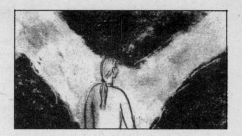

SINGLE LIFE

THIRTYSOMETHING AND ALL ALONE

*J*oanna Russell is 38 and has never been married, a fact that places her in what is becoming one of the least exclusive clubs in America: Single and Living Alone.

According to the U.S. Census, the Family of One has grown by more than 25 percent over the last decade, making it the fastest-growing household type in the United States. There are 23 million of them, and 61 percent are women.

How does it feel to be part of a trend? "It stinks," says Joanna, who lives and owns a business in Washington, D.C., a town of up-and-coming transients who, she says, make the dating scene feel "like you're swimming in a shark tank."

"Actually," she says, "life as a single person can be very full, especially when you've reached an age where you've achieved career fulfillment and some financial security. On one hand, I love the freedom the single life offers. On the other hand, not having a soulmate is terrible. Being single doesn't stink. Trying not to be single stinks."

YOU AND YOUR MARITAL STATUS

Although she says it never bothers her, Joanna says most of her single friends think the rest of the world looks at them judgmentally. "They think that as soon as someone finds out you're single, especially if you're over 30 and have never been married, they think, 'What's wrong with you?' "

In her Manhattan practice, psychiatrist Carol Weiss, M.D., also a clinical assistant professor of psychiatry and public health at Cornell University Medical College in New York City, says this is an attitude common among older singles she sees. "They're embarrassed to be single and sometimes even lie about it. They feel freakish. 'What's wrong with me that I haven't met somebody?' They think they will not be viewed highly by others, that people would respect them more if they had a mate. I don't know whether society really feels that way about them, but that's certainly the way they feel about themselves."

An article in the *New York Times* in February 1991 certainly helps foster this notion. Headlined "Society Looks Askance at Family of One," the article implied that being on the "single track" makes you an also-ran. The article quoted one expert who said that, although there's a greater acceptance today of the single lifestyle, marriage is still perceived as part of the "success ethic" and being single is perceived as "flawed."

Such social values, notes Dr. Weiss, do nothing to help single people feel the way they should about their marital status. "You don't need to be in a relationship to feel like a valid person," she says. In fact, feeling flawed about singlehood may actually reflect a more fundamental problem: low self-esteem. "Not having a mate in and of itself is not a reason to feel freakish," says Dr. Weiss. "If you're feeling that way, it may be a reflection of feelings of inadequacy for some other reason, which need to be explored."

THE KATHARINE HEPBURN ATTITUDE

Support groups—even informal groups, like your single friends—can be very helpful in combating any uncomfortable feelings you have about being single, not to mention offering companionship to battle the loneliness you may sometimes feel. "One of the treatments for alienation is to learn you aren't alone. Once you see other capable, lovely people in the same boat as you, you realize they don't look like freaks, they don't look like 'poor things,' " says Dr. Weiss.

Role models can help, too. One woman says she admired actress Katharine Hepburn, who, after a brief early marriage, has been single her whole life. "I saw you could be happy, successful and loved without a husband," she says.

Some women find role models in their own lives. "When I was in college, I was fascinated by one of my professors who was gorgeous, 30 and not married," says one happily single woman. "She had a beautiful apartment, lots of friends, men falling at her feet and a glamorous life. My life isn't quite so glamorous, but she offered me a viable option if Mr. Right didn't come along. I saw that life didn't start at marriage."

SINGLE-MINDED THINKING

In fact, that's the way many unhappy singles think: Life begins at marriage. And marriage is something that happens to you when you're young. What they fail to see, says Dr. Weiss, is that life is full of interesting, often undreamed-of possibilities.

"Some single women think that the end of their lives are right around the corner if they don't get married soon," says Dr. Weiss. "They worry they're going to end up old and wrinkled and never be attractive enough to find a mate. They can't see ahead into the different life phases that await them. They think the only person who will be interested in them is a 30-year-old single male. They don't realize that as they grow older, they can be attractive to other people in different life stages. They don't realize that not everyone's life runs the traditional course."

Many women are limited by their childhood dreams, which called for a beautiful white wedding to the human equivalent of Prince Charming while they were still young enough not to worry about crow's-feet and gray hair. When it doesn't happen, they put their lives on permanent hold.

"They thought they would be married by the time they

were 30 and when it doesn't happen, then they think that's it, life is over, 'I'm a failure,' " says Dr. Weiss.

But that's narrow-minded thinking, she says. "You need to be able to see diverse ways of living. There is a very full life ahead of you, no matter how it pans out. Whether you remain single forever, whether you get married, or get married and get divorced. There's richness in every aspect of your life. But you become fixated on one way of doing it and see all the rest as darkness. You need to get out and learn how to enjoy yourself and how to enjoy life."

Allison Harvey learned the importance of keeping an open mind. Instead of waiting for marriage to become a homeowner, she bought an old house, which she is renovating. She spends weekends haunting garage sales or at car races. And the man she is seeing isn't the figure of her childhood dreams. For one thing, he's 24 and she's 39.

Allison says she turned down two marriage proposals before she was 30 because "until I was 35 I was terrified of getting married." But once she decided getting marriage seemed like a good idea, all of the marriageable men her age had disappeared. So she expanded her horizons to include younger men.

"The truth is, I thought he was older and he thought I was younger, but the age difference isn't much of a problem," she says. "We do have an experience difference, but that has made it very interesting."

THE LAW OF DIMINISHING DATES

Like Joanna Russell, many single women say the worst thing about being single is dating. "How many frogs do you have to kiss before you discover the Prince?" Joanna jokes. Psychologist Marion Frank, Ph.D., says many of the single women she sees in her private practice in Philadelphia complain the men they meet are "inappropriate."

"As a feminist and a psychologist, I'm afraid I believe there's some truth in that," she says. "As women become more successful careerwise, there are fewer and fewer available men."

Not that there aren't men. But traditionally, women

marry men who are older than they are and men marry younger women. Allison's situation notwithstanding, it rarely works the other way around.

And, says Dr. Frank, men and women *are* different, particularly when it comes to sexuality. While a woman might be proud of her career success and independence, there are a lot of men who find it daunting. Success in a man is sexy; in a woman, it can be a turnoff.

"That means men have a lot of pickings and ours are slim," says Joanna. "There are always younger women around to be infatuated with them. If a man has anything at all going for him, there will always be some younger women around to say, 'Oh, wow!' The older a single woman gets, the less we say, 'Oh, wow!' "

That doesn't mean it's hopeless. "I see some women who get so tired of dating, they feel it's a lost cause and stop," says Dr. Frank. "You need to keep yourself open to possibilities, otherwise it becomes a self-fulfilling prophecy. It's still possible to find a man who will understand and care and will not be intimidated."

CHAPTER
82

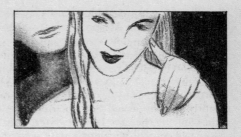

STERILIZATION

CALLING IT QUITS

*Y*ou've talked to your husband, your doctor, your friends. And you've decided that the time for having children has passed. You're moving in other directions, which are going to demand all your time, energy and concentration.

You don't need the monthly am-I-or-am-I-not seesaw swinging through your emotions at just the wrong time, nor do you need the aggravation of remembering to squirt, insert, swallow or otherwise appropriately apply contraception.

So you've decided that either you or your husband should write *finis* across your reproductive lives.

That's pretty much what Suky Webster decided. Suky had grown up the oldest in a dollar-stretching house overflowing with brothers and sisters, and she vividly remembers how her father—who earned a decent income—would moan and groan over how he was going to feed six children. He did manage to do it, she says, but because of the drain six children placed on the family's resources, Suky lacked three things in particular that a child needs: clothes, attention—and love.

By the time she was 28, however, Suky had rectified the situation. As a successful executive, she had more exquisite clothes than many women see in a lifetime and a bank account to match. She was involved with a tight circle of friends and colleagues, and she was practically worshipped by her husband, Aaron.

The only thing that could sabotage the nurturing life Suky had built was a baby. A baby would drain both personal and financial resources, Suky reasoned, and limit her freedom to travel. Suky was not willing to have that happen, nor did she want to deal with the am-I-or-am-I-nots every month. So she asked her doctor to tie off her fallopian tubes and, as she says 14 years later, "put our birth control on cruise control with not a nanosecond of regret."

THE PROCEDURE

Once you and your husband have decided to put childbearing on ice, the next question is *who* should be sent to the freezer?

And that depends. For a man, the procedure—a vasectomy—is a safe, simple, minor operation that takes 15 minutes in a doctor's office under local anesthesia. The surgeon either makes a tiny incision or puncture through the scrotum, reaches in with an instrument and cuts and seals the vas deferens—the narrow tube through which sperm travel to the testes. The sealed vas deferens no longer lets the sperm cells reach the ejaculate. Sperm cells made by the testicles are harmlessly reabsorbed by the body. A man should not notice any difference in the amount or appearance of his ejaculate.

On the other hand, the procedure for a woman is a lot more complicated. Tubal sterilization involves blocking the fallopian tubes that carry an egg from the ovaries to the uterus. It usually means an operation, done under sedation and local anethesia, during which a small incision is made in the abdomen. The surgeon inserts an instrument called a laparoscope that allows him to see, sever and tie off the fallopian tubes.

The "tying" is done with absorbable sutures, rings or clips, although occasionally the ends of the tubes are cauterized. Once in a while the operation is performed through the vagina.

The most common time for female sterilization is within

48 hours of giving birth. About 40 percent are done at that time, doctors report, largely because it's convenient and the surgery is technically simpler.

WEIGH THE EVIDENCE

Both vasectomies and tubals are highly effective, which is probably why sterilization is the most popular contraceptive method among married couples. The pregnancy rate is 0.2 percent with a vasectomy, 0.5 percent with a tubal.

But how do they affect your health? For women, complications from voluntary sterilization surgery occur in less than 1 percent of cases, doctors report. Fatality rates are about 3 per 100,000, so the operation itself is considered relatively safe by professionals. One major long-term physical complication is a higher risk of ectopic pregnancy.

Vasectomy is even safer, with less chance of serious complications. Mortality is rare—one in 300,000 procedures—as are complications, such as infection or bleeding. As many as two-thirds of all men who have a vasectomy develop sperm antibodies, but there's no evidence that this has any adverse effects. There is some evidence, in fact, that a woman whose husband has had a vasectomy is protected against cervical cancer.

IS IT REVERSIBLE?

Although doctors encourage men and women to think of sterilization as a permanent decision, on occasion the procedure can be reversed. About half of those men who have had vasectomies reversed do go on to impregnate their wives, doctors report, but most of those who had their vas unclipped did so within ten years of the initial procedure. After that, the success rate drops off dramatically, partly because a vasectomy tends to lead to decreased sperm counts.

Some surgeons have bragged about pregnancy rates as high as 60 to 80 percent in women who have had tubes reconnected, but most experts believe that typical numbers are much lower. The reversal operation is a tricky piece of microsurgery—under general anesthesia—to rejoin the severed ends of the fallopian tubes. It is a much riskier operation than the sterilization procedure itself.

HOW DO YOU REALLY FEEL?

Before you make a decision, you should know that of those who have undergone sterilization, some women regret the decision. So the most important task for anyone contemplating the procedure is to take some time and find out how you really feel about permanently ending your reproductive ability.

The following questions developed by researchers at the University of Texas Health Science Center in San Antonio and the Transactional Research Institute in Palo Alto, California, can help clarify some of the issues involved and evaluate the emotional impact such a decision will have on your life.

Does your husband want this more than you do? In one study, women whose husbands wanted sterilization more than they did were more likely to be uncomfortable with the decision to be sterilized.

Are you feeling social pressure to be sterilized or not to be sterilized? In one study, women who felt pressured either way were the most likely to regret their decision.

Have you reached your ideal family size? The smaller a woman's ideal family size, according to researchers, the more certain she was that she was making the right decision. If you have two but think four is the ideal family size, you may have mixed feelings. Couples who decided to be sterilized because they thought their families were big enough were more likely to be comfortable with their decision.

Have you considered your decision for a long time, or is it based on a recent experience? Researchers found that the longer a couple considered their decision, the more certain they were that they were doing the right thing. The more they based their decision on a recent experience— such as a health problem during pregnancy—the more uncertain they were.

Is this a decision you and your husband made together? A decision made exclusively by one spouse can leave the other feeling uncomfortable, according to one study. It also found that women who had argued with their husbands over the decision—or who simply had a contentious relationship with them to begin with—were also uncomfortable with the decision once it was made.

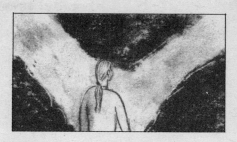

SUPERWOMAN SYNDROME

IS HAVING IT ALL WORTH IT ALL?

When Marjorie Hansen Shaevitz wrote *The Superwoman Syndrome* in 1984, hundreds of women flocked to her workshops to find out how they could have it all. But six years later, something changed. "The woman of the 1980s wanted to have it all," says Shaevitz, a marriage and family counselor in La Jolla, California. "The woman of the 1990s has just had it."

What happened in those half-dozen years? It's quite simple. Reality set in. Today, women who envisioned themselves in tailored suits carrying a briefcase in one hand and a baby in the other have learned the valuable lesson of experience: What is possible is not always easy. "In real life, having it all means being it all, means doing it all," says one executive, the mother of a rambunctious toddler. "And, believe me, it's exhausting."

Janet Loeb, 38, went back to her publishing job when her son was 4 months old. She says she was ill-prepared for Superwomanhood, an image she, like most women, gleaned from the media. Movies like *Baby Boom*, in which single mother Diane Keaton raised a daughter while simultaneously launching a multimillion dollar baby food company, and ads showing executive women bringing home the bacon and cooking it, too, are "the untouchable fantasies," Shaevitz, of the Institute of Family and Work Relationships, says. Such images contribute to a woman's sense that having it all is a cinch.

BACK TO REALITY

"It all looked so easy," says Janet. "You had this great career, you had this great baby and you had this great caregiver who tended to his every need while she taught him to speak French. Nobody talked about what it would be like to go to high-level meetings on 4 hours' sleep because your great baby didn't know night from day. Do you know how brilliant you can be on 4 hours' sleep? You're lucky if you remember you name. I had a great caregiver, but nobody talked about what it was like to be away from your baby 8 hours a day. To hand him over to someone else, however wonderful, was a wrenching experience. All I kept thinking to myself was, 'Why didn't anybody tell me?'"

In her book, *Sequencing*—which promised women could have it all, but not all at once—Arlene Rossen Cardozo turned her introduction into an obituary. The Death of Superwoman, she called it. Joining the funeral cortege was San Francisco-based public relations executive Carol Orsborn, founder of Superwomen's Anonymous, a self-help group for refugees from the fast track, and author of *Enough Is Enough: Exploding the Myth of Having It All*.

But if Superwoman is dead, where was she born? Cardozo, an authority on women's issues, says Superwoman sprang full-blown from the women's movement, which, in its campaign to liberate women from home and hearth in the 1960s and 1970s, assured women they could have children and careers, too. "They told us we could do it all," observes Janet. "They just didn't tell us how to do it."

THE POSITIVE SIDE: SUPERMOM, SUPER HAPPY

That's not to say all Superwomen are unhappy. "There's nothing inherently wrong with wanting it all," says Shaevitz. On the contrary, a number of studies show that women who combine family and career—what the researchers call multiple roles—are happier and healthier than traditional housewives. "Although people with multiple roles have a lot of different demands, they're able to cope better, perhaps because of the satisfaction they're getting from work," says Sharon A. Lobel, Ph.D., assistant professor of management at the Albers School of Business and Economics at Seattle University.

One of the benefits of having a family and working outside the home are greater opportunities for fulfillment and enhancing self-esteem. You run a big risk, as the old cliché goes, when you have all your eggs in one basket. When your child throws a tantrum in a supermarket, you may be less likely to think of yourself as a worthless human being if you've just been made sales manager. Conversely, a bad day at work can be soothed by a heart-melting "I love you, Mommy."

Dr. Lobel, who combines her career with marriage to a physician and raising a 4-year-old son, says she never has to ask herself, "What's my purpose in life?"

"There are so many answers—maybe too many," she says, laughing. "But having a lot of different ways to fulfill myself is better than not having a sense of self-worth."

Also, there's a big psychological payoff for "doing it all." When it works, you get to take the credit. But when it doesn't, you're like the juggler spinning plates on poles. When one plate tumbles, they all go.

SUPER STRESS

Many women are coming to the new realization that they have limits, says Dr. Lobel. "Probably we can handle two intense roles fairly well, perhaps parenting and one other, but we need to realize that other things are going to suffer."

For some women, juggling career, home and children means they cut back—on housework, on their relationships with their husbands, or frequently, on themselves. Shaevitz, who counsels working women, says the women she sees exhibit a plethora of physical and psychological stress symptoms, from irritability to ulcers, from disinterest in sex to insomnia. "The most frequent complaint I hear is insomnia. Sleep disturbances among American women are so rampant as to be epidemic," she says.

In fact, a study by the University of Washington's Marcia Killien, R.N., Ph.D., and Marie Annette Brown, R.N., Ph.D., noted that many women deliberately cut down on their sleep in order to get more things done or, perhaps more important, to get some time alone. Many working women regard lack of personal time as a prime stress factor in their lives, studies have shown. "Without some time to yourself," says Janet Loeb, "you never recharge."

(The Killien/Brown study also pinpointed which women are the "most hassled" on a daily basis: married working mothers. At the top of the "hassle" hit parade are physical and emotional symptoms, children's behavior and transportation problems, with work-related problems coming in dead last.)

Part of the problem for women is that they are, in effect, doing two full-time jobs, both demanding. The women's movement intended to offer us choices, but the term *choice* implies either/or. Today, it's not a matter of career *or* motherhood, accounting *or* vacuuming. Women are expected to do it *all*—and they're starting to question why.

DOUBLE DUTY AND DISINTEREST

In her landmark book *The Second Shift*, Berkeley professor Arlie Hochschild, herself a dual-career parent, found to no one's surprise that married women who work also do the bulk of the housework. Thus, they work a "second shift." Although studies show that more men are pitching in on the homefront, it's usually to take over some of the more social and rewarding jobs such as bathing or entertaining the kids.

Hochschild says that both women and men tend to see this double duty as the woman's problem, although the impact on men is undeniable. A woman working a double shift is tired, and fatigue makes for estranged bedfellows. Disinterest in sex can just as likely be the result of resentment, too, and there may be a significant amount of marital tension in a household where a working woman never stops working.

There are studies that show a husband's lack of involvement in household tasks and child care has led to divorce or at least thoughts of divorce. In one study, the researchers were able to quantify the effect of the husband's household help on his wife's satisfaction with their marriage. They found that for each household task a man performed at least half the time, his wife was about 3 percent less likely to think about divorcing him.

IRREPLACEABLE YOU

Even when men do help, the woman is just as likely to still think she's responsible for it all—meaning she's always on call. As Shaevitz points out, while contraception has made motherhood voluntary, the actual job description hasn't changed. Many women still expect to be responsible for the same functions their mothers were—in the audience of the school play, driving the car pool, making and keeping doctors' appointments—while, unlike their mothers, holding jobs outside the home.

Women, Shaevitz points out, have grown up "other-oriented," feeling compelled to fulfill the needs of the other people in their lives, often at the sacrifice of their own. The impulse comes naturally. After all, most of us were raised by women who were probably the last to sit down to dinner, the last to go to bed, the last to get a new winter coat.

Women are also the keepers of family traditions—who else remembers birthdays and anniversaries?—and the managers of the household even when their spouses and children "help out." Mothers tend to be the hub of the family, prompting one T-shirt manufacturer to note on one popular product, "When Mama ain't happy, ain't nobody happy."

But is caring for others so bad? No, says researcher Nancy Fugate Woods, R.N., Ph.D., of the University of Washington. In fact, for most women, it is a nurturing source of pleasure. It's what makes life worth living. But caring is not without its costs, including burden, conflict and guilt. Burden occurs when the caring person is overwhelmed, notes Dr. Woods.

The fact is, the only Superwoman who may be dead is the one who died of exhaustion. Notes Shaevitz: She is "the woman who is trying to be everything to everybody and denies her own needs."

HAVING IT ALL MADE EASIER

"Some things have to go if you're trying to combine a career with home life," says Dr. Lobel. "You may say, 'well, we can't afford hired help' or 'I can't impose on someone.' Decide what you *can* afford and whom you can impose on and do just that. The idea of being a Superwoman is workable, if you have support."

Depending on the size of your home, it may cost you as little as $25 a week to have a cleaning service help you keep up with the dust. "We have lived in the same place for six years and have never mowed our lawn," brags Janet. "A retired man in our neighborhood does yard work for extra income and he only charges us $12. It's worth it. It's one less thing we have to do."

Don't look at hiring help as wasted money; look at it as buying time.

Women, especially working women, have a tough time asking for help, largely, says Shaevitz, because they don't have the time to reciprocate. But friends and family might be happy to pitch in—if you'd only ask.

"When I was working on a nine-month project at home, I needed someone to watch my son one day a week, but I couldn't afford a babysitter," says Janet. "I got up my courage and asked my aunt if she'd be willing. Not only was she willing, she was thrilled. It turned out to be the highlight of her week."

There's no reason your spouse and children can't make some contribution to the running of the household. Dr. Lobel suggests that you make it clear to the rest of the family "what you really need." Shaevitz goes a step further. Become the household manager, she says. Like any manager, you'll set goals, organize household activities and delegate tasks. It will help if you eliminate some tasks that aren't absolutely necessary ("When in doubt, dump it,"

SUPERWOMEN ANONYMOUS: ONE REFORMER'S STORY

Susan Ashton is a freelance writer, married to an attorney, who calls herself a reformed Superwoman.

"When I had one child, I really could do it all and, in fact, I was pretty smug about it," she confesses. "When my son was born, that all changed. I got 'second childitis.' I was working full-time, caring for a 3-year-old and an infant and commuting an hour each way to work. It wasn't just that I couldn't do it all. I didn't have time to do anything."

Susan solved at least part of her problem by following some advice that counselors like Marjorie Hansen Shaevitz, author and family and marriage counselor in California, give to other recovering Superwomen. She asked herself, "What is essential? Who is important?"

Once she came to terms with these feelings, she was able to winnow out of her life the things that were dragging her down. In doing so, she warns, you've got to be ready to make some sacrifices.

In Susan's case, both she and her husband felt their relationship and their children were more important to them than the annual vacations and gift blitzes at Christmas that their considerable salaries bought them. So they both quit their full-time jobs to work part-time, sharing child care and household duties equally.

"The chief benefit is that our children have finally realized that they have both Mom and Dad as resources," says Susan, who admits the solution has its own problems. "To have less money and not be able to afford to do leisure things now that we have leisure time is one big problem," she laughs. "But you do find out how to do leisure things without spending a lot of money. And when you read all those articles ruminating about the real meaning of Christmas, that it's not all in big gifts, you can say, 'Yeah, that's right!' It fits in perfectly with our plan because we have no money."

The Ashtons have not found it easy to lower their expectations or their standards. When vacation time rolls around, Susan says, "it's hard to settle for day trips when you're used to two weeks in the sun."

For some families, accumulation has become a way of life. But the trappings of success—the big house, the emblem cars, the Ivy League preschools—have a price. There's always a trade-off.

The Ashtons saw the toll their previous lifestyle was exacting: no time for the kids, no time for each other. "I've finally concluded there's no easy way to do it," says Susan. "You've simply got to decide what you can live with and what you can live without. If financial security means a lot to you, then you stay in your job. If being with your children means a lot to you, then you stay home if it's a financial option. You find your own solution. What we're doing is rough, but I've just accepted that it's going to be rough. You just have to find the least-rough way for you personally."

says Shaevitz) and set a time limit for ordinary chores and errands.

What if someone says no? It happens. Simply make it worth their while. Point out that the more people who pitch in, the quicker the job gets done and the more time you'll all have to spend together pleasurably, says Shaevitz.

Are you still responsible? Yes, that hasn't changed. But you may be less busy.

"I" IS IMPORTANT, TOO

One of the biggest reasons you need help around the house is because it gives you time to take care of yourself. When you establish your priorities, make sure one of the "important" people in your life is you, says Shaevitz. "Don't think you're being selfish," she says. "You've been selfless for too long." Many women pay so little attention to their own needs, she says, that the only way they feel they can legitimately rest or ask to be cared for is by getting sick. "But why wait until you get ill?" she says. "Give yourself permission to take care of yourself. It's in your best interest and that of your family."

Take some time off. Pencil yourself in. Schedule a pleasurable activity for yourself a couple of times a week, be it a bubble bath or a dinner out with a friend. Don't forget to schedule in some open time for doing nothing.

THE 2 FACES OF SUPERMOM

You don't have to work outside the home to be Superwoman. You may simply go by another name: Supermom.

Marjorie Hansen Shaevitz, family and marriage counselor in California, sees two distinct varieties of these Type-A moms. Supermom Number One may have worked at one time and, although she's home, she hasn't given up her well-stoked ambition. Life is still run by her file organizer. There's the PTA Monday night, Junior League Tuesday morning, ballet lessons and soccer for the kids a couple of nights a week and Jazzercize for her on Wednesday night. Most nights she's on the phone organizing charity bazaars or school programs. This Supermom is a victim of the continued devaluation of "women's work."

"Most women won't admit it, but they feel they must do these things because they don't work outside the home," says Shaevitz, author of *The Superwoman Syndrome*. "They feel they need to justify their existence."

Supermom Number Two is what Shaevitz calls the Everything-from-Scratch Mom. She's as chained to the kitchen or her sewing basket as any pioneer woman, whipping up homemade bread and soups and Halloween costumes in a frenzy of domesticity.

Although they express it differently, both versions of Supermom are struggling with low self-esteem, says Shaevitz. "When you're employed, your weekly paycheck is a testament to your worth. When you're not employed outside the home, you need to find other sources of self-esteem. You need to do something that makes you feel useful, that taps the energy and talents you have."

She suggests avoiding the shotgun approach of these Supermoms whose energy is dissipated over a wide range of activities. Don't try to do everything. Pick your shots. Do the things that "give you a sense of satisfaction and peace," Shaevitz says.

Like mothers who work outside the home, stay-at-home moms need a few hours to themselves in order to recharge their energy. "We tend to give out energy until we reach the point of exhaustion or illness," says Shaevitz. "When you take a look at healthy people, they have an array of special things that help them feel balanced."

Kathy Scott reads. "Everything. Mysteries, biographies. I

do it during my kids' naps or after they go to bed, instead of watching TV. I feel like it keeps my mind sharp in a way having tea parties with my daughter or playing Legos with my son doesn't. Not that I don't enjoy playing with the kids, but a steady diet of that turns your brain to strained plums."

If reading isn't your secret pleasure, decide what is, even if you have to grope in the back of your mind for what you used to do BB—before baby. "Some women like gardening, others like to cook, some enjoy art," says Shaevitz. "Do something that makes you feel good."

Pay special attention to your marriage or significant relationship. There's a subset of Supermom who hasn't given up her version of the having-it-all fantasy. She and her spouse want it all—the house, the cars, the vacations—and they're trying to do it on one salary. That often means long hours away from home for the working husband—and long hours at home alone for the wife.

The key word here is time. "Successful marriages involve three kinds of time—time to have fun together, time to talk with one another and time to be sexual with one another," says Shaevitz. Ask yourself where you put your marriage on this list of priorities.

"Sure, I'd love to have a big house and all the conveniences," says Kathy, who, with her engineer husband and two children, lives in a three-bedroom townhouse on a quiet suburban cul-de-sac. "But when we decided that I would stay home with the kids, we sat down and drew up a budget that would enable us to live comfortably with time and money left over to enjoy ourselves. Rob and I both wanted our kids to be at home with a parent and not in day care, but we weren't going to accomplish our goal at the expense of our marriage. Our relationship came first—and it still does. Without it, everything else falls apart."

You can also take some of the load off if you lower your expectations. Forget trying to be "a 10 in everything," says Dr. Lobel. Perfectionism is the antecedent of failure. Unfortunately, women have been convinced—by their upbringing and some realities of the marketplace—that good enough isn't good enough. They believe they need to be perfect.

Women, taught to "look for needs and fill them," may feel they can win the approval they desire by being perfect, says Shaevitz. The solution, she says, is not to look to others for approval. "If you don't meet your own needs directly, you become dependent on others for positive feedback. You need to take responsibility for your own life."

WORK: DOUBLE STRUGGLE

At work, says Dr. Lobel, women have learned that "they have to do 150 percent to be considered average. Studies have shown that women get fewer promotions and lower salary increases than men even though they're getting the same perfect ratings, so there are less returns for a good performance."

In fact, a study comparing working men and working women found that women tend to have higher standards for themselves than men. They also feel so stressed trying to meet those standards they are more likely to suffer physical symptoms and seek help from a mental health professional.

There's some evidence that the atmosphere of the workplace is changing—slowly. There are, however, ways to help speed it up.

ENLIGHTEN YOUR EMPLOYER

One of the biggest stresses on women in multiple roles is the dissonance between working women and motherhood. Being Mommy is quite different from being Manager. But even that seems to be changing.

"We're just starting to read and hear about how people are now applying parenting skills to the workplace," says Dr. Lobel. "I'd like to see a lot more of that happening. You get a lot of basics with a 2- or 3-year-old: patience, good listening and people skills. One executive interviewed said he learned from raising five kids that it's better to get cooperation from his employees by fostering mutual respect than by giving orders. As another manager put it, 'Counting to 10 works everywhere.'"

If your employer needs to become a little more parent-friendly, offer to provide supporting evidence that programs like on-site or company-supported day care, maternity/paternity leave and flexible hours are in the best interest of both the company and its employees. There is some evidence that companies that offer good work and family programs have a competitive edge in attracting and retaining working mothers.

POSTPONING IT ALL

If you have already met some of your career goals and are financially able, you may want to consider taking a career break.

Arlene Rossen Cardozo calls it sequencing, a way to have it all, but not all at once. Simply put, you take a brief vacation—one, two, even five years—to be with your children when they are young, then reenter the job market. This is an option that's probably best done if you already have a fairly impressive résumé. You don't want any regrets—and you want to jump back into your career with some ease.

Carol Marden became president of a marketing research firm at the age of 33. She became a first-time mother a year later. Married to another marketing executive, she and her husband had a commuter marriage for a year. "Every weekend, the baby, the au pair we hired to care for the baby and I would drive to Baltimore from Philadelphia to be with my husband," she explains. "We had a rather nice income, but our lives were hectic."

But she wasn't willing to give it up then. "My career was still a priority at the time," she explains. "I have a Master of Business Administration and it was a goal of mine to become president or CEO of a company. Fortunately, I reached my goal early. That was one of the reasons I was able to leave it after our second son was born. I wasn't on the verge of getting something I always wanted. I had it."

Her role model, she says, was Supreme Court Justice Sandra Day O'Connor, who took a five-year hiatus from her career when her children were young to be a full-time mother.

"She didn't do so badly taking time off, so I thought it might work for me," says Carol. "I have 20 or 30 more years of work left. In 5 years, I think some employer might be interested in a 40-year-old former company president with an MBA."

WORTH MORE THAN MONEY

Taking a hiatus from a successful career is a gamble, of course. In some professions, a five-year absence can leave your skills rusty or even outdated. That's easily remedied by keeping up with the latest technology and trends by reading professional journals or taking occasional courses, or perhaps doing consulting or volunteer work in your profession as well as keeping in touch with former coworkers.

There's also a sacrifice. You'll be going from two salaries to one. You may want to make your big purchases—the house, the car, the essential furniture—well in advance of your leave-taking. That's what the Mardens did. Their advance planning allowed them to continue to live comfortably in a nice house they could afford on one salary with enough left over to enjoy a few simple pleasures.

But the real pleasure, says Carol, is being able "to sit down as a family every night at dinner. That's worth more than what money could buy us. The truth is, I have it all *now*."

See also Dual Careers, Housework

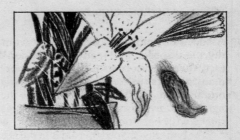

THYROID PROBLEMS

ENERGY REGULATION ON THE FRITZ

Connie Kriegler was sick for two years before doctors could finally point to an underactive thyroid—hypothyroidism—as the source of her numerous symptoms. "Through the whole ordeal," says the 61-year-old respiratory therapist, "and as miserable as I was, it hurt worst of all that the doctors thought my complaints were completely in my head. What did they think, that I waited until I was 59 years old to become a hypochondriac? Did they think I suddenly discovered that being sick was fun?"

Majorie Chase, on the other hand, discovered she had an overactive thyroid—hyperthyroidism—almost by accident. "I'm an insulin-dependent diabetic and had just walked into my endocrinologist's office for a checkup, when the secretary noticed the change in my appearance," says Marjorie, a 37-year-old saleswoman. "Suddenly, I realized she was right. My eyes had been looking kind of bulgy, and I had lost about 15 pounds, although I wasn't dieting. Since the secretary often sees patients come into the office with these symptoms, she made the diagnosis before the doctor had a chance to—Graves' disease." Graves' disease is the most common form of hyperthyroidism.

THE THYROID SNAFU

When it comes to thyroid problems, Connie and Marjorie have lots of company. According to the American Thyroid

Association, millions of American women suffer from a thyroid disorder, and many of them don't even know it. In fact, thyroid disorders occur much more often than even many doctors realize. They're particularly common among middle-aged and older women, where they often go unrecognized or are mistaken for something else. Connie's experience with her doctors, unfortunately, was not unusual.

The butterfly-shaped thyroid is in the neck, its two "wings" wrapped around the windpipe just below the Adam's apple. This vitally important gland normally weighs less than an ounce, but it can have an enormous impact on your health. Think of it as the body's metabolism regulator. It does the job by releasing two hormones, most of which is the iodine-containing hormone thyroxine. The hormones help regulate your heartbeat, body temperature, the smooth working of your muscles, how quickly you burn calories, how swiftly food moves through the digestive tract and more.

Normally, the thyroid doles out just the right amount of hormone to keep these processes humming smoothly. But, as in Marjorie's case, it may turn overactive and pump out too much hormone. Or, as in Connie's case, it may become underactive and pump out too little. Either way, the abnormal hormone level can profoundly affect the body's metabolism, either slowing it way down, or speeding it way up.

Most thyroid problems—involving either overactive or underactive glands—are caused by an autoimmune reaction. Normally the immune system functions to defend the body from invading microbes. In an autoimmune reaction, however, the immune system unaccountably turns against the body itself and goes on the attack.

In the case of hypothyroidism, the immune system produces antibodies that attack and damage thyroid cells, progressively reducing the thyroid's hormone output, says Kay McFarland, M.D., an endocrinologist and professor of medicine at the University of South Carolina School of Medicine in Columbia.

In Graves' disease, on the other hand, the antibodies attach to the thyroid cell receptors and stimulate the thyroid to produce excessive amounts of thyroid hormones, explains Dr. McFarland. In both instances serious imbalances in the body's energy regulation system occur. The good news is that both kinds of thyroid problems respond well to treatment once they are diagnosed.

HYPOTHYROIDISM: THE BIG SLOWDOWN

Before Connie's doctor discovered her hypothyroidism, she had experienced just about every symptom. "I was like a textbook case," she says. "My skin was dry, my hair was falling out, I was cold all the time, and I was tired and achy all over. Why none of the doctors I went to couldn't just look at me and see these signs—which I later found out were classic for hypothyroidism—is beyond me."

But hypothyroidism can be difficult to recognize, especially in older people, says Dr. McFarland. "The symptoms are so nonspecific that they could point to any number of possible conditions."

For example, the symptoms closely resemble those of advancing age, which is why hypothyroidism is frequently overlooked by the patient's doctor, according to the American Thyroid Association. In fact, a woman herself is often fooled since the symptoms usually come on gradually over a period of months or years. Thyroid deficiency can cause muscle stiffness, spasm and pain. These symptoms are frequently overlooked by physicians.

A hypothyroid condition can also raise the levels of cholesterol in the blood and thus increase the rate of hardening of the arteries (atherosclerosis), says Dr. McFarland.

That's just what happened to Connie. "I developed a high cholesterol level, chest pains, dizziness, difficulty in breathing and heart palpitations. My heart doctor discovered I had two blocked coronary arteries. I had a procedure called balloon angioplasty to correct it. I was sure that that would be the end of my problems," she says, "but instead, the chest pain and other symptoms continued. It took a tremendous effort to simply get out of bed in the morning. As the months wore on and my symptoms worsened, I thought I was dying."

But she got better.

POSITIVE OUTCOMES

Uncovering hypothyroidism is as easy as doing a few simple blood tests, the most important of which are measuring the level of TSH (thyroid-stimulating hormone) in the blood and the level of thyroxine in the blood. TSH is produced by the pituitary gland and does what its name suggests—stimulates the thyroid to release its hormone. The pituitary sends out TSH in response to the amount of thyroid hormone it senses in the blood. The less thyroid hormone the body produces, the higher the level of TSH circulating in the bloodstream.

When Connie was tested, her TSH level was found to be about seven times higher than normal. She was started immediately on a synthetic thyroid hormone to compensate for the thyroid's diminished output. "After taking just one pill I felt a tremendous difference," says Connie. "In a matter of *hours*, I could feel that my heart had stopped skipping beats, my circulation had improved and the aching stopped."

Physicians agree that there is a spectacular response to treatment. As one doctor put it, "It's like giving insulin to a diabetic, because you're giving the body exactly what it needs."

Doctors at the National Institutes of Health now believe that one in ten women over age 40 has some degree of hypothyroidism. Since women develop the condition four times more often than men, many experts recommend a thyroid examination as part of every gynecological checkup.

HYPERTHYROIDISM: ALL REVVED UP

The diagnosis of an overactive thyroid may be easier than diagnosing hypothyroidism because the symptoms are so obvious.

Picture yourself sitting in a car that's idling quietly in the driveway. If you press your foot on the accelerator the engine idles faster—too fast if the car is just sitting there.

About two million Americans are similarly revved up, and most of them are women aged 30 to 55. Their thyroids pump out excess hormones, which push their metabolisms into overdrive.

By far the most common type of hyperthyroidism is Graves' disease. It produces such diverse symptoms as frequent loose stools, heightened sensitivity to heat, bulging eyes (due to a thickening of certain tissues behind the eyeball), excessive sweating, weight loss, fatigue, muscle weakness, nervousness, irritability, insomnia and hand tremors. Another symptom—a rapidly pounding heart when you're at rest—can be especially serious. It can intensify chest pain in people with heart disease and even cause a heart attack. Left untreated, it can be fatal.

Marjorie Chase says she had experienced most of the symptoms common to the condition by the time it was finally brought under control. "Hardest of all to deal with, however, was the change in my appearance," she admits. "It's one thing to have a disease that no one knows you have. It's quite another to have people look at you and say, 'What's wrong? You look different. Your eyes look funny.'

"What's more, I had to alter my lifestyle. I couldn't do anything that required a lot of walking, and I wasn't able to exercise the way I used to. I was simply too tired, and my heart wasn't able to take it."

COOLING AN OVERACTIVE THYROID

It takes several different types of blood tests to diagnose Graves' disease. There are three different options for treating it: drugs, radioactive iodine and surgery.

Antithyroid drugs are taken not only to stop overproduction of thyroid hormones, but also with the hope that the condition will go into remission. In the majority of adult cases, however, permanent remission does not occur, and the next recourse is radioactive iodine therapy—an "atomic cocktail" taken by mouth. The hormone-producing cells of the thyroid absorb the iodine and are killed by the radioactivity. The result: a decreased secretion of thyroid hormone. If there is a reason not to use radio-iodine therapy, surgery is used to remove part of the thyroid.

It sounds drastic, but radioactive iodine has been a standard treatment for hyperthyroidism for more than 50 years. Medical experts view the treatment as safe—it causes few ill side effects. After treatment, the resulting underfunctioning thyroid gland can be corrected with daily doses of replacement hormone, just as it is for those with hypothyroidism, says Dr. McFarland. In both conditions, treatment involves taking a single, inexpensive pill every day.

Marjorie tried initial treatment—the antithyroid medication. But she had an undesirable reaction to it. She soon moved on to radioactive iodine.

"Before I had the radioactive iodine treatment, I barely had enough energy to go to work," she remembers. "Forget about straightening the house. And I always felt like I was on the verge of breaking—you know, wired, high-strung. After therapy with radioactive iodine, I started to recover immediately. It still took a year or more, though, until the dose of hormone was properly regulated and I felt completely back to normal."

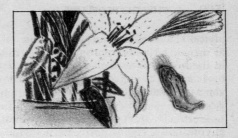

VAGINAL INFECTIONS

GETTING AN EDGE OVER YEAST

"The first time I got a yeast infection I had no idea what it was," says Beth Hyland, a 46-year-old medical secretary. "I was 18 and had just started having sex with my steady boyfriend. I thought it was some kind of punishment from God. When I finally got up the nerve to tell my mother, the itching and burning were so bad that I was in tears. She took me to our family doctor and he immediately diagnosed it as a yeast infection, no doubt brought on by an antibiotic I had just taken for strep throat.

"I was so relieved that its cause was not something sexual in nature that I didn't even complain about the messy cream I had to insert for a week," says Beth.

Yeast infection is not a sexually transmitted disease, although it is *possible* to be infected by a partner. Nor is it a punishment from God. It is, however, a frightfully common torment for an astounding number of women.

Between four and seven million women each year experience the itching, burning and white, cottage-cheese-like discharge that signal a yeast infection. In fact, it's so common that about 75 percent of American women will suffer at least one attack during their childbearing years.

FROM NORMAL TO OVERGROWN

It's no wonder that yeast infection is so universal. The main culprit behind all this itching and burning is *Candida albicans*, a fungus found in everyone to some degree. It's all around us in the environment, it often takes up residence in the human intestinal tract, and researchers have found that at least 20 percent of women carry the yeast in their vaginas. That figure climbs to 40 percent in pregnant women.

Normally, yeast exists in harmony with other organisms in your body, says Dorothy Barbo, M.D., professor of obstetrics and gynecology at the University of New Mexico School of Medicine and medical director of the university's Center for Women's Health in Albuquerque. "But when something comes along that changes the usually acidic environment of the vagina, it can cause the yeast organisms that are already there to grow at an unusual rate," she explains. "It literally takes over, and that's when you get symptoms."

And apparently all kinds of things can happen to trigger that change in the vaginal environment. Often, antibiotics used to treat other infections also eradicate the competing bacteria and other micro-organisms that keep the vagina acidic. The balance is disturbed. The result—a yeast infection. Indeed, "antibiotic use is believed to be one of the most common precipitants of this infection," according to Terry Kriedman, M.D., director of the Obstetrics and Gynecology Department at Chestnut Hill Hospital in Philadelphia.

But that's far from the only cause. Some women are particularly susceptible at the end of each month's menstrual flow, says Dr. Barbo. Low estrogen levels accompanying menopause can trigger vaginal infections, too. So can pregnancy, where the prevalence of a yeast infection is as high as 20 percent toward the end. What's more, women under a great deal of stress, those who use oral contraceptives or corticosteroids and women who have diabetes are also at an increased risk of developing a yeast infection.

Even diet can affect your risk, according to research done by Barbara Reed, M.D., assistant professor in the Department of Family Practice at the University of Michigan. Dr. Reed and her colleagues found in their study of 373 women that those who ate high-calorie diets were more likely to report past vaginal infections than those whose diets were lower in calories.

Marsha Ellis would agree with that. "I noticed that I always came down with a vaginal infection right after a vacation," says the 37-year-old accountant. "One year we had three vacations and I had three vaginal infections. After I thought about it for awhile, it dawned on me that on vacation I tend to pig out on rich, sweet desserts—far more often than I ever would at home. When I cleaned up my vacation eating habits, I stopped getting yeast infections."

SOMETIMES IT'S NOT YEAST

Candida, however, is not the only culprit behind those tormenting symptoms. Both trichomonas and bacterial vaginosis (caused by a *Gardnerella vaginalis*) can mimic the symptoms of a yeast infection, but the treatments for the infections caused by these three organisms are different, says Dr. Barbo. That's one of the reasons you need to let your physician make the initial diagnosis.

Certain chemicals can also cause what appears to be a vaginal infection, says Dr. Barbo. "Some women become allergic to douches or the perfumes or deodorants that they contain," she says. "Occasionally, I've seen women who have developed an allergy to tampons, to latex condoms or to the spermicide that's used with a diaphragm. Although the symptoms may feel like a yeast infection, there is no sign of the fungus upon examination. What you've got then is an inflammation of the vaginal area. Simply eliminating what's triggering the inflamation will often solve the problem."

TREATMENT STRATEGIES

So, when that infernal itching and burning announces the beginning of a possible yeast infection, what do you do?

Take heart. It's easier than ever to counteract an overgrowth of yeast. But first you have to be sure it *is* yeast. If it's your first infection, you should see a doctor to pin down the exact cause of your symptoms. On the other hand, if

REDUCING YOUR RISKS OF REINFECTION

As if yeast infections aren't unpleasant enough, they have a regrettable tendency to pay repeat visits.

Learning what sets off an infection in *your* body is the first step in reducing your chances of getting another one, say the experts. Meanwhile, try these tips to help prevent future attacks.

- Always wear cotton or at least cotton-crotch underwear, which "breathes" by allowing air to circulate.
- Avoid pantyhose or any tight-fitting clothing in the summertime, for the same reason as above.
- Don't sit around in a wet bathing suit for hours at a time. It creates a moist, warm environment that yeast adore.
- Don't overwhelm your body with too many sweets, which can alter the vaginal pH, making it a breeding ground for yeast.
- Try a vinegar-and-water douche to help acidify your vagina. Changing the pH at the first sign of a yeast infection may be enough to stop it in its tracks.
- You might also try a povidone-iodine douche (Betadine Disposable Medicated Douche), which may destroy many yeast organisms. This product is available without a prescription.
- Keep a tube of anti-yeast medication on hand for those times when you must take an antibiotic for another ailment.
- Abstain from sexual intercourse during treatment for a yeast infection.
- Eat a cup of yogurt every day. But not just any yogurt, notes Eileen Hilton, M.D., an infectious disease specialist at Long Island Jewish Medical Center in New Hyde Park, New York. She conducted a study that showed that yogurt that contained active *Lactobacillus acidophilus* cultures reduced the incidence of yeast infections three-fold in women with a history of recurrence. Not all brands of yogurt contain these beneficial organisms. Dannon is one national brand that does. To find out if your favorite brand does, you'll have to call the company. Ask a public- or consumer-relations representative this question: What is the viable count (in cells per gram) of culture in your frozen yogurt? If the answer is 10 to the eighth or ninth power (one billion) cells per gram, you've found an excel-

lent source; 10 to the fifth to seventh powers would be pretty good; below that is poor.

- Dry the genital area thoroughly after showering, bathing or swimming.
- Don't share towels with others. Damp towels can harbor infection.
- Wipe from front to back to keep from transporting anal bacteria into the vagina.
- Avoid products such as bath oils, feminine hygiene sprays and powders, which can irritate the skin around the vulva.
- Keep stress under control, always a good idea, but especially if you notice your infections coincide with particularly stressful events. Deep breathing exercises and meditation may help.

you've had yeast infections many times and are sure you have it again, then treatment is as close as your nearest drugstore. That's because the two most common medicines for yeast—miconazole (Monistat) and clotrimazole (Gyne-Lotrimin)—are both available over-the-counter now. That means that you don't have to wait to get a prescription from your doctor, says Dr. Barbo, and you can start your course of treatment at the first inkling of infection.

Both of these medicines are used for seven days. If you want to try the three-day dose or the newer one-day dose, you'll still have to get a doctor to prescribe it.

"The shorter-duration medicines don't work for everybody," says Dr. Barbo. "For some, medication simply doesn't get rid of enough of the yeast, and infection can recur. Still, it's worth a try, especially if it's your first infection. A cortisone preparation is often prescribed for those with more severe symptoms."

If this is your second or third yeast attack within a few months, however, your sexual partner may need to be treated as well, according to Felicia Stewart, M.D., gynecologist in Sacramento, California, and coauthor of *Understanding Your Body: Every Woman's Guide to Gynecology and Health*. Although this is not a common cause of yeast infection, you can be reinfected by yeast from your partner's mouth or semen, she notes.

CHAPTER 86

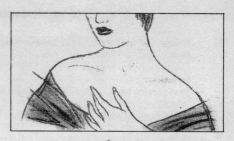

VARICOSE VEINS

MORE THAN SKIN DEEP

Twisted, ropey, knotted, engorged—it's no wonder that women with varicose veins hide their legs beneath tights, slacks or long skirts, no matter how hot the weather.

Forget shorts. "Most of the women who come to me don't own a single pair of shorts," says Deborah Foley, M.D., a staff physician at the Vein Clinics of America in Chicago. "We like to have our patients wear shorts for the examination—we think they'll feel more comfortable than walking around in their underwear—so now we stock disposable shorts at the clinic for those that don't have any of their own to bring along," she says.

Often a woman will put on the shorts and just be horrified by what she sees, says Dr. Foley. "She'll try to cover her legs with her arms as if she were standing there stark naked. I find it helps tremendously to point out the many before and after treatment pictures that we have hanging on the walls of the clinic. No matter how bad you think your legs are, you can see there's someone else who looked as bad or worse than you."

FEELING PAIN AND SHAME

Normally, tiny valves within the veins permit the blood to flow in only one direction. When those valves lose their function, the blood that should be moving upward toward

GET A LEG UP ON TROUBLE

Varicose veins that have been treated are unlikely to reappear, but because this is a chronic progressive disease, it is necessary that you stay on a follow-up program. The tendency to develop new, troublesome veins doesn't go away. It's likely that sometime in the future, veins that are currently normal are likely to become varicosed. "The potential is there," says Deborah Foley, M.D., staff physician at Vein Clinics of America in Chicago. Here's what you can do to help slow the progression of the disease.

- Elevate your feet whenever you can to drain pooled blood.
- Wear compression stockings. They put pressure on the vein walls, which then force the blood from the superficial varicose veins back into the deep veins.
- Get into an exercise program. Walking or swimming are particularly good for increasing circulation in the legs, a sure way to prevent complications such as ulcers.
- Avoid long periods of standing in one place or sitting still. This causes blood to accumulate in the lower legs and puts added pressure on the weakened veins.
- Wear loose-fitting clothes. Tight garments restrict circulation.
- Stretch frequently when taking a long trip, whether in a plane, train or automobile.
- Go on a reducing diet if you are overweight. The heavier you are, the worse it is for your varicose veins.
- Be aware that increased levels of estrogen associated with pregnancy, birth control pills and menstruation can worsen the symptoms of varicose veins.

the heart pools and presses on the surface vein walls, causing them to bulge. The result of this is aching, swollen, heavy and tired legs. And the more you're on your feet, the more aggravating the symptoms get. Some sufferers complain of night cramps.

Interestingly, the size of the varicose vein does not determine the degree of symptoms. Indeed, the veins that look the worst may hurt the least.

"Women often suffer for years with their varicose veins before they seek help," says Dr. Foley. Nancy Strackany, a 42-year-old housewife and mother of five, says that she has always cared about her appearance, but it wasn't until after her third child was born that her varicose veins started to bother her. "That's when I noticed a large, unsightly vein in my pubic area," she says. "That groin vein prevented me from feeling sexy. It was so big that I could even see it through the leotards that I wore for my exercise class. I also had spider veins that had spread over my lower leg and foot, which created an overall bluish tinge to my skin."

Still it wasn't until after the birth of her fifth child that Nancy decided to seek help. By that time the varicose veins had spread to her inner thighs and calves. "There was a lot of pain and pressure, and it became increasingly difficult to stay on my feet for any length of time," she says. "What's more, they were so unsightly. I didn't feel comfortable wearing anything that exposed my legs."

ODDS: 1 OUT OF 5

Seventeen percent of all adults in the United States are plagued with some form of vein disease, with women affected seven times more often than men. "So when you think of your own group of friends, that means about one out of five probably has a significant amount of vein problems, and you may not even know about it," Dr. Foley says. Varicose veins often appear or become more pronounced after a pregnancy. But they can show up in the teen years or even earlier.

Beverly Sedlacek, a 37-year-old secretary, says she first noticed hers at age 12. "I used to dread putting on a bathing suit," she says, "especially after a huge vein developed near my groin. No one ever said anything rude to me, but I could see people looking at my legs. I tried wearing white hose with my skirts, because I though that would camouflage them. But you could still see them bulging through."

IN HARM'S WAY

Unfortunately, there is a prevailing myth that varicose veins are harmless, that the biggest problem is the unsightliness and embarrassment they bring. But this simply isn't so.

Varicose veins are not a normal variance of your anatomy. They are abnormalities with the potential for some very serious medical complications, says Dr. Foley. "Over time varicose veins can become inflamed (a condition known as phlebitis), or they may lead to chronically swollen legs and skin ulcers that never heal. At their worst, blood clots can form in an inflamed vein (called thrombophlebitis), and engorged veins can hemorrhage.

"Our physicians have treated people who suffered with leg ulcers for as long as ten years before seeking help," Dr. Foley says. "One woman had an ulcer that had been open on her leg for years. Do you know how painful that is? She was spending $40 a week in dressings just to keep the drainage from getting on her clothes. And she hadn't been out of her home for two years. How the family got her to us is a miracle. We were able to get the ulcer to close completely. Granted," admits Dr. Foley, "her leg will never look beautiful after what it's been through. But this woman is now able to walk everywhere. She goes to the grocery store and goes out with her grandchildren. She feels that her entire life has been changed."

Even if varicose veins were harmless, Dr. Foley feels that the overwhelming embarrassment they cause is reason enough to warrant treatment. "The one thing I hate to see more than anything else," she says, "is a woman who comes in and apologizes for seeking treatment. She'll say she knows it isn't a serious problem (because that's often the way it's been portrayed by the medical community, believe it or not). People like this actually feel that they don't have the right to have it treated, that it's frivolous. Well, even if their appearance were the *only* reason they sought help, even if they weren't in any pain, they should be able to feel good about having their veins corrected."

PRETTY LEGS AGAIN

For most women treatment of even the largest varicose veins can create legs they don't mind revealing in shorts and miniskirts. What's more, say the experts, all the uncomfortable physical symptoms associated with the condition generally disappear completely following treatment—and that includes eliminating the potential for complications. There are three types of treatment: compression, sclerotherapy and surgery. Sometimes the three methods are used in combination.

COMPRESSION. If you have mild pain and discomfort, and especially if your varicose veins are small, over-the-counter support hose are often enough to achieve comfort. If you have more severe symptoms, your doctor might prescribe individually tailored hose of light to medium compression. These compression stockings generally improve symptoms, reduce the risk of thrombosis and can be used indefinitely.

SCLEROTHERAPY. Probably the treatment of choice today, it's the nonsurgical alternative to "vein-stripping" surgery. Today, sclerotherapy can be performed even on the largest varicose veins, says Dr. Foley. A special solution is injected into the vein, irritating it to the point where it shrivels up and closes off. On large veins and even on smaller spider veins, the effect is quite dramatic.

Beverly says she went to eight treatment sessions over a period of six months per leg to achieve her final results. Each treatment session consisted of multiple injections. "It hurt a bit the first time, probably because I was scared. But once I knew the outcome, I looked forward to each treatment. The veins practically disappeared before my eyes. There was a little bruising, which cleared up in no time. The best thing with this treatment," says Beverly, "is that you're on your feet right away. In fact, part of the program is that you must walk 3 miles every day." Walking is important for the circulation, explains Dr. Foley, and helps keep the veinous system healthy.

Nancy Strackany had sclerotherapy, too, and says she noticed an 80 percent improvement in the looks of her legs even before her treatments were complete. "It's a long procedure," she points out. "You have to be willing to go back for treatments for several months and to wear the compression stockings during recovery. But it's worth it. It's not painful and there's no recuperation period. I'm a very busy person, on my feet a lot. Even before the treatments were complete, I found my legs could already keep up with the rest of me. At the end of the day, they still felt just fine." Strackany reports that her ugly groin vein is almost completely gone. She's wearing shorts again.

SURGERY. Once the procedure of choice for severe problems, surgery is far less popular today. Incisions are made at the top and bottom of the leg and the large varicose vein is literally "stripped," or pulled out of the leg. It requires general or regional anesthesia, a hospital stay of a day or two and a few weeks' recovery time. Surgery can eliminate the large ropey vein, but usually leaves small scars at the ankle and upper medial thigh.

One woman who had her varicose veins removed surgically felt that the pain, scarring and time off from work were real disadvantages. Three years later, when she needed treatment again, she opted for sclerotherapy with a much better outcome.

CHAPTER
87

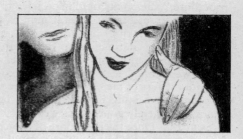

VIRGINITY

ALL YOU NEED IS LOVE

*I*t was a conscious decision," says Sarah Gold, recalling the first time she had sex at age 17. Sarah admits she was more curious than in love.

"I wasn't even aroused at the time. The boy was someone I had known for a long time and had been dating, but he wasn't the love of my life. We'd make out but always stop short of sex because he knew I was a virgin.

"Afterward, I remember walking into my house thinking I should feel different somehow. That it should feel like a tremendous occasion. But all I felt was empty, even a little ashamed. The whole thing was a disappointment."

That was ten years ago—and very typical of the way a girl might feel after her first sexual encounter. But what was typical ten years ago was also typical ten years before that. And it's also typical today, according to Lillian B. Rubin, Ph.D., author of *Erotic Wars: What Happened to the Sexual Revolution?* and senior research associate at the University of California in Berkeley. While social mores and attitudes about having sex have greatly changed over the last generation, feelings about having sex for the first time haven't. Losing their virginity is, always has been and probably always will be an unsettling experience for most girls.

IS THAT ALL THERE IS?

These are some of the words girls have used to describe lovemaking after just one experience: Overrated. Disappointing. A waste. Just awful. Boring. Stupid. Empty. Ridiculous. Awkward. Miserable. Unmemorable. Those are mighty depressing words for describing the event that's supposed to make the world go round! So what goes wrong?

Experts say it's normal to think about having sex and wonder what it's like. But having sex too young, before you're emotionally ready, can be disappointing. In Dr. Rubin's survey, those who found it rewarding—who could speak positively about it—were girls who almost always shared it with someone they cared about a great deal. Often this someone was older and more experienced.

Unfortunately, notes Dr. Rubin, some teenagers think that sex the first time is what sex will be like all the time—an impression that can make it harder for them to develop a good sexual relationship when they are older.

NO, NO, NOT YET

Teenagers need to consider some important issues before they make the decision to have sex. Will you disappoint your family, friends, and most of all, yourself? Will you compromise your values? Will you feel guilty? In effect, you really have to be able to handle the variety of emotions "giving in" for the first time brings. Some know they can't. So they don't.

Laura Pinto, a 24-year-old graduate student, says that when she was 17 she "refused to have sex with the biggest hunk" she ever dated. Although she was extremely attracted to him, she sensed he was only interested in her for sex, not a real relationship. "I knew having sex with him would have made me feel cheap," she says. "I wanted sex to be the extra bonus to a loving relationship. So I said no. The funny thing is, it's many years since that happened and we're still in touch, still friends."

BABES IN BOYLAND

Just like their mothers and their mothers before, the teens of the 1990s may be finding sex a little disappointing the first time—but they're finding it out sooner.

A survey conducted by the Centers for Disease Control of teenage girls between the ages of 15 to 19 found that 51.5 percent were no longer virgins, nearly double the 28.6 percent reported in 1970—around the time their mothers were the same age.

Another study, reported in *Family Planning Perspectives*, showed that even younger kids are losing their virginity almost as frequently. This survey of 14-year-olds, who were from three rural counties in Maryland, revealed that 47 percent of the girls (and 61 percent of the boys) had already experienced sex.

Before you take these numbers at face value, consider this. While statistics may not lie, "they often leave us with a distorted version of the truth," states Dr. Rubin. Yes, these kids have had sex, but for many it did not make them sexually active. In fact, after trying it, many decided that once was enough—for a while. Sarah Gold, for example, says that it was two years before she had sex again after her first experience. "I don't regret what I did," she says. "I just felt it had been too early for me. When I had sex again, it was for the right reason. I was head over heels in love with someone who felt the same way about me."

A MOTHER'S PERSPECTIVE

If you're a mother of a teenage daughter, statistics such as these can be a little startling—even if they are not surprising. So how do you handle a subject your mother may not have handled very well where you were concerned—or more likely may not have handled at all?

"Most people today understand that the insistence on celibacy before marriage is little more than a nostalgic dream," says Dr. Rubin. But it's not unnatural for mothers—even those who lived through and dabbled in the Sexual Revolution—to feel some discomfort at the thought of their own daughter's impending sexuality, says Lonnie Barbach, Ph.D., a psychologist and sex therapist in San Francisco and author of *For Yourself: The Fulfillment of Female Sexuality*. "It's mostly because everything is happening faster, at a younger age," she explains.

"A mother who tells her daughter that she absolutely cannot have sex before marriage is putting up a barrier to all potential communication," warns Dr. Barbach. Instead, it's better to be an "askable parent."

"In this way you can help your daughter navigate life as best she can, knowing that the decisions she makes are ultimately her own," says Dr. Barbach. "She also needs to know that once a relationship becomes sexual, she becomes more vulnerable to being deeply hurt."

Laura Pinto had an "askable mother." She remembers having a heart-to-heart talk with her mother about sex before her experience with "the hunk."

"My mother and I have always had the kind of open relationship that my friends envied," says Laura. "So I naturally turned to her for advice. She told me that she couldn't give me 'permission' to have sex, which I wanted, of course. But, she said she trusted me to know when it would be right. She said not to be afraid to tell this boy no if in my gut I felt uncomfortable with the idea. She also said she hoped I would wait, but that if I decided the time was right, to make sure I understood about and used birth control. I thought long and hard about that decision before I turned him down. But it was *my* decision to make."

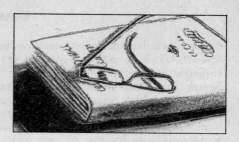

WIDOWHOOD

ACCEPTING THE UNACCEPTABLE

*W*hen Melissa Madenski's husband died of a congenital heart ailment at the age of 34, she found herself a young widow with two children, ages 6 and 18 months. A teacher and writer, she had worked since she was 16. She had always thought of herself as self-reliant, independent, "a survivor." But after Mark's death, she found herself stricken by "pure terror."

"For the first time in my life I didn't know if I could handle it," recalls Melissa. "I felt like I was trapped in a little box with no door and I couldn't see my way out of it. There were times I thought I couldn't breathe. The sky, the trees, everything lost its essence. It's as if somebody throws you up in the air and you hit the ground, dazed."

MULTIPLE LOSSES

Every year, hundreds of thousands of American women lose their husbands. And many of them, like Melissa, find they have lost even more.

The loss of a spouse has a far-reaching impact that can even threaten your sense of who you are, says Houston grief researcher Elizabeth Harper Neeld, Ph.D., author of *Seven Choices: Taking the Steps to New Life after Losing Someone You Love* and herself a young widow. "A relationship is gone that helped identify who you were and what you did each day," she points out. In an instant, you stop being a wife and become a widow. You may have lost your best friend, the person you turned to for comfort and support. If you have children, you are now a single parent. If you are childless, you have lost the children you planned to have. You lose "your assumed future," says Dr. Neeld. All your mutual plans and hopes and dreams are buried with the man you love. You have not only lost your husband, you have lost part of who you are. It is as if your life has been pulled up by its roots.

As time passes, you continually see new, basic ways in which your life has been irrevocably changed. "At the beginning you have no idea how extensive and deep are the patterns that you and your husband had created together: how much milk you buy at the store, what you do after work, how many Christmas cards you order, how the income tax is handled, what you do on birthdays and anniversaries," says Dr. Neeld. "There's no one to call out, 'I'll get it,' when the telephone rings and nobody to help bring in the groceries."

Experts assert that losing a spouse is one of the most stressful events that can occur in our lives. Because, in general, women outlive men, widowhood is an inevitability for a significant number of women. And while you might anticipate this devastating event, there is really no way to adequately prepare for it.

IT TAKES TIME

As with other griefs, this one follows no particular path or timetable. Though your friends and loved ones may expect you to be "over it" in a year, your experience may be very different. One study of 300 people who had lost their spouses found that the course of grief was much longer than expected. Most of the widows, the researchers said, were "relatively well-adjusted" after four years.

Your own mourning time will be dictated by your personality—how you respond to change, for example—the centrality of your spouse to your life, the circumstances of his death (whether it was sudden or occurred after a long illness), your support system of friends and relatives, even past losses, which may be churned up by this new bereavement.

The younger widow has an additional jolt—the injustice of it. "This is not supposed to happen," says Philadelphia psychologist Marion Frank, Ph.D., who was widowed at 23 when her husband was killed in a plane crash. "This is totally outside the realm of expectation. You may experience a huge sense of injustice, bordering on rage."

But for each woman, the experience is unique.

In the days, weeks and months following her husband's death, Melissa's life virtually stopped. She couldn't eat and had trouble sleeping. She was either caught up in frenetic activity or was too exhausted to move. She cried all the time. Sometimes she was surprised at the ferocity of the anger she felt toward strangers, she remembers, "because they could go on living untouched by this tragedy that had so changed my family's lives."

In the midst of her grief, she had to cope with practical matters. She was suddenly the single mother of two children, one in diapers, the other mourning the loss of a beloved father. Though her husband had left some money, Melissa knew she would have to find some way to supplement her income. "At three A.M. I would sit bolt upright in bed and think, 'My God, how am I going to do this?' "

And she learned that while "it's the natural state of affairs to heal, you move forward imperceptibly." Four years after his death and "still on the razor's edge financially," she is finally able to think about Mark "without pain." But, she confesses, "I can hear a song on the radio— our song was 'My Funny Valentine'—and I'll burst into tears."

CONFLICTING EMOTIONS

Older widows also may find their mourning prolonged by their uncertain futures. "An older woman may never have worked outside the home, and if not left with sufficient income, may be forced to go into the work force where she may face age discrimination or not have the skills in the first place," says Midge Marvel, senior program specialist for the Widowed Persons Service of the American Association of Retired Persons in Washington, D.C., who was herself widowed at 58. "It can be devastating. If you're in a panic because you don't have sufficient money, it will affect everything you do."

Some women even feel angry at their husbands. "You may be angry because you feel you've been abandoned, which indeed you have," says Marvel. It's not unusual to resurrect every argument, every slight, every cross word you and your spouse exchanged. "Some people even become angry with God," says Marvel. It's also not unusual to focus your anger on others, as Melissa found herself doing.

You may feel guilty, not only for your angry thoughts but because you may wonder if—and wish—there was something you could have done. "You think, 'If only I had taken better care of him, if only I'd been there at the time. I could have done a lot more,' " says Marvel.

You may ask yourself what Melissa came to call the questions of futility: Why me? Why him? What does it mean?

"You'll find yourself talking about it all the time," says Dr. Frank. " 'I can't believe it happened. It hasn't happened.' One of the reasons you need to repeat the story over and over is to get it into your head that it really did happen."

In the beginning, there may be a sense of unreality about the death. You may expect to see your spouse at the door, you may dream about him alive or even see him in hallucinations. "I had to tell the story over and over again, it was so unreal," says Melissa, whose young husband died suddenly after a family dinner out. "I'd heard people in the throes of grief say, 'Maybe he didn't die. Maybe someone came and took him away.' I understand now why they felt that way."

LEARNING TO SURVIVE

There's no handy prescription for dealing with widowhood, but the experts offer some suggestions to help you survive.

At the top of the list is getting professional help to see you through the worst. Even if you feel you're handling things pretty well and are surrounded by loving friends and family, the course of grieving for a lost spouse and rebuilding a new life can be long and rocky. "I made sure I went to the hospice and saw a counselor once a month for two years," says Melissa. "I didn't want to wear my friends out. You need to tell your story so many times. Though I knew I had a few friends who would still be listening, I had to tell someone else."

Many widowed persons develop some symptoms of severe depression, such as insomnia, weight loss, withdrawal or crying spells that go on for a year or more after their loss. Studies have found that widows who suppress their emotions have more physical and psychological problems than those who don't, which is why it's so important to have someone who is understanding to talk to.

A counselor or a support group for widowed persons can be very helpful during the rough times, particularly in dealing with loneliness. "I found myself working later and later," says Marvel. "The only reason I came home was because I knew I had to feed the dog. The idea of coming home to an empty house was unbearable."

If you have younger children, you will need to deal with their grieving at a time when your resources are few. A counselor or support group can help you learn how to comfort your children, whose reaction to death may be very different from your own.

REACHING OUT

You also may need help with practical matters. Some bereavement counselors and support groups can help you with everything from managing your finances to uncovering job and educational opportunities.

Unfortunately, in some cases you may need help in making new friends, especially ones who understand what you're going through. "One of the most difficult things, although you don't believe it will happen to you, is that a lot of your couple friends will fade away," says Marvel.

"They don't know what to do with you. Some women will be afraid you're interested in their husbands. Sometimes people will try to match you up. It can be awkward. You feel like a kid."

Often, old friends, trying to make you feel better, will make you feel worse instead. "You're going to run into people who don't know what to say or who say things like, 'You're young enough, you'll get married again,' or 'It's long enough now—pull yourself up by your bootstraps,'" says Marvel.

If you don't want to talk to others, and even if you do, keeping a journal of your thoughts and feelings may be helpful. Melissa, a freelance writer and children's book author, wrote in her journal every day. She found it comforting, she says, particularly when she felt she was struggling and never gaining any ground. "I could look back at my journal entries and see how far I'd really come," she says.

TAKE CARE OF YOURSELF

A certain amount of turning inward and self-examination may, in fact, be an important tool for survival. That's because as a widow, you may be at greater risk of becoming ill or having accidents. According to one study, within a year of bereavement, the health of about 67 percent of widows declined. And, though it's rare, there seems to be an increased death rate among those who have lost a spouse. A study done by researchers at several California medical centers found that the immune systems of widows were impaired, possibly putting them at increased risk of illness.

That's why it's important to eat a balanced diet and fit some exercise into your life, even if you've never exercised before. Studies have shown that, along with contributing to your overall good health, exercise can elevate the mood.

"I exercise because with two children I lived in absolute terror of getting sick," says Melissa. "I ride my bike every day, and I jump rope at 10 at night. I know it saved me; I'm rarely sick."

She also heeded the warning of a friend, who lost her

husband in Vietnam, to be extra careful, particularly when she was driving or doing something potentially dangerous, such as climbing a ladder.

"When you've lost someone, you tend to live more on the edge of the world. You take more risks," explains Dr. Marion Frank. "You have to be careful and think, 'Is what I'm doing rational or not?' You may tend not to care."

ALLOW YOURSELF TO GRIEVE

During the grieving process you're vulnerable in a number of ways. It's important to recognize that and allow yourself adequate time to heal.

Don't try to hurry your recovery or fill the void in your life too soon, says Dr. Frank. Grieving takes time and it's rarely, if ever, a straight, level path.

Some women make the mistake of falling into new relationships too soon, warns Dr. Frank. "There's no sense in making a commitment when you're still in heavy mourning," she says. "It's usually a form of escape, which doesn't work."

As you resume your life, you'll find yourself making small changes that, while painful, will be part of the new life you're building. "Of necessity, you become a new person," says Marvel.

But it's a process that can take months, even years. Give yourself that gift of time to get accustomed to life without your husband. Getting over the rough spots may take some forethought.

PLAN THOSE SPECIAL OCCASIONS

Some of the toughest aspects of widowhood are the special occasions you once spent with your spouse and must now spend without him.

For Marvel, those times were particularly painful because her husband "made a big deal of special occasions. He always had all kinds of surprises planned. He wrote poetry. The first birthday I had after he died was just terrible. What we suggest is that people plan for special occasions like Christmas and anniversaries and start new traditions."

It may also be helpful to establish rituals to remember your spouse, something that is very helpful for young children who need to come to grips with the loss of their father at each new developmental stage. "Every year, we have a ritual celebration of Mark's life," says Melissa. "One year, we attended a game of the Portland Beavers baseball team. At the stadium, the scoreboard read, 'In memory of Mark and the years he lived.' My son, Dylan, asked me, 'Aren't we celebrating Dad's death?' I said, 'No, we're celebrating his life. That's always been very important to us.' "

THIS, TOO, SHALL CHANGE

During the most painful moments, it's hard to believe that your life will be better. "It's just plain hard to face, the pain is incredible," says Marvel. "And nobody can go through it for you. You have to go right through the middle of it yourself."

But you do come out on the other side, perhaps stronger, perhaps wiser. "You never forget those feelings," says Dr. Frank, "but they become further and further apart."

Says Melissa: "I tell Dylan it's like a cut that scars over, but sometimes it still hurts. You don't get over it, but you adapt to it. If someone asked me if I were healed, I would say, 'Yes, but it was a long road.' Today, it's not terrible because I lost him, but wonderful because I had him."

See also Grief

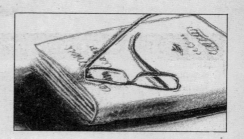

WRINKLES

TRYING TO BUY TIME IN A BOTTLE

*R*emember that sunlit day at the beach with your very first boyfriend? Or how about that daylong hike at the edge of the desert with your brother?

Surely you remember? If you don't, just look at your face. Because just in case you've forgotten all the fun you've had in the sun, your face has kept a permanent scrapbook to remind you.

Yes, it's time that you, er, face it.

The accumulation of time spent in the sun over your lifetime is what you're wearing on your face today in terms of lines and wrinkles.

Unfortunately a little bit of sun *does* hurt, explains Nia Terezakis, M.D., a clinical professor of dermatology at Tulane University School of Medicine in New Orleans. It damages the skin and accelerates the normal process of skin aging that causes wrinkles, crow's-feet and age spots. And it frequently does it long before you're old enough to know better.

SUNSCREEN: NUMBER ONE DEFENSE

"By the age of 15 or 20, you've already gotten about 80 percent of your lifetime exposure to the sun," says Dr. Terezakis. And if you doubt the effects it has on your body, just peel off your clothes and stand in front of the mirror.

WRINKLE PREVENTION

Although most wrinkles are etched by the sun, some are formed by personal habits such as wrinkling your nose. Here are a few ways dermatologists suggest you can help prevent these woman-made wrinkles.

- Avoid frowning and "contorted" face patterns such as wrinkling your nose, raising your forehead and making faces.
- Sleep on your back. Sleeping on the side of your face can cause diagonal wrinkles on your cheeks or forehead.
- Don't smoke cigarettes. After a number of years, smokers develop tiny wrinkles that spread out from the upper and lower lips. They also have accentuated crow's-feet around their eyes, deep lines on their cheeks and leathery-looking skin with a tinge of gray.
- Don't do facial exercises. It's a myth that they prevent wrinkles. Fact is, most of these exercises can accentuate wrinkles because they use the very muscles that cause wrinkling.

"Look at your face," says Dr. Terezakis. "Now turn around and look at your fanny. "Both those areas have had the same number of birthdays, yet the difference is unmistakable.

"That's why, as far as I'm concerned, there's only one wrinkle cream—sunscreen.

"I tell my patients they should use sunscreen every single day even if they don't think they're going to go out," she adds. "Of course, I get an argument. 'I'm only running to the store.' Or, 'I was just coming here,' they'll say.

" 'So how did you get to my office,' I'll ask them, 'by tunnel?' The point is that every ray of sunshine affects your skin."

RETIN-A: THE RESCUE CREAM

But what if you've fried your skin for years and are now faced with the weathered results?

You could opt for a face-lift, chemical peel, or even have your wrinkles filled out with collagen injections. Or you could ask your doctor about the possibility of trying a topical cream like Retin-A, a less-drastic, less-expensive and quite promising alternative.

Retin-A is the same drug—topical tretinoin, a derivative of vitamin A—that doctors have been using for years to treat acne. But applied diligently to the face, hands or forearms it has been shown to slough off the dead cells that frequently give your skin an "old" look, reduce wrinkles, decrease pore size, fade age spots, counteract the dermal thinning that occurs with age and increase blood flow to give you that rosy glow most of us associate with youth. Indeed, doctors say Retin-A can actually *reverse* at least some of the sun's damage to the skin.

Retin-A must be prescribed and monitored by a doctor, says Dr. Terezakis, since everyone has different degrees of damage and different types of skin. But it's not without some side effects. Redness, irritation and occasional peeling can occur. And because Retin-A can make the skin ultrasensitive to the sun, you *must* use a sunscreen with an SPF of at least 15 every day without fail. One thing's for sure: Once you start on Retin-A, your days of sporting a tan should be over.

You should also be aware that Retin-A is a long-term treatment, adds Dr. Terezakis. It's not an overnight miracle. Although you may begin to see some improvement within 8 to 16 weeks, full effects may not be seen for a year but continue the longer you use it. And if you stop the treatment at any time, your skin may very gradually go back to the way it was.

A NATURAL ALTERNATIVE

Another anti-aging skin treatment that helps reduce wrinkles involves the use of alpha hydroxy acids—five different acids found in common foods such as sugar cane, sour milk, apples, pears, oranges, mangoes, grapes and lemons.

Studies show that all these acids help reduce fine lines

and wrinkles, fade age spots, improve dry skin and even help reduce acne and acne scarring.

Eugene J. Van Scott, M.D., a clinical professor of dermatology at Hahnemann University in Philadelphia, is one of the leading researchers on alpha hydroxy acids. He's used them for 15 years to treat acne and ichthyosis—a disorder characterized by extremely dry, scaly skin. He noticed that, during the course of these treatments, some of his patients began to look younger. Their age spots faded, and in some cases, wrinkles seemed to disappear.

What was going on?

In many skin conditions, dead skin cells don't slough off as they should. They accumulate on the surface, forming a thick outer layer and making the skin look dull and old. If this buildup can be eliminated, the skin improves, according to Dr. Van Scott. And that's how alpha hydroxy acids help. They soften the "physiological glue" that holds the dead surface cells together and allow them to be removed. What's left underneath is baby-soft skin.

The treatment for removing fine lines and wrinkles is a simple office procedure. A concentrated solution of alpha hydroxy acids is applied to the skin for a few minutes, then rinsed off with water. The patient may feel a little sting, which indicates that a certain amount of the concentration is getting through the skin and having its effect, according to Dr. Van Scott.

Further research is necessary to determine just how effective these acids are. But if we're lucky, they may provide a natural alternative to face-lifts.

See also Aging, Cosmetic Surgery

INDEX

Note: Page references in **boldface** indicate tables.